Gynecological Imaging: A Reference Guide to Diagnosis and Surgery

Gynecological Imaging: A Reference Guide to Diagnosis and Surgery

Edited by Elizabeth Elliott

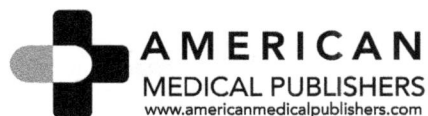

AMERICAN
MEDICAL PUBLISHERS
www.americanmedicalpublishers.com

American Medical Publishers,
41 Flatbush Avenue,
1st Floor, New York,
NY 11217, USA

Visit us on the World Wide Web at:
www.americanmedicalpublishers.com

ISBN: 978-1-63927-071-2

Cataloging-in-Publication Data

Gynecological imaging : a reference guide to diagnosis and surgery / edited by Elizabeth Elliott.
    p. cm.
Includes bibliographical references and index.
ISBN 978-1-63927-071-2
1. Generative organs, Female--Imaging--Guidebooks. 2. Gynecology--Diagnosis--Guidebooks.
3. Generative organs, Female--Surgery--Guidebooks. I. Elliott, Elizabeth.
RG107.5.I4 G96 2022
618.107 5--dc23

Table of Contents

Permissions

List of Contributors

Index

Preface

Gynecological imaging encompasses a full range of gynecological technologies for detecting pathologies and conditions of the female reproductive organs. Gynecological conditions are usually diagnosed using magnetic resonance imaging (MRI), ultrasound, computed tomography (CT) and fluoroscopy. Medical imaging is also vital in infertility investigations, gynecological oncology and diagnosis of Mullerian duct anomalies. Gynecological ultrasonography allows the visualization of the ovaries, the uterus and the fallopian tubes, as well as the adnexa, bladder and the recto-uterine pouch. It also facilitates the diagnosis of gynecologic cancers, assessment of pelvic organs, diagnosis of acute appendicitis, diagnosis and management of endometriosis, leiomyoma, ovarian cysts and lesions, etc. MRI, X-ray CT, projectional radiography and nuclear medicine are employed for investigating pregnancy related complications and intercurrent diseases, or for routine prenatal care. This book discusses the fundamentals as well as modern approaches of gynecological imaging. It strives to provide a fair idea about the diverse gynecological imaging techniques and to help develop a better understanding of their diagnostic and therapeutic applications. A number of latest researches have been included to keep the readers up-to-date with the global concepts in this area of study.

This book unites the global concepts and researches in an organized manner for a comprehensive understanding of the subject. It is a ripe text for all researchers, students, scientists or anyone else who is interested in acquiring a better knowledge of this dynamic field.

I extend my sincere thanks to the contributors for such eloquent research chapters. Finally, I thank my family for being a source of support and help.

Editor

Hysteroscopic sterilization with Essure® device in situ: a challenge?

Michel P. H. Vleugels · Sergine Heckel ·
Sebastian Veersema · Jean Bernard Engrand ·
Vincent Villefranque · Hervé Fernandez · Pierre Panel

Abstract Hysteroscopic sterilization through the Essure® method is preferably performed in the outpatient department without any form of anesthesia. This approach requires the hysteroscopic skills of the gynecologist to use the vaginoscopic route. Initially, the manufacturer advised to remove any type of intrauterine device (IUD), 1 month before the procedure, to prevent difficult procedures and also to increase the success rate of placement. This observational prospective study analyzed the outcome in women in where the IUD was left in the uterus during the sterilization. During a period of 2 years, all women have been included consecutively in seven public hospitals located in France and the Netherlands. During this procedure, 32 out of 239 IUDs had to be removed to finish the sterilization successfully. The placement success rate was 97%. Placement failures were not related to the IUD being present at the time of the procedure. At confirmation tests 3 months after insertion of the Essure®, only five tubes were still patent. No complications were registered. Pain was recorded, and women responded well on oral nonsteroidal anti-inflammatory drug medication. The IUD did not need to be removed before the start of the hysteroscopic sterilization; only in case the procedure could not be completed, the IUD had to be removed during the sterilization itself. Placement rate was 97.1%.

Keywords Essure · IUD · Sterilization

M. P. H. Vleugels (✉)
Rivierenland Hospital,
Tiel, Netherlands
e-mail: wings.michael@wxs.nl

S. Heckel
Centre Hospitalier St. Joseph St. Luc,
Lyon, France

S. Veersema
St. Antonius Hospital,
Nieuwegein, Netherlands

J. B. Engrand
Centre Hospitalier Général,
Dunkerque, France

V. Villefranque
CHG René Dubos,
Pontoise, France

H. Fernandez
CHU Kremlin Bicêtre,
Paris, France

P. Panel
CHG André Mignot,
Versailles, France

Introduction

Female sterilization by the hysteroscopic route has been pioneered for many decades. The first commercially available method (Ovabloc®) was introduced in Europe in 1988, but never outside Europe. Since the introduction of the micro-insert "Essure"®, the hysteroscopic sterilization became a real option for women [1] worldwide. Sterilization by this device Essure® is meant to be performed in the outpatient department without spinal or general anesthesia.

The hysteroscopic approach is done preferably according to the vaginoscopic approach as has been promoted by Stefano Bettocchi [2]. After the placement of the device in both tubal ostia, the presence of the nitinol spring and its inner coil of polyethylene terephthalate fibers provokes a

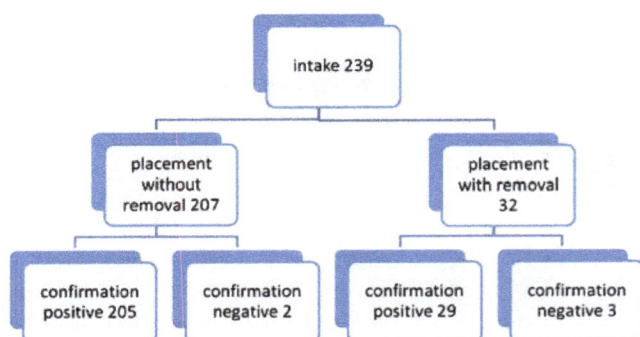

Fig. 1 Study design

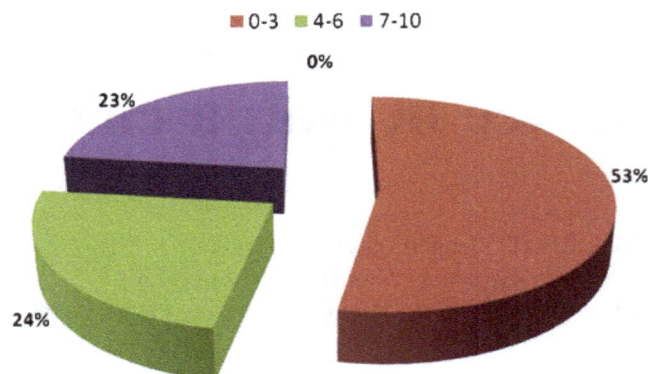

Fig. 2 Outcome of the pain score list (visual analogue score)

tissue reaction. Fibrotic tissue is formed in the proximal tube. This chronic fibrotic reaction will be completed in all patients after 3 months after the placement of the device and will block both tubes in all patients: 96.5% at 3 months and 100% at 6 months [3].

For 12 weeks after the placement of the device, an alternative form of contraception is necessary. Women are advised to continue their usual method of contraception. In case the woman is using an intrauterine device (IUD), it is advised by the marketing company to remove the IUD preferably one cycle before the placement of the device. The reason for the removal of the IUD is the fear that it can hamper a quick hysteroscopic procedure and might interfere with proper placement of the device in the tubes.

The disadvantage of this advice is the need to rely on an alternative contraception for the duration of 3 months. This increases the risk of an unreliable contraception.

In this multicenter prospective observational study, the surgeons left all the IUDs in place and tried to insert the devices. Once they succeeded, this IUD was removed after the confirmation test at 3 months. Patients' characteristics and procedures were recorded; the outcome measurements were the placement rate of the devices, the number of IUDs which had to be removed during the procedure, and the outcome of the confirmation test at 3 months.

Materials and methods

This prospective observational study has been performed by seven study centers spread out over France and the

Netherlands. The study setup is shown in Fig. 1. All gynecologists used this sterilization method for more than 1 year. In all patients, the vaginoscopic approach according to Bettocchi was used.

The procedures were performed ambulatory, either on the outpatient department or in the clinical theater. All gynecologists advised their patients the use of nonsteroidal anti-inflammatory drug (NSAID) premedication before the start of the procedure.

The endpoints were defined as the placement rates of Essure devices in those women who had an IUD in place at the moment of the hysteroscopy. The acceptance of the patients measured by pain scores during the procedure, their voluntary use of NSAID medication, and the complication rate were recorded. Sedation, local, or general anesthesia was only given in specific situations at the decision of the surgeon and on request of the patients. In case of local anesthesia, cervical clockwise injections were given.

From November 2006 till January 2009, all 239 consecutive women who requested sterilization through this method of Essure and who were using an IUD have been included.

Three months after the sterilization, the confirmation was done according to the protocol chosen by the

Table 1 Type of analgesia

General anesthesia	15
Intravenous sedation	45
Oral sedation	6
Local anesthesia	3
No anesthesia	170

Table 2 Visual analogue score (VAS) pain registration related to the use of nonsteroidal anti-inflammatory drug (NSAID)

VAS score	NSAID premedication	No premedication
0–3	72 (57%)	40 (47%)
4–6	27 (21.5%)	24 (28%)
7–10	27 (21.5%)	21 (25%)
	126	85

p value=0.206; Mann–Whitney U test

Table 3 Problems encountered

1 breakage of device; replacement
1 none expenditure; replacement
2 lost in cavity to shallow placements replaced
1 migration, i.e., perforation into the abdominal cavity
2 incorrect placement without any further information

gynecologist, either the protocol based on the plain X-ray of the abdomen or the transvaginal ultrasound. A hysterosalpingogram was done on the judgment of the gynecologist to exclude patent tubes.

Results

The majority of the procedures, 136 of 239 (57%), were done on a day care unit, while a smaller group of 103 of 239 (43%) was performed in the outpatient department.

All surgeons used the vaginoscopic hysteroscopic approach, so called Bettocchi hysteroscopy: no use of disinfectants, speculum, or tenaculum. Overall, there was no use of anesthesia; only in a few exceptional cases, sedation, local, or general anesthesia was given (Table 1).

Pain has been scored during the procedure using the visual analogue score (VAS) listed in 211 of 239 patients; the procedure was very well accepted (Fig. 2).

Most patients used the prescribed premedication of NSAID drugs, which is suppose to influence the pain, although the comparison of the VAS scores for premedication versus no premedication did not show a significant difference (p value=0.206 Mann–Whitney U test; Table 2).

The devices could be placed in 232 of 239 (97%) of all women; the presence of the IUD was not registered by the surgeons as the cause of failure. In all these patients, the IUD was left in place.

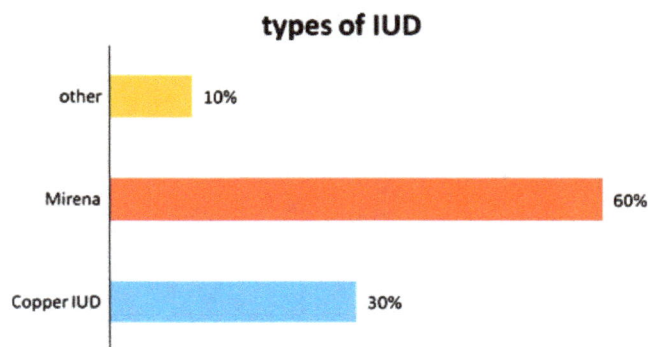

Fig. 4 Rates of removal of intrauterine device type

An overview of the different causes of placement failure is given in Table 3. Except for one perforation, all other problems were resolved.

Mirena IUD was used in 60% (144/239), a copper IUD in 30% (71/239), and other types of IUD in 10% of patients (24/239; Fig. 3).

During the procedure, 32 IUDs had to be removed to successfully insert Essure®; in these women, no placement failure occurred. There was no relation between the type of IUD and the rate of removal during the sterilization: p value=0.6267 (Fig. 4). For the comparison of the removal rate by type of IUD, we used the Chi-square test.

An overview of placement failure rates and removals of IUD in order to succeed the procedure related to the different gynecologists is given in Table 4.

The confirmation test at 3 months after placement of the devices was done by transvaginal ultrasound, plain X-ray, or hysterosalpingogram (Fig. 5).

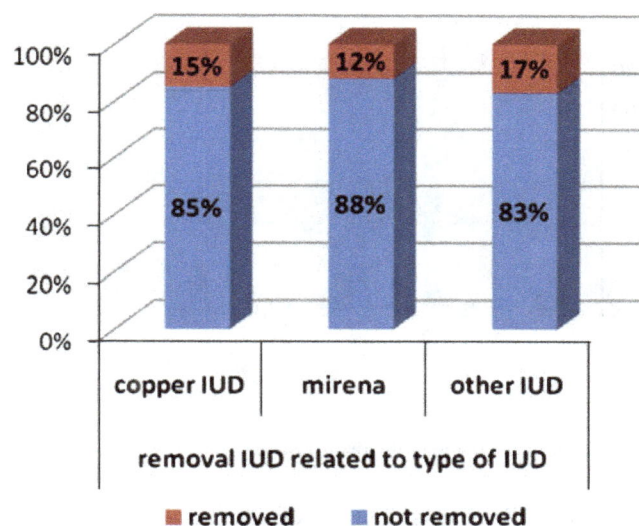

Fig. 3 Types of intrauterine device used in this group

Table 4 Removal of intrauterine device during placement and placement failure rate (divided by gynecologist)

	Total/removal	Placement failure
Panel	22 (7; 31.8%)	1 (4.5%)
Fernandez	36 (4; 11%)	3 (8.3%)
Engrand	95 (11; 11.6%)	3 (3.2%)
Heckel	27 (2; 7.4%)	0 (0%)
Villefranque	15 (0; 0%)	0 (0%)
Vleugels	22 (1; 4.5%)	0 (0%)
Veersema	22 (7; 31.8%)	0 (0%)
Total	239 (32; 13.4%)	7 (2.9%)

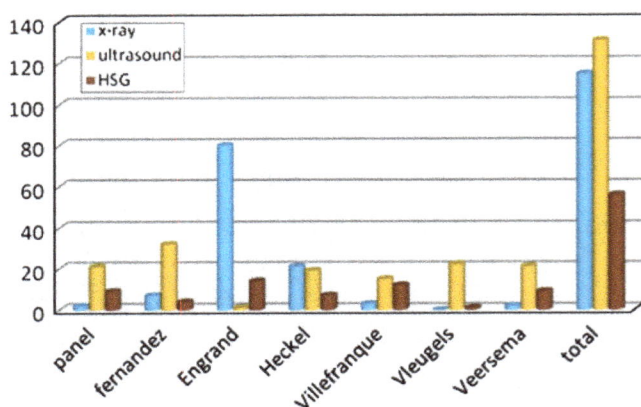

Fig. 5 Confirmation tests divided by surgeon

Almost all patients, 236 out of 239, turned up for their checkup at 3 months, including all patients from whom the IUD had to be removed during the procedure to succeed the placement. Ten patients received one device inserted on one side, since they had a registered tubectomy in the past.

The overall success rate of the sterilization procedure at 3 months was 98% (231/236; Table 5).

Discussion

Any IUD in the cavity of the uterus may hamper a good visualization of the whole cavity. Especially, the view on both tubal ostia is sometimes more difficult with an IUD with long arms like the Mirena®. Thereby, due to avascular fibrotic synechia, a clear view is often not possible, especially in case of atrophic endometrium due to the local progesterone release by the Mirena® IUD. These difficulties can prolong the hysteroscopic approach to the tubal area, and in combination with the inevitable manipulation of the IUD, spasm of the uterus and the tubes might be induced. The risk of placement failures increases.

In case the micro-inserts were placed correctly, some patients required a confirmation test by hysterosalpingo-gram instead of ultrasound or plain X-ray according to the Dutch confirmation protocol due to a difficult procedure that lasted longer than 15 min [4]. This protocol has been accepted by most European gynecologists. Due to all above-described difficulties, an increased risk of non-placement or displacement has been assumed. So, the product instruction for use advises to remove the IUD before the procedure.

In this study, we analyzed the outcome of all conse-quently performed sterilizations by seven surgeons who documented their experience with the IUD in place at the moment that they started the procedure.

The data are too small to analyze any relationship for each surgeon between the placement failure rate and removal of IUD during the procedure to succeed. The placement failure rate was very low in this group of patients.

Placement could be achieved in 97%, which is even higher than the overall success rates in the normal population [3, 5]. A few small retrospective feasibility studies elucidated the advantage to leave the IUD in place, but their outcomes were also less successful [6, 7].

Failure of placement was not related to the presence of the IUD. Eleven times (9.8%), the IUD had to be removed during the procedure since placement of the Essure® device might have been impossible. In all these women, the sterilization could be completed. Although the IUD may jeopardize a quick performance, the average procedure time did not exceeded 15 min. In spite of the preoccupation of more pain, the VAS did not show more pain compared to the literature; hence, most sterilizations were done without general or spinal anesthesia.

We concluded that every gynecologist who has experi-ence with this hysteroscopic sterilization can perform this procedure without removal of the IUD beforehand. The outcome during sterilization, like the placement rate, pain,

Table 5 Patency of tubes at HSG=failure rate according protocol

Surgeon	Success		Failure		Control	Total treatments
	Bilateral	Unilateral	Bilateral	Unilateral		
Panel	21		1		22	22
Fernandez	31	3	1	1	36	36
Engrand	88	6	1		95	95
Heckel	24				24	27
Villefranque	15				15	15
Vleugels	22				22	22
Veersema	20	1	1		22	22
	221	10	4	1	236	239

Success=blocked tubes, 231=98%; Failure=open tubes, 5=2%

complications, and as well as the confirmation test at 3 months, does not differ from the normal population. Since we have the policy to leave the IUD in place, we know that it might be a little more painful and might create more discomfort in an individual case, but the consulting gynecologist has to counsel the patient about these items. The woman herself has to make the decision to leave the IUD in or not. The advantage is clear: a reliable contraception will be continued during the waiting period of 3 months.

Acknowledgements The authors would like to thank Mr. J.C. Kelder Msc, epidemiologist at the St. Antonius Hospital Nieuwegein, for his statistical analyses.

Conflict of interest Dr. Michel Vleugels is a member of the advisory medical board. He is a consultant. A group of gynecologists together is advising critical studies. The travel/accommodation expenses are covered or reimbursed in case the medical advisories organize a meeting abroad.

References

1. Kerin JF, Carignan CS, Cher D (2001) The safety and effectiveness of a new hysteroscopic method for permanent birth control: results of the first Essure pbc clinical study. Aust N Z J Obstet Gynaecol 41:364–370
2. Bettocchi S, Selvaggi L (1997) A vaginoscopic approach to reduce the pain of office hysteroscopy. J Am Assoc Gynecol Laparosc 4:255–258
3. Valle RF, Carignan CS, Wright TC (2001) Tissue response to the STOP microcoil transcervical permanent contraceptive device: results from a prehysterectomy study. Fertil Steril 76:974–980
4. Veersema S, Vleugels MPH, Timmermans A, Brölmann H (2005) Follow-up of successful bilateral placement of Essure® micro inserts with ultrasound. Fertil Steril 84:173–176
5. Vleugels MPH, Veersema S (2005) Hysteroscopic sterilization on the outpatient department without anesthesia. Gyn Surg 2:155–158
6. Mascaro M, Mariño M, Vicens-Vidal M (2008) Feasibility of Essure placement in intrauterine device users. J Minim Invasive Gynecol 15:485–490
7. Tatalovich J, Anderson T (2010) Hysteroscopic sterilization in patients with a Mirena intrauterine device: transition from extended interval to permanent contraception. J Minim Invasive Gynecol 17:228–231

2

Endoscopic management of a sebaceous carcinoma arising in a mature cystic teratoma of the ovary

Daniele Bolla · Arthur von Hochstetter · René Hornung

Abstract Malignant transformation of a mature cystic teratoma (MCT) of the ovary is extremely rare. Squamous cell carcinoma is the most common malignancy, which occurs in MCT and accounts for ~80% of all cases. We describe the eighth undisputed case of a pure sebaceous carcinoma arising in a teratoma of the ovary. A 45-year-old woman underwent laparoscopic hysterectomy, bilateral salpingo-oophorectomy with pelvic and paraaortic lymphadenectomy. The final stage was pT1a, pN0 (0/30), M0, G2. The carcinoma was localized within a dermoid cyst not involving the capsule or adjacent abdominal structures. Complete tumor excision without iatrogenic tumor cell dissemination and proper staging are important for the prognosis and treatment and should be performed as soon as possible after diagnosis. Unfortunately, the very small number of cases published does not allow an evidence-based therapeutic management.

Keywords Mature cystic teratoma · Sebaceous carcinoma · Ovary · Endoscopic surgery

Introduction

Mature cystic teratomas (MCT) of the ovary, also known as dermoid cyst, represent 44% of ovarian neoplasms. They are benign tumors containing mature tissue of any of the three germ-cell layers. MCT represent up to 58% of benign ovarian tumors and typically occur in young women [4]. Malignant transformation is rare and occurs in 1–3% of cases [12]. It usually arises in postmenopausal women and can develop from any element of the dermoid cyst, but mainly from the ectodermal tissue. Squamous cell carcinoma is the most common malignancy that occurs in dermoid cysts and accounts for 75% to 88% of all cases [6, 9].

To the best of our knowledge, there are only seven reports of pure sebaceous carcinomas arising within a benign teratoma of the ovary [1–3, 6, 7, 11, 12]. We present the first case of this rare neoplasm managed by endoscopic surgery only.

Case report

A 45-year-old gravida 15 para 12 was referred to our hospital with a histological diagnosis of a sebaceous carcinoma within a mature cystic teratoma of the ovary and a TNM score of pT1a, pNX, M0, G2, and R0. Two months earlier, the patient had undergone a laparoscopic left-sided salpingo-oophorectomy in another clinic for an adnexal mass suspicious for a dermoid cyst. During this operation, the ovary was removed entirely using an endobag without rupturing the capsule. After the diagnosis of sebaceous carcinoma was rendered, an abdominal PET CT abdominal scan was performed. No metastatic lesions were found.

By admission in our hospital, physical examination revealed no peripheral lymphadenopathy or hepatosplenomegaly. The complete blood count was normal. The tumor marker CA125 was within a normal range. Past and family history was unremarkable.

D. Bolla (✉) · R. Hornung
Department of Obstetrics and Gynecology,
Kantonsspital St. Gallen,
Rorschacher Strasse 95,
CH- 9007, St. Gallen, Switzerland
e-mail: daniele.bolla@kssg.ch

A. von Hochstetter
Pathology Institute Enge Zurich,
St. Gallen, Switzerland

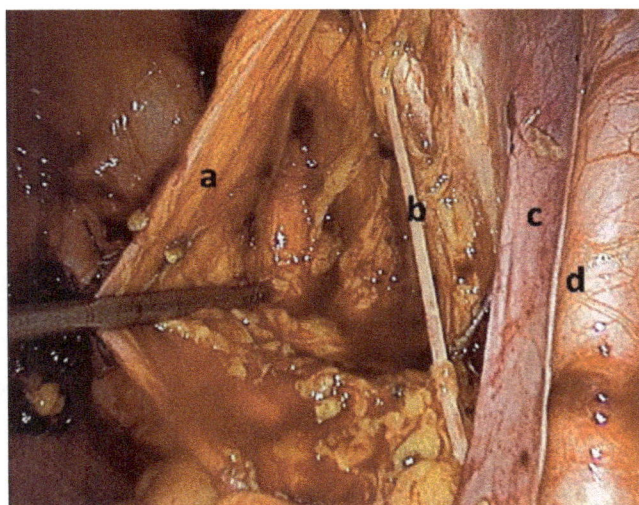

Fig. 1 Laparoscopic pelvic lymphadenectomy: **a** right lateral umbilical ligament, **b** right obturator nerve, **c** right external iliac vein, **d** right external iliac artery

An exploratory laparoscopic with surgical staging was undertaken. The uterus and the right adnexa were unremarkable. There was no ascites. No tumor implants were found in the peritoneal cavity. A total laparoscopic hysterectomy, right-sided salpingo-oophorectomy and laparoscopic pelvic and paraaortic lymphadenectomy were performed (Figs. 1, 2). The patient made an uncomplicated postoperative recovery.

At the tumor conference in our clinic we recommended no further treatment but only close follow-up gynecological examinations.

The patient is alive without evidence of recurrence 23 months after diagnosis.

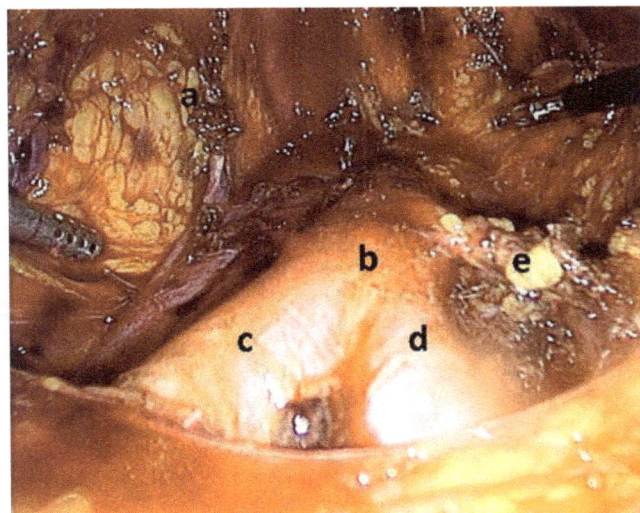

Fig. 2 Laparoscopic pelvic lymphadenectomy: **a** right ovarian vein, **b** aorta, **c** right common iliac artery, **d** left common iliac artery, **e** inferior mesenteric artery

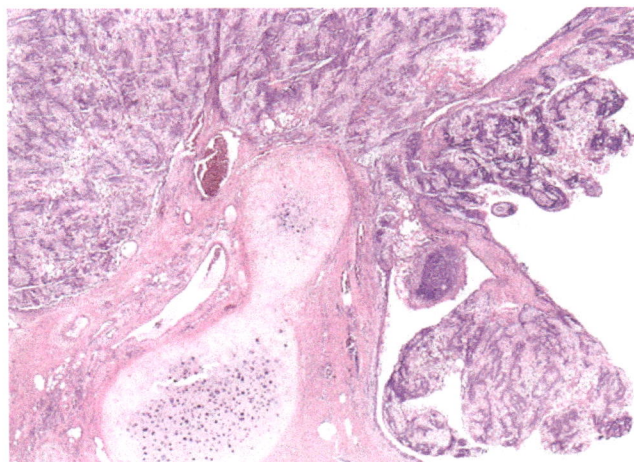

Fig. 3 Massive polypoid proliferation of basaloid epithelial cells with sebaceous differentiation within the lumen of a cystic teratoma. Nodules of mature cartilage tale up the base

Pathological findings

The cyst is lined by respiratory and squamous epithelium, the wall containing mature tissues including islands of cartilage, inflammatory infiltrates and foreign body giant cells.

In addition, the intraluminal tumor consists of polypoid confluent masses of dark basaloid cells showing varying degrees of sebaceous differentiation, the latter forming at times masses of parakeratotic debris (Fig. 3). The basaloid sheets contain prominent round to oval nuclei with finely granular chromatin and small- to medium-sized nucleoli. In some areas, nuclei and nucleoli are prominent and mitotic activity is brisk (Fig. 4). The pattern of growth is largely by pushing borders, but less circumscribed in areas, showing microscopic penetration into the ovarian stroma. Vascular invasion is not seen. The ovarian surface is not involved,

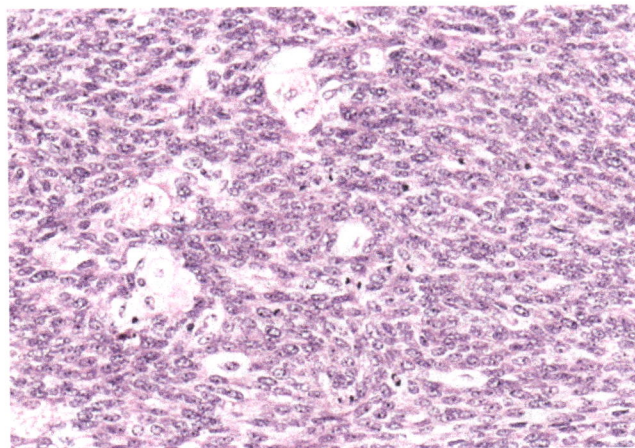

Fig. 4 In some areas, sebaceous differentiation was very focal, within sheets of poorly differentiated, highly proliferative basaloid cells

intervening stroma remaining at least 2 to 3 mm wide. In analogy to sebaceous neoplasms of the skin, the features of hypercellularity, nuclear atypia, mitotic activity, and micro-invasion were considered evidence of malignancy. Hence, the diagnosis of sebaceous carcinoma arising in a mature teratoma was rendered and subsequently confirmed in consultation by the AFIP (Washington, DC) and by Dr. A. Talerman (Thomas Jefferson University Hospital, Philadelphia). Tumor stage was determined as pT1a R0.

Discussion

Malignant transformation of a dermoid cyst of the ovary is rare and occurs in less than 3%. It usually arises from the ectodermal tissues and occurs almost exclusively in postmenopausal women with a mean age of 50 years [11].

Squamous cell carcinoma is the most common compo-nent (~80%) in malignant transformation in teratomas. However, several other malignancies have also been reported.

We report the eighth undisputed case of a pure sebaceous carcinoma arising in a mature teratoma of the ovary. In our case, the carcinoma was localized in a dermoid cyst without involving the capsule or adjacent abdominal structures.

Teratomas with malignant transformation are usually larger than ordinary dermoid cysts (10–20 cm) [9]. Clinical findings are often unspecific like abdominal distension, lower abdominal pain associated with bowel or bladder symptoms. Notwithstanding this, a diagnosis of malignancy in teratoma can only rarely be made preoperatively [5].

The histogenesis of sebaceous carcinoma is still poorly understood. Some authors believe that they originate from pluripotent stem cells, while other suggested that they may originate from more differentiated sebaceous cells in mature teratomas, which undergo malignant transformaton rather than from stem cells [10].

In general, sebaceous carcinomas of the skin often cause regional metastasis, but seldom spread to viscera [10]. In fact, none of the seven sebaceous carcinomas reported in literature, in different stages at diagnosis, developed a recurrence or metastasis. This favorable outcome is sup-ported by the findings by Ribeiro-Silva et al. of a low proliferation rate of Ki67 associated with an inactivation of p53 gene in the sebaceous carcinoma [9].

For this reason, the role of chemotherapy and radiother-apy in sebaceous carcinomas arising from teratomas is unclear. Neither postoperative radiation nor adjuvant chemotherapy in patients with extracapsular disease has shown to improve survival time.

Hence, debulking surgery remains crucial for patient survival. Petterson et al. described a 75% 5-year survival

rate for unruptured stage I tumors [8]. Kashimura et al. showed a 50% 5-year survival rate in stage 1 versus 25% in stage 2 [5]. This referred to all types of teratomas with malignant transformation, showing that an improved surgi-cal management of ovarian cancer is the single most important factor.

The utility of node dissection as well is controversial since the mode of spread is generally by direct extension or peritoneal seeding, but it may influence treatment planning, especially in early stage of disease.

In our case, the patient underwent laparoscopic hyster-ectomy, bilateral salpingo-oophorectomy with pelvic and paraaortic lymphadenectomy according the staging proce-dure for ovarian neoplasm (Figs. 1, 2 and 3). Omentectomie was omitted as peritoneal washing during the first surgery had been negative. The final stage was pT1a, pN0 (0/30), M0, G2. No further treatment was recommended. The patient is in excellent condition 23 month after diagnosis without evidence of local recurrence or metastasis.

Unfortunately, the very small number of cases published does not allow an evidence-based therapeutic management and prognosis. In our case, the therapeutic strategy proved effective. However, whether the patient was over-treated or not remains speculative.

In conclusion, a complete tumor excision and proper staging are important for prognosis and treatment planning and should be performed at the time of initial surgery or as soon as possible following pathologic diagnosis. In early tumor stage, a laparoscopic approach can be justified and midline laparotomy avoided.

Declaration of interest The authors report no conflicts of interest. The authors alone are responsible for the content and writing of the paper.

References

1. Betta PG, Cosimi MF (1984) Sebaceous carcinoma arising in benign cystic teratoma of the ovary. Case report. Eur J Gynaecol Oncol 5(2):146–149
2. Changchien CC, Chen L, Eng HL (1994) Sebaceous carcinoma arising in a benign dermoid cyst of the ovary. Acta Obstet Gynecol Scand 73(4):355–358
3. Chumas JC, Scully RE (1991) Sebaceous tumors arising in ovarian dermoid cysts. Int J Gynecol Pathol 10(4):356–363
4. Comerci JT Jr, Licciardi F, Bergh PA, Gregori C, Breen JL (1994) Mature cystic teratoma: a clinicopathologic evaluation of 517 cases and review of the literature. Obstet Gynecol 84(1):22–28
5. Dos Santos L, Mok E, Iasonos A, Park K, Soslow RA, Aghajanian C, Alektiar K, Barakat RR, Abu-Rustum NR (2007) Squamous cell carcinoma arising in mature cystic teratoma of the ovary: a case series and review of the literature. Gynecol Oncol 105(2):321–324, Epub 2007 Jan 22

6. Kontogianni E, Koukoura E, Christopoulou E (2001) Squamous cell carcinoma arising in mature cystic teratoma of the ovary: a case report. Eur J Gynaecol Oncol 22(3):238–239

7. Papadopoulos AJ, Ahmed H, Pakarian FB, Caldwell CJ, McNicholas J, Raju KS (1995) Sebaceous carcinoma arising within an ovarian cystic mature teratoma. Int J Gynecol Cancer 5(1):76–79

8. Peterson WF (1957) Malignant degeneration of benign cystic teratomas of the overy; a collective review of the literature. Obstet Gynecol Surv 12(6):793–830

9. Ribeiro-Silva A, Chang D, Bisson FW, Ré LO (2003) Clinico-pathological and immunohistochemical features of a sebaceous carcinoma arising within a benign dermoid cyst of the ovary. Virchows Arch 443(4):574–578, Epub 2003 Jun 27

10. Rim SY, Kim SM, Choi HS (2006) Malignant transformation of ovarian mature cystic teratoma. Int J Gynecol Cancer 16(1):140–144

11. Vartanian RK, McRae B, Hessler RB (2002) Sebaceous carcinoma arising in a mature cystic teratoma of the ovary. Int J Gynecol Pathol 21(4):418–421

12. Venizelos ID, Tatsiou ZA, Roussos D, Karagiannis V (2009) A case of sebaceous carcinoma arising within a benign ovarian cystic teratoma. Onkologie 32(6):353–355, Epub 2009 May 25

3

Video endoscopic-assisted inguino-femoral lymphadenectomy (VEIL) in squamous cell invasive vulvar carcinoma

Daniela Huber · Damien Robyr · Nicolas Schneider

Abstract Inguinal lymphadenectomy is a part of the surgical treatment of invasive perineal cancers and lower extremities and inferior trunk melanomas. Inguinal node metastasis represents a major prognostic factor; therefore, inguinal lymphadenectomy has a central role in oncological patient management. Nevertheless, inguinal node dissection is associated with significant morbidity such as lymphedema, wound dehiscence, flap necrosis, infection, seroma, femoral hernia, and deep venous thromboembolism. Recently, several publications have reported experiences with video endoscopic-assisted techniques attempting to reduce the high morbidity related to open inguinal lymphadenectomy. The primary results are promising in terms of feasibility, oncological survey and goals, postoperative complications, and esthetic results. We discuss here our initial experience with video endoscopic inguino-femoral lymphadenectomy (VEIL) in a patient with invasive vulvar carcinoma. To our knowledge, this is the first report of a bilateral VEIL in vulvar carcinoma.

Keywords Invasive vulvar carcinoma · Inguinal lymph node dissection · Inguinal lymphadenectomy · Video-assisted surgery · Video-assisted inguino-femoral lymphadenectomy (VEIL) · Minimal invasive surgery

Background

Vulvar carcinomas represent the fourth most common gynecological malignancy, accounting for 4% of all female genital tract cancers [1]. Inguinal nodal metastasis is the essential independent prognostic factor. Predictors of metastasis in inguinal lymph nodes are: histological grade, extent of tumor stromal invasion, capillary-like space involvement with the tumor, clinically suspect regional nodes, and clitoral or perineal location. In pT1 vulvar tumors, the survival rate is reduced from 90% to 55% in cases of nodal metastasis [1]; therefore, the lymphadenectomy has a major role in surgical management with prognostic and potentially therapeutic implications [2, 3]. Traditional single extended incision for bilateral inguinal node dissection and radical vulvectomy has a reported morbidity of up to 76% [4, 5] including infections, flap necrosis, wound dehiscence, chronic lymphedema, lymphocyst formation, femoral hernia, and deep venous thromboembolism [4–9]. The mortality related to classical lymphadenectomy is as much as 3%.

In response to this morbidity, several less invasive surgical techniques were developed: separate incisions for inguinal lymphadenectomy, unilateral inguinal node dissection for lateralized lesions, saphenous vein preservation [9], and sartorius muscle transposition. Superficial lymphadenectomy was also proposed as a less invasive alternative to complete inguinal node dissection in order to diminish local complications. This procedure excludes the inguinal deep nodes located beneath the cribriform fascia and medial to femoral vein (including the Cloquet node). However, excessive nodal recurrences were reported in the literature [10, 11] with this technique.

One of the most interesting approaches to reduce the morbidity of extensive inguinal lymphadenectomy in vulvar cancer is the sentinel lymph node biopsy. This minimally invasive procedure allows selective ablation of the first draining tumor node, thereby permitting a less aggressive inguinal surgery. Published results are promising [12–15].

D. Huber (✉) · D. Robyr · N. Schneider
Obstetrics and Gynecology, CHCV Sion Hospital,
Rue Champsec 80,
Sion 1950, Switzerland
e-mail: ghetudana@gmail.com

In 2008, the GROINSS-V study concluded that the sentinel lymph node procedure in early stage unifocal vulvar cancer reduces morbidity without increasing groin recurrence or compromising overall survival.

The newest minimal invasive procedure—video endoscopic inguino-femoral lymphadenectomy (VEIL)—was developed by Bishoff [16], an oncological urologist who demonstrated its feasibility by dissecting two cadaveric models in 2003. In 2006, Tobias-Machado et al. [17] published an initial case report of video endoscopic inguinal lymphadenectomy compared with a controlateral open radical procedure. VEIL continues to evolve: single site and robotic variants were recently presented [18–20].

Material and method

A 55-year-old postmenopausal female presented with an exophytic and ulcerated mass in both the minor labia and clitoris. A preoperative biopsy suspected a VIN III lesion. The superficial anterior vulvectomy established the diagnosis of invasive vulvar carcinoma, pathological stage pT1b with no carcinomatous lymphangitis. A CT scan infirmed pelvic and inguinal nodes involvement. Video-assisted inguino-femoral lymphadenectomy was scheduled 5 weeks after the vulvectomy.

Preoperative vascular Doppler ultrasound mapping was performed to identify the internal saphenous vein, its accessory vein, and the femoral vessels projection on the femoral triangle. The landmarks of the femoral triangle, the course of femoral vessels, and the saphenous veins were traced with indelible ink before prepping and draping (Fig. 1). This allows the correct placement of trocars outside the perimeter of the femoral triangle and permits the constant survey of the extent of subcutaneous dissection by transillumination during the endoscopic procedure.

The patient was placed in a supine position on a regular table with split movable footrests, which allowed abduction and external rotation of the thighs. The surgeon was positioned between the legs of the patient and the assistant was positioned lateral to the operated groin. The monitor was opposite the patient's shoulder. A Foley catheter was placed in the bladder.

A 15-mm incision was made 2 cm below the vertex of the femoral triangle. After the incision of Camper's fascia, scissors and digital blunt dissection were used to develop a space beneath it. The second and the third 10-mm incisions were placed at 6 cm external and 6 cm internal to the vertex of the femoral triangle. Three 10-mm Hasson trocars were placed in these incisions and fixed to the skin with nonresorbable sutures. A zero-degree laparoscope was inserted through the first trocar. CO_2 insufflation pressure was started at 15 mmHg for 15 min to help the dissection

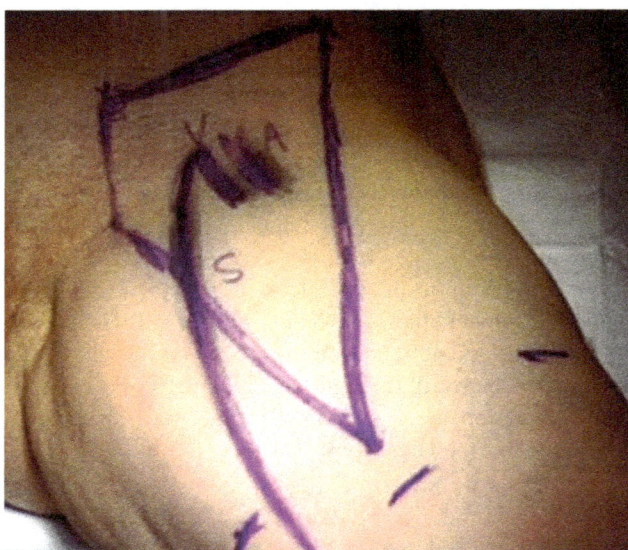

Fig. 1 The landmarks of the femoral triangle, the course of the femoral vessels and saphenous veins traced with indelible ink before prepping and draping

and was subsequently reduced to 5 mmHg during the rest of the procedure.

The retrograde dissection beneath the Camper fascia was continued until clear identification of the inguinal ligament (Fig. 2). Selective electrocoagulations or clip ligations were necessary before division of several saphenous veins and femoral artery branches. Early identification of the internal saphenous vein is needed for a precise and bloodless technique.

The distal lymphatic tissue and saphenous veins were divided at the vertex of the femoral triangle with the Endo GIA Roticulator™ 45-2.5-mm endovascular stapler and a harmonic scalpel. The lymphatic tissue was lifted from the

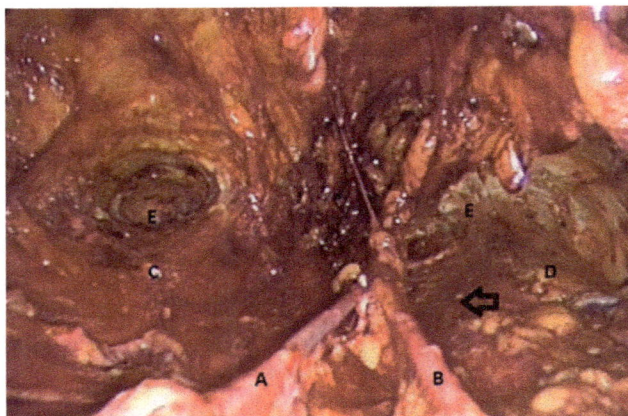

Fig. 2 Retrograde dissection with development of anterior space beneath the Camper fascia. *A* and *B* saphenous veins and their respective accessories; *C* sartorius muscle; *D* adductor longus muscle; *E* inguinal ligament

fascia lata by a combination of blunt and sharp dissection up to the fossa ovalis. The femoral sheet was carefully dissected and opened at the inferior limit of the fossa ovalis. The femoral vessels and the saphenofemoral junction were identified and skeletonized up to the femoral channel. The same Endo GIA endovascular stapler was used to transect the saphenous arch. Inguinal lymphadenectomy was continued medially to the femoral vein to harvest the deep inguinal nodes up to the Cloquet node. At the level of the inguinal ligament, the lymphatic tissue was divided with the harmonic scalpel and completely liberated. The nodal tissue was removed through the lateral 10-mm incision using an endobag. A suction drainage was placed and exteriorized at the lateral port incision.

Findings

The total operative time for the bilateral inguinal lymphadenectomy was 260 min. The estimated blood loss was less than 50 ml on each side. No subcutaneous CO_2 emphysema was observed beyond the upper thighs. Prophylactic 1.5 g intravenous cefuroxime was administered at the anesthetic induction and a second equivalent dose after 180 min. An adapted compression stocking was applied immediately post-intervention. Postoperative pain control was achieved with oral nonsteroidal anti-inflammatory drugs. Early ambulation was encouraged. The inguinal drainage was maintained until the 24-h output was less than 50 ml (seventh postoperative day for both sides). On the right side, acute lymphangitis occurred on the fifth postoperative day and successfully managed by oral antibiotics for 1 week (Fig. 3). The definitive pathological stage was pT1bN0M0 (eight negative nodes on each side).

An external vulvar radiation therapy and a close clinical follow-up were recommended to the patient. The patient was satisfied with both the functional and esthetic results 4 months after the procedure.

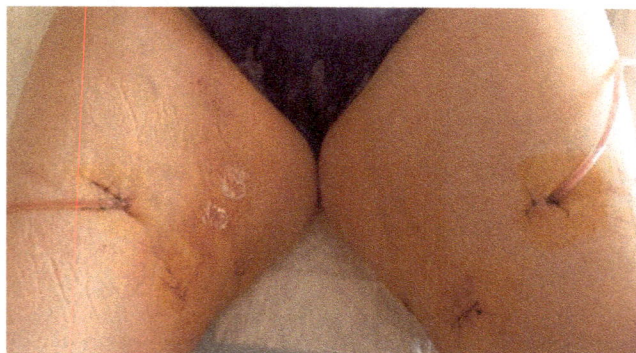

Fig. 3 Postoperative aspect on the fifth day after surgery

Conclusion

The video-assisted approach follows the same main steps as those for the open technique but in a reverse manner as lymphadenectomy is started caudally and continued up to the saphenous arch and the inguinal ligament. Inguinal lymphadenectomy is a challenging surgical procedure with a high complication rate even for skilled surgeons and in the most recent series [9, 21, 22]. This can be related to the devascularization of skin flaps, the disruption of lymphatic afferents, concomitant medical conditions that predispose to poor wound healing, and simultaneous septic operative steps as ablation of a potential necrotic and infected primary tumor. Since the first description of an endoscopic approach by Bishoff in 2003 [16], Tobias-Machado et al. have published a consistent comparison with the open procedure on the same patient [17, 23–26] demonstrating a significant reduced morbidity for the video-assisted approach (70% versus 20%) [23–25]. Other published series have consistently reported fewer skin postoperative events and lymphatic morbidity [27–29].

VEIL appears attractive in current oncological practice. The number of lymph nodes harvested is comparable with open inguinal lymphadenectomy [18, 23, 26, 29, 30] and with the advantage of less subcutaneous flap injuries and attendant complications, shorter hospitalization, and early patient ambulation and recovery [17, 23–26, 29–31]. Our operating time was significantly longer compared to classical surgery, but we believe that standardized surgical procedures, improvements of endoscopic instrumentation, and a dedicated trained surgical team could considerably improve this aspect. Reports indicate that operating time significantly decrease with the learning curve [32]. Our feeling is that the learning curve is not steep for a trained oncologist surgeon with experience in laparoscopic techniques as the main principles of endoscopic surgery apply. In addition there are the advantages of enhanced visualization of anatomical structures and optical magnification.

In 2009, Master et al. developed a modified endoscopic approach permitting completion of a lymphadenectomy even for large or adherent inguinal adenopathy, in cases of previous groin surgery and for obese patients expanding the indications for this minimally invasive technique. Thus, VEIL has the potential to replace open inguinal surgery for a large panel of patients. The middle-term outcome of the initial series seems to fulfill the oncological objectives [25], but extended follow-up is needed for more definitive conclusions and a better patient selection. To our knowledge, this is the first report of a video endoscopic bilateral inguinal lymphadenectomy in a patient with low genital tract malignancy.

Acknowledgments Many thanks go to M.E. Visher for her essential and gracious support in revising the manuscript's English.

Conflicts of interests The authors report no conflicts of interest. The authors alone are responsible for the content and writing of the paper.

References

1. Jemal A et al (2010) Cancer statistics. CA Cancer J Clin 60 (5):277–300

2. Courtney-Brooks M et al (2010) Does the number of nodes removed impact survival in vulvar cancer patients with node-negative disease? Gynecol Oncol 117(2):308–311

3. Butler JS et al (2010) Isolated groin recurrence in vulval squamous cell cancer (VSCC). The importance of node count. Eur J Gynaecol Oncol 31(5):510–513

4. Nelson BA et al (2004) Complications of inguinal and pelvic lymphadenectomy for squamous cell carcinoma of the penis: a contemporary series. J Urol 172(2):494–497

5. Gaarenstroom KN et al (2003) Postoperative complications after vulvectomy and inguinofemoral lymphadenectomy using separate groin incisions. Int J Gynecol Cancer 13(4):522–527

6. Han LY et al (2004) A gelatin matrix-thrombin tissue sealant (FloSeal) application in the management of groin breakdown after inguinal lymphadenectomy for vulvar cancer. Int J Gynecol Cancer 14(4):621–624

7. Magrina JF et al (1997) Femoral hernia: a complication of laparoendoscopic pelvic lymphadenectomy after groin node dissection. J Laparoendosc Adv Surg Tech A 7(3):191–193

8. Senn B et al (2010) Period prevalence and risk factors for postoperative short-term wound complications in vulvar cancer: a cross-sectional study. Int J Gynecol Cancer 20(4):646–654

9. Zhang SH et al (2000) Preservation of the saphenous vein during inguinal lymphadenectomy decreases morbidity in patients with carcinoma of the vulva. Cancer 89(7):1520–1525

10. Iyibozkurt AC et al (2010) Groin recurrence following stage IA squamous cell carcinoma of the vulva with negative nodes on superficial inguinal lymphadenectomy. Eur J Gynaecol Oncol 31 (3):354–356

11. Gordinier ME et al (2003) Groin recurrence in patients with vulvar cancer with negative nodes on superficial inguinal lymphadenectomy. Gynecol Oncol 90(3):625–628

12. Radziszewski J et al (2010) The accuracy of the sentinel lymph node concept in early stage squamous cell vulvar carcinoma. Gynecol Oncol 116(3):473–477

13. Cabanas RM (2000) The concept of the sentinel lymph node. Recent Results Cancer Res 157:109–120

14. Levenback CF et al (2009) Sentinel lymph node biopsy in patients with gynecologic cancers Expert panel statement from the International Sentinel Node Society Meeting, February 21, 2008. Gynecol Oncol 114(2):151–156

15. Van der Zee AG et al (2008) Sentinel node dissection is safe in the treatment of early stage vulvar cancer. J Clin Oncol 26(6):884–889

16. Bishoff JA, Lackland A, Basler JW et al (2003) Endoscopic subcutaneous modified inguinal lymph node dissection (ESMIL) for squamous cell carcinoma of the penis. J Urol 169(4):78

17. Tobias-Machado M et al (2006) Video endoscopic inguinal lymphadenectomy (VEIL): initial case report and comparison with open radical procedure. Arch Esp Urol 59(8):849–852

18. Tobias-Machado M et al (2011) Single-site video endoscopic inguinal lymphadenectomy: initial report. J Endourol 25(4):607–610

19. Josephson DY et al (2009) Robotic-assisted endoscopic inguinal lymphadenectomy. Urology 73(1):167–170, discussion 170–171

20. Tobias-Machado M, Neto AS (2009) Re: Josephson et al.: robotic-assisted endoscopic inguinal lymphadenectomy (Urology 2009;73:167–170). Urology 73(6):1424–1425

21. Manci N et al (2009) Inguinofemoral lymphadenectomy: randomized trial comparing inguinal skin access above or below the inguinal ligament. Ann Surg Oncol 16(3):721–728

22. Micheletti L, Bogliatto F, Massobrio M (2005) Groin lymphadenectomy with preservation of femoral fascia: total inguinofemoral node dissection for treatment of vulvar carcinoma. World J Surg 29(10):1268–1276

23. Tobias-Machado M et al (2008) Can video endoscopic inguinal lymphadenectomy achieve a lower morbidity than open lymph node dissection in penile cancer patients? J Endourol 22(8):1687–1691

24. Tobias-Machado M et al (2007) Video endoscopic inguinal lymphadenectomy: a new minimally invasive procedure for radical management of inguinal nodes in patients with penile squamous cell carcinoma. J Urol 177(3):953–957, discussion 958

25. Walter F, Correa MT-M (2010) Video-endoscopic inguinal lymphadenectomy. Eur Oncol 6(2):80–84

26. Tobias-Machado M et al (2006) Video endoscopic inguinal lymphadenectomy (VEIL): minimally invasive resection of inguinal lymph nodes. Int Braz J Urol 32(3):316–321

27. Machado MT, Molina W Jr, Tavares A et al (2005) Comparative study between video-endoscopic inguinal lymphadenectomy (VEIL) and standard open procedure for penile cancer: preliminary surgical and oncological results. J Urol 173:226

28. Thyavihally Y, Tongaonkar H (2009) Video-Endoscopic inguinal lymphadenectomy (VEIL): our initial experience. J Urol 72:181 (4):427

29. Master V et al (2009) Leg endoscopic groin lymphadenectomy (LEG procedure): step-by-step approach to a straightforward technique. Eur Urol 56(5):821–828

30. Sotelo R, Sanchez-Salas R, Clavijo R (2009) Endoscopic inguinal lymph node dissection for penile carcinoma: the developing of a novel technique. World J Urol 27(2):213–219

31. Sotelo R et al (2007) Endoscopic lymphadenectomy for penile carcinoma. J Endourol 21(4):364–367, discussion 367

32. Tobias-Machado M, Starling ES, Oliveira ABP, Pompeo AC, Wroclawski ER (2009) 5-years experience with video endoscopic inguinal lymphadenectomy (VEIL): learning curve and technical variations of a new procedure. J Androlog Sci 16:25–32

4

Constructing a protocol for the evaluation of residents' competency with office hysteroscopy

Charalampos S. Siristatidis · Dimitrios S. Miligkos ·
Igor V. Klyucharov · Nikos Vrachnis · Zoe Iliodromiti ·
Charalampos Chrelias · Johannes Bitzer ·
Dimitrios Kassanos · Stefano Bettocchi

Abstract There is an increasing need for clinician self-evaluation. The need becomes bigger when it comes to assess residents in operative procedures; office hysteroscopy in its current form is one of the best examples to teach and to assess them. We propose a simple protocol for the evaluation of residents in office hysteroscopy that can be used as a platform for future improvement. This will improve their learning experience and ensure that they do not miss any steps of the procedure. As each task is outlined on the evaluation checklist, it is easier to objectively demonstrate the strengths and deficiencies of each one with respect to the given procedure. This can be the basis for application of extra attention and highlights the areas in which each individual needs to improve. The advantage of recording parameters, such as duration of the procedure and pain scores, is that they can serve as tools that demonstrate acquisition of experience and of confidence.

Keywords Office hysteroscopy · Training ·
Residents' training · Education · Protocol

C. S. Siristatidis (✉)
Assisted Reproduction Unit, 3rd Department
of Obstetrics and Gynecology, University of Athens, Athens,
Attica, Greece
e-mail: harrysiri@yahoo.gr

D. S. Miligkos
Department of Obstetrics and Gynecology, Princess Anne
Hospital, Southampton University Hospitals, Southampton, UK

I. V. Klyucharov
Department of Obstetrics and Gynecology No. 1, Kazan State
Medical University, Republican Clinical Hospital, CCCH No. 18,
CAC No. 2,
Kazan, Russia

N. Vrachnis · Z. Iliodromiti
2nd Department of Obstetrics and Gynecology, University of
Athens Medical School, Aretaieio Hospital, Athens 11528, Greece

C. Chrelias · D. Kassanos
3rd Department of Obstetrics and Gynecology, University of
Athens Medical School, Attikon Hospital, Athens, Greece

J. Bitzer
Department of Obstetrics and Gynecology, University Hospital
Basel, Spitalstrasse 21,
CH-4031, Basel, Switzerland

S. Bettocchi
First Unit of Obstetrics and Gynecology, Department of
Biomedical Sciences and Human Oncology, University "Aldo
Moro", Bari, Italy

Introduction

Ambulatory procedures are currently a significant part of the obstetrician/gynecologist's diagnostic and therapeutic armamentarium [1]. In this context, hysteroscopy has gained considerable popularity among clinicians, replacing traditional approaches in many cases. Its advantage lies in the capacity for the direct visual assessment of the cervical canal and uterine cavity and, depending on the case, the possibility for surgical intervention at the time of diagnosis ("see and treat" technique) [2]. Advantages offered by instrumentation, refinement of the technique and adequate training, have led to the development of office hysteroscopy employing the "no-touch" (or vaginoscopic) approach; no cervical dilatation or any kind of anesthesia/analgesia is needed [2]. Its chief importance stems from the fact that the patient is awake and a minimal intervention can solve the problem at the time of diagnosis without generating marked discomfort or complications. The latter are reported as extremely rare [3]. There are reports pointing out that the anxiety of an outpatient treatment can affect tolerance of the procedure. However, this is counterbalanced by the reduction of waiting time and number of clinic visits as well as results in *n* overall increased patient satisfaction [4]. However, it is imperative that a physician perform this type of advanced hysteroscopy only after demonstrating competency in the accredited setting with standardized assessment instruments [1].

Training of young physicians in new modalities remains a crucial step in optimizing health care services. This process encompasses the provision of adequate levels of knowledge and skills, without simultaneously placing the patients' health at risk. A major issue in postgraduate medical education is that trainees are often deemed competent to act as primary surgeons based on self or supervisors' global assessments and case logs which lack the appropriate validity and reliability [5, 6]. Therefore, the challenge still exists for development and testing of more robust methods for documenting the residents' competency to perform a procedure in a highly accurate manner.

The construction of protocols/algorithms of the competency of a trainee is essential for both himself/herself and the tutors. Such methods have been developed, but they largely remain as research tools and have yet to be widely accepted and applied to current surgical practice. The technical skills required for endoscopic surgery differ from open surgery due to the lack of perception of depth, tactile feedback, and the necessary hand–eye coordination when operating by looking at a TV screen [7]. These skills are even more imperative for outpatient endoscopic surgery where the patient is awake and surgical accuracy and efficiency are of major significance for minimization of patient discomfort.

The objective of this article is to describe the construction of a protocol for the evaluation of residents in performing outpatient office hysteroscopy.

Skills assessment scales

In general, there are three types of skills assessment tools currently used: (a) rating scales for the assessment of generic skills (Global Rating Scale, Objective Structured Assessment of Surgical Skills, Global Operative Assessment of Laparoscopic Skills, etc.): they aim to evaluate generic technical abilities, not necessarily linked to a specific procedure; (b) procedure (task)-specific skills assessment (procedure-specific checklist, error scoring system, observational clinical human reliability analysis, etc.): they are characterized by a breakdown of a procedure into tasks (task analysis), though the type of scoring may differ; and (c) a combination of generic and procedure-specific assessment tools [8].

The concept of objective structured assessment of surgical skills was first pioneered by Reznick et al. to assess general surgery residents [9]. In hysteroscopy, various examples have been reported [10–12]. Now, more than ever, it is common sense—and there is also a pressing need—for trainees to be assessed as concerns their technical skills in an objective way targeted to the procedure under assessment. With regard to minimally invasive surgical skills, there is an increasing shift to training outside the operating room by using models and simulators. Surgeons can improve their performance by repeated practice, feedback, and learning without concerns of causing any harm [13]. Different tools have been applied to evaluate either overall operative performance, as for example, the Contrasting Group Method [14] and the Global Rating Scale of operating performance [9] or to assess specific procedures, such as the Vaginal Surgical Skills Index [15] and laparoscopic, open abdominal, and hysteroscopic procedures [10, 16].

Outpatient hysteroscopy setting and procedure

Since 2005, we have developed an outpatient hysteroscopy service in a specialized treatment clinic, which is adequately equipped and staffed. We provide a "see and treat" service when this is deemed appropriate and after the patient's full counseling regarding the procedure. Our standard technique is the vaginoscopic approach with insertion of the hysteroscope through the cervical canal and into the uterine cavity without the need for a vaginal speculum, cervical manipulation, or local anesthesia. This technique has been described by Bettochi et al. [2, 4].

We use a rigid single-flow mini-hysteroscope with a final diameter of 3.4 mm with an oval profile to match the shape of the cervical canal (Bettocchi Office Hysteroscope; Karl Storz GmbH & Co., Tuttlingen, Germany). The scope is based on a rigid rod lens system with a diameter of 2 mm and a 30° view and armed with an incorporated 5-Fr. working channel. Only mechanical instruments are used, including sharp scissors and crocodile grasping forceps (Karl Storz GmbH & Co.). A 250-W xenon light source is used to offer a high performance in optimal visualization and image quality.

We use normal saline (N/S 0.9 %) as the distension medium instilled from a 1,000/3,000-ml bag wrapped in a pressure bag connected to a manometer and pumped to 120–140 mmHg. For tissue biopsy, we use the grasp technique, as it is safer and easier for inexperienced surgeons to remove lesions and provide the pathologist with the necessary amount of tissue for histologic examination [17].

Detailed patient counseling takes place before the procedure with regard to the technique itself, the feeling of the uterine distension, and potential adverse effects. Patients are reassured that the procedure will stop as soon as the patient feels dizziness or the pain becomes intolerable.

Basal blood pressure and heart rate are monitored before and after the procedure by an attending staff nurse. Apart from a bimanual vaginal examination performed prior to hysteroscopy, no other preoperative investigations are needed. Intrauterine lesions, such as polyps, fibroids, and synechiae, and simple targeted endometrial biopsies are removed at the time of diagnosis, provided that their diameter and location permit. Our criteria for removal in the outpatient setting are polyps less than 1 cm, G0 submucosal fibroids (completely within the uterine cavity), small uterine septae, and endometrial biopsies. Larger polyps, G1 and G2 submucosal fibroids, and extensive intrauterine synechiae are scheduled for hysteroscopic resection under general anesthesia. During an operative procedure, there is continuous monitoring of the fluid deficit.

Exclusion criteria for the procedure are acute pelvic inflammatory disease, severe active vaginal bleeding, positive pregnancy test, cardiovascular disease (active or history, concerning arrhythmias and ischemia), and suspicion of uterine malignancy.

Failure of the procedure is defined as the following:

(a) When no diagnosis can be made due to poor visualization
(b) Failed access into the cavity
(c) Or patient discomfort of "5" or more on the visual analog score

Training before evaluation

Trainees undergoing a rotation in the outpatient treatment clinic have to attend four theoretical training sessions organized by specialists in operative hysteroscopy, who run outpatient treatment clinics on a regular basis. The curriculum of these sessions includes:

(a) A comprehensive theoretical program of the principles of diagnostic and operative hysteroscopy, instrumentation, complications, equipment troubleshooting, and electrosurgery principles in minimal access surgery.
(b) Video demonstration of diagnostic and operative hysteroscopic procedures is covered in the third session.
(c) In the fourth session, the trainee has the opportunity to practice the resection of endometrium, polyps, and submucosal fibroids in a hysteroscopic simulator.

Upon completion of the four sessions, each trainee participates in a minimum of five outpatient hysteroscopic procedures performed by trainers. Ideally, all trainees should have had prior experience in operative hysteroscopy under general anesthetic. We suggest differentiating groups of trainees based on existing experience in performing hysteroscopy: the first group: inexperienced and the second group: experienced

trainees. We also take into account the ESGE classification of the hysteroscopy complexity [18].

Evaluation tool

The tool is constructed as a checklist with the aim of assessing four dimensions (Table 1):

(a) Preoperative communication
(b) Technical procedure including the steps to establish a diagnosis (clear visualization) and effectiveness of eventually necessary therapeutic steps
(c) Interpretation of the findings and information of the patient
(d) Tolerability for the patient

Appropriate patient counseling and consent, documentation, equipment assembly, and the different steps of each procedure are marked on a "0–1–2" scale. Mark "0" relates to a task incorrectly performed or not performed at all, mark "1" to a task where help is needed, and mark "2" to a task performed correctly and independently. The operative technique (resection of lesion or biopsy) is rated on a "0" to "2" scale to allow more flexibility for the assessment of the trainee.

Each trainee is further assessed as to his ability to interpret findings and effectively communicate these to the patient as well as the need for the trainer's contribution to the safe completion of the procedure. The duration of the procedure is recorded and measured from the time of the insertion of the hysteroscope into the vagina until termination of the flow of the distension medium.

To assess the patient's tolerance of the procedure, we use a visual analog score with a 0–10 scale (Table 2). Score "0" suggests no discomfort at all and score "10" suggests the worst pain the patient reports ever having experienced. Patients are asked to rate the pain score during the procedure and 15 min after the end of the procedure. Intraoperatively, if the pain score is 5 or more, the procedure is discontinued. The intra- and postoperative pain scores are recorded in the trainee's evaluation form.

Evaluation procedure

The supervising trainer in the clinic performs all markings. Post-procedure discussion of the trainee's performance is undertaken to provide feedback and areas where improvement is needed. A higher score indicates a better performance. Success rate is defined as an overall score of 18/24 points or more. Trainees are deemed competent to perform a

Table 1 Task score list for performing office hysteroscopy

Task scores		0: not done or incorrect	1: needs help	2: done independently
1	Proper consultation of the patient on procedure, risks, and benefits, before and after	0	1	2
2	Exact knowledge of instruments/system and fitting	0	1	2
3	Discovery and identification of the external cervical os	0	1	2
4	Entrance into the cervical canal/rotation of the scope by 90°	0	1	2
5	Passage through the canal/appearance of the canal has to be at 6 and 12 o'clock positions (ante- or retroverted uterus)	0	1	2
6	Inspection of the intrauterine cavity/rotation of the body of the scope by 90° (right and left) for the examination of the tubal ostia	0	1	2
7	Pulling back of the scope at the level of the internal cervical os to obtain a panoramic view of the uterus	0	1	2
8	Recognition and/or selection of appropriate findings to operate (synechiaes, polyps, fibroids, uterine septum)	0	1	2
9	Operative technique/grasp technique/biopsy/polyp removal	0	1	2
10	Complications: recognition/treatment	0	1	2
11	Patients' compliance[a]	0	1	2
12	Pain scores[b]	0 (above 5)	1 (4–6)	2 (below 5)
Total:		0	12	24

[a] Refers to patient's general acceptance of the procedure and cooperation with the clinician/performer

[b] Refers to pain scores during (a) and 15 min after (b) the procedure. If it has to be discontinued, scoring falls to 0. The mean pain score is calculated as follows: mean PS $= [2(a) + (b)]/3$

certain procedure when they have successfully completed ten assessments. With increasing experience, we expect that trainees will demonstrate improvement of their performance among cases of similar complexity. For those who consistently fail to improve their score, we recommend that they observe additional procedures in the outpatient clinic, performing more frequently under general anesthetic and carrying out further practice in using the hysteroscopic simulator.

Discussion

We propose a protocol of training in office hysteroscopy, which we believe to be advantageous for both trainees and trainers. It can be used as a platform with all the tasks that need to be performed by the trainee during outpatient hysteroscopy, necessitating that the trainee focus on all the relevant surgical steps. This improves the learning experience and ensures that the trainee does not miss any steps of the procedure. Furthermore, as each task is outlined on the evaluation checklist, it is

easier to objectively demonstrate the strengths and deficiencies of the trainee with respect to the given procedure. This can be the basis for application of extra attention and highlights the areas in which each individual needs to improve. The advantage of recording parameters, such as duration of the procedure and pain scores, is that they can serve as tools that demonstrate acquisition of experience and of confidence.

For the trainer, these structural assessments help to gain an overview of the overall performance of each trainee, indicate areas of concern, and aid the feedback process. This is all the more important in busy departments with large numbers of residents/inexperienced surgeons [19].

The protocol has certain limitations. First, the fact that both trainers and trainees work in the same institution can bias the assessment and thus reduce its validity [10, 20]; unfortunately, in most departments, the organization of blinded assessments, and especially in an outpatient setting, is difficult. Second, the nature itself of an outpatient setting is a difficult environment for trainees to develop their surgical skills: anxiety that the patient might not tolerate the procedure due to unnecessary movements or inadvertent

Table 2 Pain classification and action taken

Pain score	0–1	2–4	5–7	8–10
Evaluation	No discomfort	Discomfort similar to menstrual pain (tolerable)	Moderate pain similar to heavy menstrual pain requiring drugs	Severe pain
Action	Continuation	Continuation, searching for autonomous nervous system symptoms	Discontinuation of the procedure	Discontinuation of the procedure

tissue damage can result in the trainer's lower threshold for intervening and taking over the procedure [20]: to overcome this, we have included participants who had some experience in operative hysteroscopy under general anesthetic. Third, we have not as yet validated this protocol, but we aim to do so 6 months after introducing it; in parallel, we are planning to obtain feedback from trainees as to whether they believe that this improves their training and learning experience.

Conclusion

The need for standardized assessment of residents in ambulatory procedures is obvious; office hysteroscopy in its current form is one of the best examples to teach and to assess the trainees [21]. We propose a simple protocol to assess residents' efficacy and competency. It provides a platform on the basis of which both trainees and supervisors can work together with the aim of transforming residents into safe and skilled primary surgeons. A subsequent step should include its testing in terms of validity and reliability.

References

1. Wortman M (2010) Instituting an office-based surgery program in the gynecologist's office. J Minim Invasive Gynecol 17:673–683
2. Bettocchi S, Selvaggi L (1997) A vaginoscopic approach to reduce the pain of office hysteroscopy. J Am Assoc Gynecol Laparosc 4:255–258
3. van Kerkvoorde TC, Veersema S, Timmermans A (2012) Long-term complications of office hysteroscopy: analysis of 1028 cases. J Minim Invasive Gynecol 19:494–749
4. Bettocchi S, Ceci O, Nappi L et al (2004) Operative office hysteroscopy without anesthesia: analysis of 4863 cases performed with mechanical instruments. J Am Assoc Gynecol Laparosc 11:59–61
5. Mandel LS, Lentz GM, Goff BA (2000) Teaching and evaluating surgical skills. Obstet Gynecol 95:783–785
6. Reznick RK (1993) Teaching and testing technical skills. Am J Surg 165:358–361
7. Palter VN (2011) Comprehensive training curricula for minimally invasive surgery. J Grad Med Educ 3:293–298
8. Ahmed K, Miskovic D, Darzi A et al (2011) Observational tools for assessment of procedural skills: a systematic review. Am J Surg 202:469–480
9. Reznick R, Regehr G, MacRae H et al (1997) Testing technical skill via an innovative "bench station" examination. Am J Surg 173:226–230
10. VanBlaricom AL, Goff BA, Chinn M et al (2005) A new curriculum for hysteroscopy training as demonstrated by an objective structured assessment of technical skills (OSATS). Am J Obstet Gynecol 193:1856–1865
11. Chahine EB, Janakiraman V, Robinson J et al (2008) An objective Structured Assessment of Technical Skills (OSATS) in operative hysteroscopy. J Minim Invasive Gynecol 15:14S
12. Bixel K, Doudge L, Hur H-C (2011) Use of an Objective Structured Assessment of Technical Skills (OSATS) tool during hysteroscopy workshop for resident's evaluation and education. J Minim Invasive Gynecol 18:S66–S67
13. Burchard ER, Lockrow EG, Zahn CM et al (2007) Simulation training improves resident performance in operative hysteroscopic resection techniques. Am J Obstet Gynecol 197:542
14. Fraser SA, Klassen DR, Feldman LS et al (2003) Evaluating laparoscopic skills: setting the pass/fail score for the MISTELS system. Surg Endosc 17:964–967
15. Chen C, Korn A, Klingele C et al (2010) Objective assessment of vaginal surgical skills. Am J Obstet Gynecol 203:79
16. Goff B, Mandel L, Lentz G et al (2005) Assessment of resident surgical skills: is testing feasible? Am J Obstet Gynecol 192:1331–1338, discussion 1338–40
17. Bettocchi S, Di Venere R, Pansini N et al (2002) Endometrial biopsies using small-diameter hysteroscopes and 5 F instruments: how can we obtain enough material for a correct histologic diagnosis? J Am Assoc Gynecol Laparosc 9:290–292
18. European Society for Gynaecological Endoscopy (2013) Classification hysteroscopy. http://www.esge.org/media/files/hystt%20identification%20form.pdf. Accessed 17 Feb 2013
19. Campo R, Molinas CR, Rombauts L et al (2005) Prospective multicentre randomized controlled trial to evaluate factors influencing the success rate of office diagnostic hysteroscopy. Hum Reprod 20:258–263
20. Goff BA, Nielsen PE, Lentz GM et al (2002) Surgical skills assessment: a blinded examination of obstetrics and gynecology residents. Am J Obstet Gynecol 186:613–617
21. Siristatidis C, Chrelias C, Salamalekis G et al (2010) Office hysteroscopy: current trends and potential applications: a critical review. Arch Obstet Gynecol 282:383–388

5

IBS® Integrated Bigatti Shaver versus conventional bipolar resectoscopy

G. Bigatti · C. Ferrario · M. Rosales · A. Baglioni · S. Bianchi

Abstract Conventional bipolar resectoscopy is widely recognized as the first choice for major hysteroscopic operations. We recently proposed an alternative approach to operative hysteroscopy called Integrated Bigatti Shaver (IBS®) that improves visualization during the procedure, reducing several problems of conventional resectoscopy such as fluid overload, water intoxication, uterine perforation and long surgeon's learning curve. In cooperation with Karl Storz GmbH & Co., we created a new shaving system that, when introduced through the straight operative channel of a panoramic 90° optic, allows performance of many major hysteroscopic operations. The present randomised comparative study was designed to compare 50 cases performed with conventional bipolar resectoscope with 50 cases performed with the IBS®. Several types of major intrauterine pathologies such as polyps and submucosal myomas (according to ESGE classification) were included in the study. Two cases of via falsa were reported. In one case, the procedure was immediately stopped with no further complication for the patient, whereas in the second patient, the complication did not compromise the operative course. Dilatation time, overall procedure time, resection time and fluid balance were carefully monitored during each procedure in the two groups. The aim of the study was to compare the two techniques to confirm several advantages offered by the IBS® such as reduced dilatation of the cervix, better visualization during the procedure because tissue chips are removed at the same time as the resection, no need for coagulation or cutting current, utilization of normal saline and a much faster learning curve.

Keywords IBS® · Hysteroscopy · Resectoscopy · Shaver

G. Bigatti (✉) · C. Ferrario · M. Rosales · A. Baglioni
U.O. di Ostetricia e Ginecologia,
Ospedale Classificato San Giuseppe Via San Vittore,
12-20123 Milan, Italy
e-mail: g.big@tiscalinet.it

S. Bianchi
Università degli Studi di Milano,
Direttore dell'Unità Opertiva di Ostetricia e Ginecologia Ospedale Classificato San Giuseppe Via San Vittore,
12-20123 Milan, Italy

Background

Presently, the double-flow bipolar resectoscope is considered the gold standard for performing major operative hysteroscopical procedures [1, 2]. The resectoscope Stern-McCarthy built in the 1920s must be considered the precursor of the tool that we use today [3–5]. Despite its versatility, many technique-related problems remain unsolved. The use of a bipolar technique does not prevent overload syndrome with water intoxication. Although the use of isotonic solutions like 0.9% sodium chloride prevents dilution hyponatriemia and hypocalcaemia [6], the risk of fluid overload is still present. In addition, several case reports have shown that massive absorption of normal saline solution results in severe hyperchloremic metabolic acidosis and dilution coagulopathy that must be resolved with diuretic therapy [7, 8]. Additionally, because a high-frequency electric current is used during resection, uterine perforation with bowel injury and internal and external burns caused by uncontrolled leakage of current can occur [9–11]. Finally, during resection of large polyps or myomas, the surgeon's visual field is impaired by the tissue chips that remain inside the uterine cavity, increasing the risk of perforation. Tissue pieces must be removed from the uterine cavity in order to continue the procedure under visual control, making the operation tiring and increasing the overall resection time, resulting in a higher risk of intravasation and cervical laceration. Another minor problem is that more than half of the uterine perforations are entry related because of the large diameter of the conventional resectoscopes [12].

Resectoscopy with the conventional bipolar technique has a long learning curve for surgeons, explaining why even today, only a few surgeons perform operative hysteroscopy [13, 14]. The Integrated Bigatti Shaver (IBS®), with a double-window blade, has been shown to improve on the results of conventional resectoscopy, reducing the complication rate and improving the learning curve time [15]. The IBS® can remove the tissue chips at the time of the resection so that the procedure, always done under visual control, becomes faster and easier. The present study compares 50 cases performed with the IBS® with 50 cases performed with the conventional bipolar resectoscope.

Materials and methods

We performed all operations using either the IBS® or the conventional bipolar resectoscope (Versapoint ® by Gynecare). The IBS® is made of 90° angulated 0° optic (Karl Storz GmbH of Tuttlingen) with a continuous flow sheath and an extra-operative channel into which a rigid shaving system was introduced (Fig. 1). The continuous flow sheath was connected to a peristaltic pump (Endomat® Karl Storz GmbH of Tuttlingen) to maintain optimal distension and visualization inside the uterine cavity. Two separate stopcocks regulated inflow and outflow. The outer sheath diameter was of 24 Fr (8 mm). The rigid shaving system consisted of two hollow reusable metal tubes fitting into each other. The

inner tube rotated within the outer tube and was connected to a handheld (Drill cut-x Karl Storz GmbH of Tuttlingen) motor drive unit (Unidrive® eco Karl Storz GmbH of Tuttlingen) and a roller pump (Endomat® LC Karl Storz GmbH of Tuttlingen) controlled by a foot pedal.

The foot pedal is activated at the same time as the shaver tip and the roller pump to maintain a continuous suction power on the window tip during the procedure. The shaver tip of the IBS® was specifically designed to be aggressive on any kind of tissue. The inner rotating tube has a double window blade provided with a row of very sharp teeth. At the outer tube's edge, there is a window, 17, 20, 25 and 25 mm^2 wider radial large openings (Fig. 2), also provided with teeth.

We used 300 to 450 oscillating rotation power per minute and a flow pressure of suction of 500 ml/min. After dilatation of the internal ostium of the uterine cervix up to Hegar number 8.5, the panoramic optic with inflow and outflow channels connected to the Endomat pump was inserted into the uterine cavity. For irrigation, we used a normal isotonic solution like 0.9% sodium chloride. The maximum flow setting was 450 ml/min with an intrauterine pressure less than 95 mmHg. Once the pathological site was visualized, we introduced the rigid shaving system connected to the motor drive unit and the roller pump into the operative channel and started the procedure. Aspiration started only when the pedal of the roller pump was pressed; this prevented the collapse of the uterine cavity due to massive outflow. The rotating and oscillating movements of the inner blade of the shaving system cut the tissue and allowed aspiration of specimens for histology directly into a glass bottle connected to the roller pump (Endomat® LC Karl Storz GMBH of Tuttlingen).

Correct fluid balance was calculated by checking the fluid aspirated by the Endomat and roller pump connected to the shaving system plus the fluid collected in a graduated plastic bag placed under the patient.

The conventional bipolar resectoscope (Versapoint ® by Gynecare) consists of a 4-mm wire loop electrode mounted on a working element with hand piece, and a 12° operative

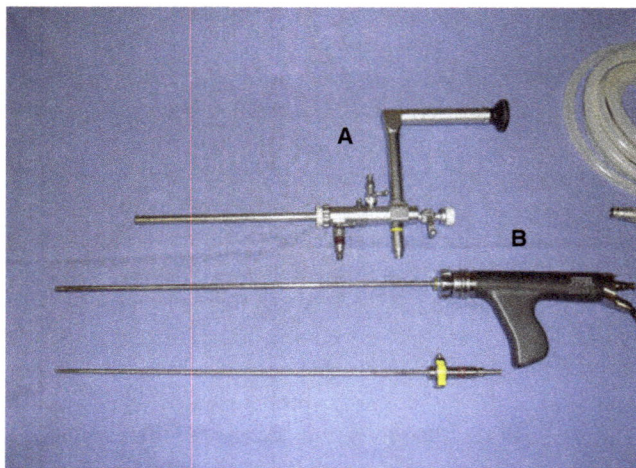

Fig. 1 Integrated Bigatti Shaver (IBS®). **a** 90° angulated 0°optic (Karl Storz GmbH of Tuttlingen) with a double flow sheath and an extra channel for the insertion of a **b** rigid shaving system

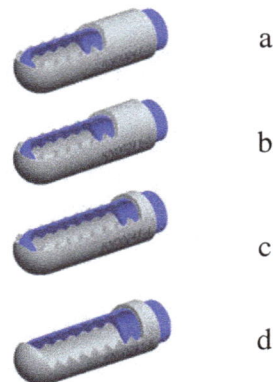

Fig. 2 Integrated Bigatti Shaver (IBS®) shaver tips: **a** 17 mm^2, **b** 20 mm^2, **c** 25 mm^2 and **d** 25 mm^2 wider radial opening

Table 1 Demographic and clinical data for Group A using Integrated Bigatti Shaver (IBS®)

	Polypectomy	Myomectomty	Polypectomy + Myomectomy	Endometrial Ablation
n (%)	31 (62)	12 (24)	5 (10)	2 (4)
Size (mm)[a]	15 (3–60), 17.5 (12.6)	20 (8–30), 20 (8.32)	Polyp 12.5 (10–40),17.5 (10.7)	
			Myoma 20 (10–25), 18 (5.09)	
Age (years) [b]	44 (84–31)	45 (35–74)	58 (46–64)	41 (36–46)
Parity(%)				
Nulliparous	16 (51.6)	5 (41.7)	2 (40)	2 (100)
Multiparous	15 (48.4)	7 (58.3)	3 (60)	0 (0)
Menopause (%)	14 (45.2)	4 (33.3)	3 (60)	0 (0)
Symptoms (%)				
None	9 (29)	1 (8.3)	3 (60)	0 (0)
Menorrhagia	9 (29)	11 (91.6)	1 (20)	2 (100)
Anaemia	0 (0)	3 (24.9)	0 (0)	1 (50)
Post Menop. AUB	3 (9.7)	0 (0)	1 (20)	0 (0)
Pelvic Pain	0 (0)	1 (8.3)	0 (0)	0 (0)
Infertility	4 (12.9)	1 (8.3)	0 (0)	0 (0)
Complications (%)	0 (0)	0 (0)	0 (0)	0 (0)

[a] Median (range); mean (SD)

[b] Median (range)

optic endoscope. The loop electrode is connected to a Versapoint® unit automatically supplying bipolar current of 170 W for cutting and 80 W for coagulation. The Versapoint® unit was set to VC1 [16]. The operative endoscope had a continuous flow sheath with separate inflow and outflow stopcocks connected to a peristaltic pump (Endomat® Karl Storz GmbH of Tuttlingen) to maintain optimal distension and visibility. The continuous

Table 2 Demographic and clinical data for Group B using the bipolar resectoscope (Versapoint®)

	Polypectomy	Myomectomty	Polypectomy + Myomectomy	Endometrial Ablation
n (%)	42 (85.7)	3 (6.1)	2 (4.1)	2 (41)
Size (mm)[a]	15 (4–55) 15.60 (9.35)	20 (10–20) 17.5 (4.33)	Polyp 8 (6–15) 9.67 (3.85)	
			Myoma 8 (8–8) 8 (0)	
Age (years) [b]	52 (29–82)	48 (43–52)	38 (37–39)	50 (39–61)
Parity (%)				
Nulliparous	16 (38.1)	1 (33.3)	2 (100)	1 (50)
Multiparous	26 (61.9)	2 (66.6)	0 (0)	1 (50)
Menopause (%)	22 (52.4)	1 (33.3)	0 (0)	1 (50)
Symptoms (%)				
None	13 (31.3)	2 (66.6)	1 (50)	0 (0)
Menorrhagia	15 (36)	1 (33.3)	1 (50)	1 (50)
Anaemia	0 (0)	1 (33.3)	0 (0)	1 (50)
Post Menop. AUB	12 (28.7)	0 (0)	0 (0)	1 (50)
Pelvic Pain	0 (0)	0 (0)	0 (0)	0 (0)
Infertility	6 (14)	0 (0)	0 (0)	0 (0)
Complications (%) [c]	2 (4.76)	0 (0)	0 (0)	0 (0)

[a] Median (range); mean (SD)

[b] Median (range)

[c] Complete perforation of the fundus (n=1) and a 5 to 10 mm false root of the fundus (n=1)

Table 3 Dilatation time

Dilatation	Group A (IBS®)				Group B (Versapoint®)				p Value
	Median	Range	Mean	DS	Median	Range	Mean	DS	
Dilatation (min)	1.5	1–18	2.14	2.7	2	1–14	2.65	2.53	0.3371

flow sheath was rotation free and had an external diameter of 27 Fr (9 mm).

After dilatation of the internal ostium of the uterine cervix up to Hegar number 9.5, the resectoscope connected to the peristaltic pump was inserted into the uterine cavity. Conventional resection technique was used. For irrigation, we used normal isotonic solutions like 0.9% sodium chloride. The maximal flow setting was 450 ml/min with an intrauterine pressure lower than 95 mmHg. Correct fluid balance was calculated by checking the fluid aspirated by the Endomat pump and by the fluid collected in a graduated plastic bag placed under the patient.

From March 2010 to February 2011, we performed 100 equally randomised either for the IBS® in Group A or the Versapoint ® Group B. The institutional ethical committee approved the research and all patients provided informed consent. Patients with several major intrauterine pathologies such as polyps as large as 6 cm, and G0, G1 and G2 submucosal myomas (classified according to the ESGE guidelines) that were up to 3 cm in diameter were included in the study [17, 18]. Uterine malformations such as partial or complete septum ablations and oncological cases were excluded from our trial. Both groups were similar with regard to age, parity and symptoms. All patients underwent general or regional anaesthesia, and a standard gynaecological setup was used in the operating room. All operations were performed by one expert surgeon and by one resident to evaluate the improvement in the surgeon's learning curve.

No statistical analysis was planned regarding preoperative therapy. Times of dilatation of the cervical canal, total operating time, resection time, fluid balance and complications were recorded. We considered the time for the procedure, without the dilatation time, as the total operative time. The time from the view of the cavity with the shaver tip or the resectoscope loop to the end of the resection was considered the resection time. Statistical analysis was performed using the Student's t test. Differences between groups were considered statistically significant at $p<0.05$. IBM SPSS Statistics 19 (©IBM Corporation 2010, IBM Corporation, Route 100 Somers, NY) statistical software package was used.

Findings

Patient collective

With the IBS®, we performed 31 (62%) polypectomies, 12 (24%) myomectomies, 5 (10%) polypectomies and myomectomies and 2 (4%) endometrial ablations (Table 1).

With the Versapoint®, 42 (85.7%) polypectomies, 3 (6.1%) myometomies, 2 (4.1%) polypectomies and myomectomies and 2 (4.1%) endometrial ablations were performed (Table 2).

The study design only randomised for major pathology but not within one group of pathology; for this reason, the myomectomies that are unequally randomised do not permit a comparative analysis.

Cervical dilatation time

As shown in Table 3, there was no statistically significant difference in the overall dilatation time between Groups A and B ($p=0.3371$). There was a statistically significantly shorter time of dilatation in the IBS® group (Group A) during myoma resection (median, 1.5 min; range, 1–2.5 min; mean, 1.37 min; DS, 0.42 min) compared with

Table 4 Polyp resection

Polyp resection	Group A (IBS®)				Group B (Versapoint®)				p Value
	Median	Range	Mean	DS	Median	Range	Mean	DS	
Dilatation (min)	1.5	1–18	2.51	3.51	2	1–14	2.5	2.33	1.0000
Operating Time (min)	5	3–13	6.76	5.21	9.75	4–21	10.5	4.51	0.0016
Resection Time (min)	2	0.16–12	2.95	3.23	5	0.33–16	5.56	3.57	0.0020
Fluid used (ml)	1500	400–5000	1845	1276.8	1550	500–5000	1697	874.9	0.5598
Fluid deficit (ml)	100	0–800	124.2	143.6	200	0–700	208.33	166.87	0.0271

Table 5 Myoma resection

Myoma resection	Group A(IBS®)				Group B (Versapoint®)				p Value
	Median	Range	Mean	DS	Median	Range	Mean	DS	
Dilatation (min)	1.5	1–2.5	1.37	0.42	1.5	1–12	4.83	5.66	0.0202
Operating Time (min)	23.25	6.5–66	27.41	18.95	8	8–13	9.66	2.34	0.1392
Resection Time (min)	15.08	0.9–50	19.92	15.29	5	2.5–9	5.34	2.7	0.1333
Fluid used (ml)	9250	2000–20.000	9925	5351.6	1700	1000–2000	1566.6	418.99	0.0208
Fluid deficit (ml)	550	100–2000	666.66	488.76	200	200–300	233.33	47.140	0.1596

Group B (median, 1.5 min; range, 1–12 min; mean, 4.83 min; DS, 5.66 min; $p=0.0202$) (Table 5).

Polyp resection

We performed 31 (62%) polypectomies in Group A (IBS®; Table 1) compared with 42 (85.7%) in Group B (Versapoint®; Table 2). The size of the polyps was similar in both groups. The median size of the polyps was 15 mm (range 3–60 mm) in Group A (Table 1) and 15 mm (range 4–55 mm; Table 2) in Group B. The median total operating time in Group A was 5 min (range 3–13 min) and 9.75 min in (range 4–21 min) Group B ($p=0.0016$) (Table 4). The median resection time in Group A was 2 min (range 0.16–12 min) and 5 min (range 0.33–16 min) in Group B ($p=0.0020$) (Table 4). In Group A, a mean of 1,845 ml of fluid was used compared with 1,697 ml in Group B ($p=0.5598$) (Table 4). The mean fluid deficit was 124.2 ml in Group A compared with 208.33 ml in Group B ($p=0.0271$) (Table 4). Our data indicate that both the operating time and resection time were statistically significantly in favour of the IBS® group. In addition, the lower fluid deficit, when the IBS® was used, was also an advantage.

Myoma resection

We performed 12 (24%) myomectomies in Group A (IBS®; Table 1) and 3 (6.1%) in Group B (Versapoint®; Table 2).

In Group A, the median size of the myomas was 20 mm (range 8–30 mm; Table 1) and the median size was 20 mm (range 10–20 mm) in Group B (Table 2). In Group A, one myoma was G0, five were G1 and six were G2, whereas all myomas in Group B were G1 (Table 6). The median total operating time in Group A was 23.25 min (range 6.5–66 min) and 8 min (range 8–13 min) in Group B ($p=0.1392$) (Table 5). The median resection time in Group A was 15.08 min (range 0.9–50 min) and 5 min (range 2.5–9 min) in Group B ($p=0.1333$) (Table 5).

A mean of 9,925 ml of fluid was used in Group A compared with 1,566.6 ml in Group B ($p=0.0208$) (Table 5).

The mean fluid deficit was 666.66 ml in Group A compared with 233.33 ml in Group B ($p=0.1596$) (Table 5).

In Group A, seven procedures were single step, two required a second operation and only the intra cavitary portion of the myoma was removed in three cases without need for a second treatment, whereas in Group B, all procedures were completed in one step (Table 6).

Apart from the total amount of fluid used, there was no statistically significant difference in favour of either of the two techniques, despite a disproportion between the number cases performed with the IBS® compared with those that underwent conventional bipolar resection (12 with the IBS® vs. three cases with Versapoint®). In addition, the longer operating and resection times, higher volumes of fluid used and the fluid deficit could be explained by the different sizes of the myomas treated: up to 3 cm in the IBS group compared with 2 cm or smaller in the bipolar group.

When myomas of 2 cm or less were considered and divided into two subgroups, Group A1 for the IBS® and Group B1 for conventional bipolar resection group (Versapoint®), the median size of the myomas in Group A1 was 15 mm (range 10–20 mm) and 20 mm (range 10–20 mm) in Group B1 (Table 8). Also, four myomas were G1 and three were G2 in Group A1 whereas three myomas were G1 in Group B1 (Table 8). The median total operating time in the

Table 6 Myoma resection by myoma type, according ESGE guidelines, and number of procedures

	Group A(IBS®)	Group B (Versapoint®)
	Myoma type	
G0	1	0
G1	5	3
G2	6	0
	Number of procedures (%)	
Single step	7 (58.3)	3 (100)
Two steps	2 (16.6)	0 (0)
Residual myoma	3 (25)	0 (0)

Table 7 Myoma resection, ≤ 20 mm

Myoma resection	Sub Group A1 (IBS®)				Sub Group B1 (Versapoint®)				p Value
	Median	Range	Mean	DS	Median	Range	Mean	DS	
Dilatation (min)	1	1–1.5	1.2	0.245	1.5	1–12	4.83	5.66	0.1009
Operating time (min)	8	6.5–13	9.1	2.49	8	8–13	9.66	2.34	0.7493
Resection time (min)	5	0.9–9	5.34	2.92	5	2.5–9	5.34	2.7	1.0000
Fluid used (ml)	2700	2000–5000	2940	1101.9	1700	1000–2000	1566.6	418.99	0.2236
Fluid deficit (ml)	300	200–400	300	89.44	200	200–300	233.33	47.140	0.2859

Group A1 was 8 min (range 6.5–13 min) and 8 min (range 8–13 min) in Group B1 ($p=0.7493$) (Table 7). The median resection time in Group A1 was 5 min (range 0.9–9 min) and 5 min (range 2.5–9 min) in Group B1 ($p=1.0000$) (Table 7). In Group A1, we used a mean of 2,940 ml of fluid compared with 1,566.6 ml in Group B1 ($p=0.2236$) (Table 7). The mean fluid deficit was 300 ml in Group A1 compared with 233.33 ml in Group B1 ($p=0.2859$) (Table 7). All procedures in the two subgroups were completed in a single step (Table 8). There was no statistically significant difference in favour of either method.

Polyp and myoma resection

We performed five (10%) polypectomies plus myomectomies (contemporary resection of endometrial polyps with submucosal myomas) in Group A (IBS®; Table 1) and two (4.1%) in Group B (Versapoint®; Table 2). The median size of the polyps in Group A was 12.5 mm (range 10–40 mm) (Table 1) and 8 mm (range 6–15 mm) in Group B (Table 2).

The median size of the myomas was 20 mm (range 10–25 mm) in Group A (Table 1) and 8 mm (range 8–8 mm) in Group B (Table 2). Three myomas in Group A

Table 8 Demographic and clinical data for patients with myomas ≤ 20 mm

	Sub Group A1 (IBS®)	Sub Group B1 (Versapoint®)
n (%)	7 (14)	3 (6.1)
Size (mm)[a]	15 (10–20) 15 (4.47)	20 (10–20) 17.5 (4.33)
Age (years)[b]	51 (44–74)	48 (43–52)
Parity (%)		
Nulliparous	3 (42.8)	1 (33.3)
Multiparous	4 (57.2)	2 (66.6)
Menopause (%)	2 (28.6)	1 (33.3)
Symptoms (%)		
None	1 (14.3)	2 (66.6)
Menorrhagia	4 (57.2)	1 (33.3)
Anaemia	1 (14.3)	1 (33.3)
Post Menop. AUB	1 (14.3)	0 (0)
Pelvic Pain	0 (0)	0 (0)
Infertility	0 (0)	0 (0)
	Myomas' Type	
G0	0	0
G1	4	3
G2	3	0
	Number of procedures (%)	
Single step	7 (100)	3 (100)
Two steps	(0)	0 (0)
Residual Myoma	(0)	0 (0)
Complications (%)	(0)	0 (0)

[a] Median (range); mean (SD)
[b] Median (range)

Table 9 Polyp + myoma resection

Polyps + myoma resection	Group A (IBS®)				Group B (Versapoint®)				p Value
	Median	Range	Mean	DS	Median	Range	Mean	DS	
Dilatation (min)	1.5	1–2	1.6	0.37	2	2–2	2	0	0.2082
Operating time (min)	17	5.33–32	19.86	9.93	12	11–13	12	1	0.3388
Polyp res. time (min)	0.5	0.16–1	0.55	0.27	4	3–5	4	1	0.0000
Myoma res. time (min)	6.89	0.16–22	8.93	8.25	5	5–5	5	0	0.5460
Fluid used (ml)	5200	1500–7500	5100	2038.6	1800	1600–2000	1800	200	0.0831
Fluid deficit (ml)	500	200–100	500	275.68	150	100–200	150	50	0.1519

were G0, one was G1 and one was G2, whereas all myomas were G1 in Group B (Table 10). The median total operating time in Group A was 17 min (range 5.33–32 min) and 12 min (range 11–13 min) in Group B ($p=$ 0.3388) (Table 9). The median resection time for polyps in Group A was 0.5 min (range 0.16–1 min) and 4 min (range 3–5 min) in Group B ($p=0.0000$) (Table 9). The median resection time for myomas in Group A was 6.89 min (range 0.16–22 min) and 5 min (range 5–5 min) in Group B ($p=0.5460$; Table 9).

In Group A, a mean of 5,200 ml of fluid was used compared with 1,800 ml in Group B ($p=0.0831$) (Table 9). The mean fluid deficit was 500 ml in Group A compared with 150 ml in Group B ($p=0.1519$) (Table 9). All procedures in both groups were completed in one step (Table 10). IBS® showed a clear superiority in terms of polyp resection time, but the time difference was not statistically significant for myomectomy.

Endometrial ablation

We performed two (4%) endometrial ablations in Group A (IBS®; Table 1) and two (4.1%) in Group B (Versapoint®; Table 2). The median total operating time

Table 10 Polyp + myoma resection by myoma type, according ESGE guidelines, and number of procedures

	Group A (IBS®)	Group B (Versapoint®)
	Myoma type	
G0	3	0
G1	1	2
G2	1	0
	Number of procedures (%)	
Single step	5 (100)	2 (100)
Two steps	0 (0)	0 (0)
Residual Myoma	0 (0)	0 (0)

in Group A was 11.5 min (range 10–13 min) and 24.5 min (range 24–25 min) in Group B ($p=0.0073$) (Table 11). The median resection time in Group A was 7.5 min (range 5–10 min) and 17.5 min (range 15–20 min) in Group B ($p=0.0572$) (Table 11). In Group A, a mean of 1,750 ml of fluid was used compared with 2,750 ml in Group B ($p=0.2473$) (Table 11). The mean fluid deficit was 200 ml in Group A compared with 150 ml in Group B ($p=0.2929$) (Table 11). The operating time was shorter with IBS, probably because the tissue chips were removed at the time of resection.

Complications

Two perforations were reported during the dilatation process in Group B (Versapoint®). In Group A, no complications were reported. Both lesions were in the fundus. The first was a complete perforation, and the second was a 5- to 10-mm false root. In the first case, the procedure was immediately stopped with no further complications for the patient. In the second case, the procedure was safely completed with complete removal of the polyp without problems for the woman. The mean complication rate in Group A was 4.76% vs. 0% in Group B. Considering that only two complications occurred during the dilatation process in Group B (Versapoint®) and no complications were reported in Group A (IBS®), it is suggested that reduction of dilatation diameter could improve patient safety.

Learning curve

Polyp resection was used to evaluate the learning curve because the number of cases was sufficiently large to reach a conclusion. We analyzed 12 cases performed by an expert surgeon and compared them with 11 cases performed by a resident in Group B (Versapoint®) and 12 cases performed by an expert surgeon and 9 cases performed by a resident in Group A (IBS®) (Table 12).

Table 11 Endometrial ablation

Endometrial ablation	Group A (IBS®)				Group B (Versapoint®)				p Value
	Median	Range	Mean	DS	Median	Range	Mean	DS	
Dilatation (min)	1.5	1.5–1.5	1.5	0	1.75	1–2.5	1.75	0.75	0.6838
Operating Time (min)	11.5	10–13	11.5	1.5	24.5	24–25	24.5	0.5	0.0073
Resection Time (min)	7.5	5–10	7.5	2.5	17.5	15–20	17.5	2.5	0.0572
Fluid used (ml)	1750	1000–2500	1750	750	2750	2300–3200	2750	450	0.2473
Fluid deficit (ml)	200	200–200	200	0	150	100–200	150	50	0.2929

In Group B, the median size of the polyps removed by the expert surgeon was 10 mm (range, 8–40 mm; mean, 15.7 mm; DS, 8.4 mm) whereas the median size of polyps removed by the resident was 15 mm (range, 7–55 mm; mean, 17.5 mm; DS, 12.7 mm) (Table 13). The median operating time for the expert surgeon was 8 min (range 5–16 min), whereas the median operating time for the resident was 14 min (range 10–20 min) ($p=0.0010$) (Table 13). The median resection time for the expert surgeon was 3.5 min (range 1–10.5 min), whereas the median resection time for the resident was 9 min (range 0.5–13.5 min) ($p=0.0371$) (Table 13).

In Group A, the median size of the polyps removed by the expert surgeon was 12.5 mm (range, 8–30 mm; mean, 15.1 mm; DS, 7.23 mm), whereas median the size of the polyps removed by the resident was 20 mm (range, 10–40 mm; mean, 21.4 mm; DS, 10.2 mm) (Table 14). The median operating time for the expert surgeon was 3.5 min (range, 2–8 min), whereas the median operating time for the resident was 5 min (range, 3–12 min) ($p=0.2167$) (Table 14). The median resection time for the expert surgeon was 1.5 min (range, 0.2–5.5 min) whereas the median resection time for the resident was 2.25 min (range, 0.5–10 min) ($p=0.2446$) (Table 14).

There was a statistically significant difference in both the operating and resection times of cases performed with conventional bipolar resectoscope, but no statistically significant difference in the cases performed with the IBS® between the expert surgeon and the resident, suggesting that the experience of the surgeon was most important when the conventional bipolar resectoscope was used. A higher number of procedures are necessary with the

Table 12 Number of polyp resection cases: expert surgeon vs. resident

	Expert surgeon	Resident
Group A	12	9
Group B	12	11

resectoscope compared with the IBS® for the surgeon to gain the same level of skill. In addition, larger-sized polyps were removed by the resident in the IBS® group than those removed by the expert surgeon, indicating that the new technique is much easier to use, even in more complicated cases.

Discussion and conclusion

This study shows that major hysteroscopic surgical procedures can be performed with the IBS® in a very easy, fast, precise and safe way. Especially for the treatment of large polyps and myomas up to 2 cm, it has several well-described advantages. As discussed by Emanuel et al., the diameter of an intrauterine pathology is strongly related to the operation time and to the complication rate [19]. Considering the volume calculation of the tissue to remove by the formula $4/3\pi r^3$, we need 8.4 min to resect 2 cm, 28.2 min for 3 cm and 67.0 min for 4 cm at a resection speed of 0.5 cm^3/min for a conventional monopolar loop. The bipolar loops are smaller and resection time should increase accordingly. In this resection time, we do not calculate the time necessary to remove the chips, a major hurdle in resection of large myomas. The first generation bipolar resectoscopes loop is even smaller than the conventional monopolar or the second generation of bipolar resectoscope resulting in a challenging situation for all pathology over 2 cm. The IBS® seems to be much faster than the Versapoint®. Probably, this is due to the fact that the continuous cutting capacity performed always under direct visual control, with immediate removal of the chips at time of resection, results in a more efficient reduction of the tumour volume. Differences in both operating and resection times were statistically significant in favour of the IBS®. No bleeding or major complication was observed in the IBS® group. Not only operation time but also total fluid loss seems to be better with the IBS® system. In fact, this study demonstrates that using the IBS® for myoma resection,

Table 13 Group B (Versapoint®)—polyp resection, expert surgeon vs. resident

Group B	Expert surgeon				Resident				p Value
	Median	Range	Mean	DS	Median	Range	Mean	DS	
Size (mm)	10	8–40	15.7	8.4	15	7–55	17.5	12.7	–
Operation Time (min)	8	5–16	9	3.59	14	10–20	15.4	3.6	0.0010
Resection Time (min)	3.5	1–10.5	4.37	2.85	9	0.5 –13.5	7.87	4.08	0.0371

the median total operating time was 23.25 min (range 6.5–66 min) with a medium resection time of 15.08 min (range 0.9–50 min). The fluid deficit was limited to 666.66 ml despite a mean of total fluid used of 9,925 ml. We could explain the better fluid deficit with a very limited bleeding we had with the use of the IBS®. While this has been proven for polyp resection, for myoma, the current study cannot make a comparative statement. Unfortunately, not enough myoma resections where allocated into the resectoscope group, and the larger myomas (>2 cm) were all treated by the IBS®. It is clear that due to the different consistency of myomas and their possible intramural location, the results of polypectomy cannot be extrapolated to the myoma resection. Anyway, all types of submucosal myomas, including G2 myomas that were excluded from similar studies with morcellators, were included in our study [14]. In addition, the main advantage of the IBS® was that the myomas were effectively enucleated from their fovea and the intramural site of insertion of the myoma was removed (Fig. 3). The surrounding healthy endometrium was avoided without any thermal injury occurring compared with the less precise behaviour of conventional resectoscopy. No coagulation was needed, and there were no excess bleeding problems. We bear in mind that myoma surgery with the resectoscope has reported complications like, major bleeding, fluid overload, two-step surgery, but even more significant postoperative adhesion formation. Deans R and Abbott J reported a 31.3% adhesion formation in a single myoma and 45.5% in multiple myoma removal [20]. Especially for the treatment of large and multiple myomas, an alternative to the conventional resectoscope could be interesting and in benefit of the patient. For very large myomas, we will possibly need to improve our blade system because the IBS® had some drawbacks also here. One of the most important finding in this study is the difference in the learning curves between the IBS® and the resectoscope. The IBS® was statistically significantly easier to learn than the resectoscope. This improvement opens a window for very common gynaecological interventions like polypectomy into the hands of less experienced hysteroscopist. Compared to other blind intrauterine applications, the IBS® has the major advantage that surgeons always perform the procedure under visual control, with automated and easy removal of tissue chips. As it has been proven in randomised control trials [21], reducing the diameter of the instrument improves the accessibility of ambulatory diagnostic hysteroscopy; the IBS® broadens the accessibility in major hysteroscopic operations. In addition, there were no complications reported in the IBS group, even if both polyps and myomas were larger than in the Versapoint ® group. The complication rate in the Versapoint ® group, although it was only related to the cervical dilatation, indicates that smaller is probably easier. Although further modifications of the IBS® will be necessary, at present, this technique has very interesting and promising features for future operative hysteroscopy, making the procedure faster, easier and with significantly fewer major complications. In conclusion, we can say that the IBS® is a very promising new instrument for the removal of polyps and myomas. This smaller instrument is easier to apply than the conventional resectoscope. For the treatment of large polyps, the IBS® seems to be superior as it works faster and at a lower risk

Table 14 Group A (IBS®)—Polyp resection, expert surgeon vs. resident

Group A	Expert surgeon				Resident				p Value
	Median	Range	Mean	DS	Median	Range	Mean	DS	
Size (mm)	12.5	8–30	15.1	7.23	20	10–40	21.4	10.2	–
Operation Time (min)	3.5	2–8	4.15	1.93	5	3–12	5.8	2.9	0.2167
Resection Time (min)	1.5	0.2–5.5	1.51	1.63	2.25	0.5–10	3.1	3.17	0.2446

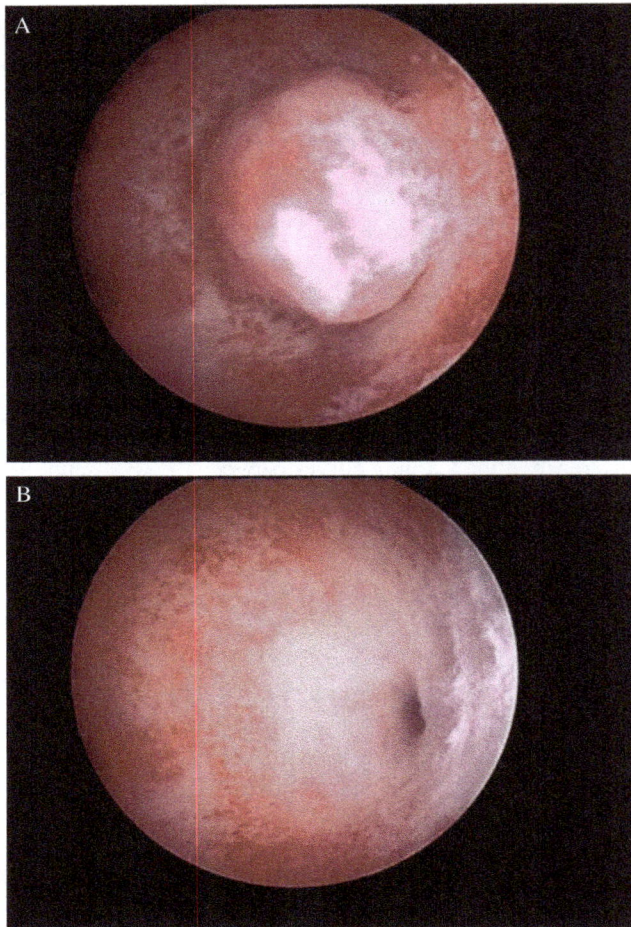

Fig. 3 Integrated Bigatti Shaver (IBS®) resection of a 2-cm G0 submucosal myoma. (**a**) Before and (**b**) after the IBS® treatment. The myoma was completely removed without damaging the surrounding healthy endometrium

profile. Very interesting is that the IBS® is able to resect also myomatous tissue, making this a very promising alternative to the resectoscope. In fact, surgery is not interrupted by tissue chips removal making total operating time shorter. It is further postulated that resection of myomas without the use of electrical current could significantly reduce the postoperative adhaesion formation and that the IBS® should preferentially be used in younger women in their reproductive age. Further studies will have to be performed to tailor the indication potential of this exiting approach.

Acknowledgment This paper is dedicated to my parents for their support throughout the years. Special thanks to Karl Storz GmbH & Co employees, Storz Italia for technical support and in particular, to Dr. H.C. Mult. Sybill Storz and Helmut Wehrstein, who believed in this project from the beginning. Special thanks go to Rudi Campo.

Declaration of interest Dr. Giuseppe Bigatti was involved in the concept and design of the IBS® with Karl Storz GmbH of Tuttlingen but received no financial compensation for this study.

References

1. Di Spezio SA, Mazzon I, Bramante S, Bettocchi S, Bifulco G, Guida M, Nappi C (2008) Hysteroscopic myomectomy: a comprehensive review of surgical techniques. Hum Reprod Updat 14(2):101–119
2. Oona Hamerlynck TW, Dietz V, Schoot BC (2011) Clinical implementation of the Hysteroscopic morcellator for removal of intrauterine myomas and polyps. A retrospective descriptive study. Gynecol Surg 8:193–196
3. Associazione Italiana di Endourologia-Da Lichtleiter ai Nostri Giorni-Segreteria Via Porrettana 76/2-40033-Casalecchio di Reno (Bo) www.ieanet.it/italiano/endourologia.php
4. Witz CA, Silverberg KM, Burns WN, Schenken RS, Olive DL (1993) Complications associated with absorption of hysteroscopic fluid media. Fertil Steril 60(5):745–756
5. Mencaglia L, Lugo E, Consigli S, Barbosa C (2009) Bipolar resectoscope: the future perspective of hysteroscopic surgery. Gynecol Surg 6(1):15–20
6. Yong Lee G, In Han J, Joo Heo H (2009) Severe Hypocalcemia caused by absorption of sorbitol - mannitol during Hysteroscopy. J Korean Med 24:532–534
7. Shaafer M, Von Ungern-Sternberg BS, Wight E, Schneider MC (2005) Isotonic fluid absorption during Hysteroscopy resulting in severe Hyperchloremic Acidosis. Anesthesiology 103:203–204
8. Van Kruchten PM, Vermelis JM, Herold I, Van Zundert AA (2010) Hypotonic and isotonic fluid overload as a complication of hysteroscopic procedures: two case reports. Minerva Anestesiol 76(5):373–377
9. Pasini A, Belloni C (2001) Intraoperative complications of 697 consecutive operative hysteroscopies. Minerva Ginecol 53(1):13–20
10. Sutton CJG, Mc Donald R (1993) Endometrial Resection. In: Lewis BV, Magos AL (eds) Endometrial ablation. Churchill Livingstone, Edinburgh, pp 131–140
11. Odell R (1993) Eletrosurgery. In: Sutton CJG, Diamond MP (eds) Endoscopic Surgery for Gynaecology. Saunders, London, pp 51–59
12. Jansen FW, Vredevoogd CB, Van Ulzen K, Hermans J, Trimbos JB, Trimbos-Kemper TC (2000) Complication of hysteroscopy: a prospective, multicenter study. Obstet Gynecol 96(2):266–270
13. Emanuel MH, Wamsteker K (2005) The intrauterine morcellator: a new hysteroscopic operating technique to remove intrauterine polyps and myomas. J Minim Invasive Gynecol 12(1):65–66
14. Van Dongen H et al (2008) Hysteroscopic morcellator for removal of intrauterine polyps and myomas: a randomized controlled pilot study among residents in training. J Minim Invasive Gynecol 15:466–471
15. Bigatti G (2011) IBS® Integrated Bigatti Shaver, an alternative approach to operative hysteroscopy. Gynecol Surg 8(2):187
16. Instruction for Use Versapoint. Official Notification 2001. Gynecare. A division of Ethicon. www.ethicon.com
17. Wamsteker K, Emanuel MH, de Kruif JH (1993) Transcervical hysteroscopic resection of submucous fibroids for abnormal uterine bleeding: result regarding the degree of intramural extension. Obstet Gynecol 82:736–740
18. Salim R, Lee C, Davies A, Jolaoso B, Ofuasia E, Jurkovic D (2005) A comparative study of three-dimensional saline infusion sonohysterography and diagnostic hysteroscopy for the classification of submucous fibroids. Hum Reprod 20:253–257
19. Emanuel MH, Hart A, Wamsteker K, Lammes F (1997) An analysis of fluid loss during transcervical resection of submucous myomas. Fertil Steril 68(5):881–886
20. Deans R, Abbott J (2010) Review of intrauterine adhesions. J Minim Invasive Gynecol 17(5):555–569
21. Campo R, Molinas CR, Rombauts L, Mestdagh G, Lauwers M, Braekmans P, Brosens I, Van Belle Y, Gordts S (2005) Prospective multicentre randomized controlled trial to evaluate factors influencing the success rate of office diagnostic hysteroscopy. Hum Reprod 20(1):258–263

6

Hysterosalpingo-foam sonography (HyFoSy) using two different balloon catheters

Dominique Van Schoubroeck · Thierry Van den Bosch ·
Lieveke Ameye · Thomas D'Hooghe · Dirk Timmerman

Abstract The purposes of this study were to evaluate and compare the technical feasibility and the patients' pain during hysterosalpingo-foam sonography (HyFoSy) using two different 2-mm balloon catheters. Randomized trial in 46 consecutive women referred for tubal patency testing by HyFoSy at the Leuven University Hospital. Six women refused to participate. Forty women were randomized and blinded as to the catheter used. The patients underwent first a transvaginal ultrasound examination to assess the uterus and the ovaries and to exclude the hydrosalpinx, and subsequently, a HyFoSy was performed using an uVue catheter (Cook Medical, Bloomington, IN, USA) or a pediatric Foley's catheter with stylet (Pediatric Folysil, Coloplast A/S; Humlebaek, Denmark) according to randomization. If the catheter could not be inserted smoothly into the uterine cavity at first attempt, transabdominal ultrasound guidance was performed. After the procedure, the patients were asked to fill in a questionnaire including a visual analog scale (VAS) score for the pain at initial ultrasound examination (VAS_{US}), used as baseline score, and at HyFoSy (VAS_{HyFoSy}). The pain related to the HyFoSy procedure was reported as ($VAS_{HyFoSy}-VAS_{US}$)/VAS_{US}. Catheter insertion failed in one patient of the uVue group (5 % failure rate) and in none of the Foley group. Ultrasound guidance during catheter insertion was performed in 68 % of the uVue group and 20 % of the Foley group. The median ratio ($VAS_{HyFoSy}-VAS_{US}$)/VAS_{US} for the uVue and the Foley group was 1.82 and 0.54, respectively ($p=0.005$). A pediatric Foley catheter was easier to insert as compared to an uVue catheter, and HyFoSy using a pediatric Foley catheter was reported by the women to be the least painful.

D. Van Schoubroeck (✉) · T. Van den Bosch · L. Ameye ·
T. D'Hooghe · D. Timmerman
KU Leuven Department of Development and Regeneration,
University Hospital Leuven, Herestraat 49, 3000 Leuven, Belgium
e-mail: Dominique.vanschoubroeck@uzleuven.be

Keywords Ultrasonography · Infertility · Female · Fallopian tube patency tests · Microbubbles

Background

Hysterosalpingo-contrast-sonography (HyCoSy) is as accurate as hysterosalpingography (HSG) in the evaluation of Fallopian tube patency and is to be preferred as it does not expose the patient nor the examiner to radiation [1–3]. Moreover, HyCoSy is reportedly less painful and better tolerated by the patients as compared to HSG. Hysterosalpingo-foam sonography (HyFoSy) is a novel variant of HyCoSy using gel foam, a mechanically mixing of water, gel, and air, as a positive contrast agent [4–8].

This study aims to evaluate and compare the technical feasibility and the patients' pain during HyFoSy using two different 2-mm balloon catheters.

Methods

We performed a randomized trial in 46 consecutive women referred for tubal patency testing by HyFoSy at the Leuven University Hospital. The study had been approved by the local ethics committee, and informed consent was obtained in all patients. Six women refused to participate. Forty women were randomized (Fig. 1) using a random number generator (https://www.random.org/). The random assignments were placed in 40 numbered, opaque, and sealed envelopes. The envelope was opened after consent was given and just prior to the HyFoSy procedure. The patients were blinded as to the catheter used, but for obvious reasons, the clinician was not blinded. The patients underwent first a transvaginal ultrasound examination to assess the uterus and the ovaries and to exclude the hydrosalpinx, and immediately thereafter, a

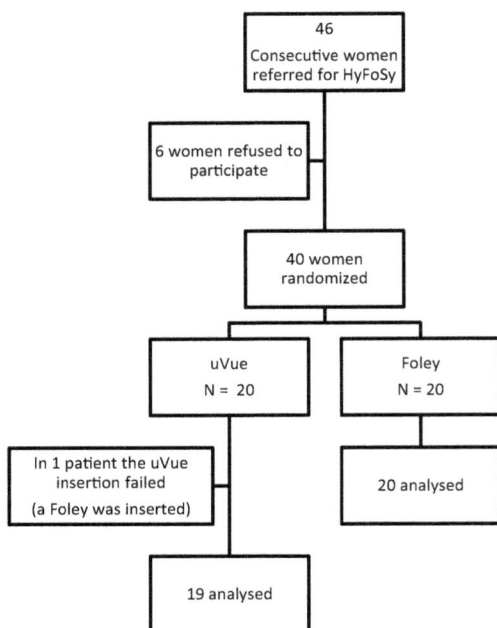

Fig. 1 Study design

HyFoSy was performed using a 2-mm uVue catheter (Cook Medical, Bloomington, IN, USA) or a 2-mm pediatric Foley's catheter with stylet (Pediatric Folysil, Coloplast A/S; Humlebaek, Denmark) according to randomization. The HyFoSy procedure was performed as outlined elsewhere [5]. An open-sided Collin speculum was inserted, the cervix disinfected with a water-based Dakin solution, and the catheter was inserted into the uterine cavity. If the catheter could not be inserted smoothly at first attempt, transabdominal ultrasound guidance was performed. Catheter insertion was performed without the use of a cervical tenaculum or a dilator. The balloon was slowly inflated with 0.5 to 1.0 ml of saline in the lower part of the uterine cavity till the patient reported a vague pressure in the lower abdomen indicating perceptible intrauterine pressure. The speculum was removed, and the vaginal ultrasound probe was reinserted. The size of the balloon was measured in three perpendicular diameters, and

Table 1 Patients' characteristics

	uVue ($n=19$)[a]	Foley ($n=20$)
Mean age	31	29
Primary subfertility	13	12
Secondary subfertility	6	8
$P \geq 1$	4	5
Unilateral block at HyFoSy	1	3
Bilateral block at HyFoSy	1	0

P parity (all nine cases had a parity of 1)

[a] In one patient randomized in the "uVue" arm, a Foley was used after uVue insertion failed

Table 2 Reported pain/discomfort during HyFoSy

	uVue		Foley	
	N	%	N	%
Neutral	1	5.3	2	10.0
Unpleasant	6	31.6	8	40.0
Painful but bearable	7	36.8	8	40.0
Really painful*	5	26.3	2	10.0
Total	19		20	

*p value 0.24

the gel foam was slowly injected under direct ultrasound control. Tubal patency was defined as a sustained and fast forward flow of the gel foam through the entire Fallopian tube.

After the procedure, the patients were asked to fill in a questionnaire including a visual analog scale (VAS) score for the pain at initial ultrasound examination (VAS_{US}), used as baseline score, and at HyFoSy (VAS_{HyFoSy}). The pain related to the HyFoSy procedure was calculated as the median ratio ($VAS_{HyFoSy} - VAS_{US}$)/VAS_{US}.

The patients were asked also to describe the pain/discomfort during HyFoSy (as "neutral," "unpleasant," "painful but bearable," or "really painful") and to compare the pain/discomfort during HyFoSy with two common minor procedures (i.e., blood sampling and cervical cytology smear) as 'less,' 'equally,' or 'more painful/causing discomfort.'

The Fisher's exact test was used to assess the differences in categorical variables, t test and Wilcoxon test were used to assess differences in continuous variables. SAS 9.4 (SAS Institute Inc., Cary, NC, USA) was used for the statistical analyses.

Table 3 Compared to blood sampling

	uVue		Foley	
	N	%	N	%
Less	0	0.0	2	10.0
Equal	4	21.1	5	25.0
More*	15	78.9	13	65.0
Total	19		20	

*p value 0.48

Table 4 Compared to cervical cytology smear

	uVue		Foley	
	N	%	N[a]	%
Less	1	5.3	2	10.5
Equal	5	26.3	7	24.1
More*	13	68.4	10	52.6
Total	19		19	

*p value 0.33

[a] One patient randomized to the Foley arm did not answer this question

Fig. 2 Pain related to the HyFoSy procedure; for each patient, the reported pain during ultrasound examination (VAS$_{US}$) and during the HyFoSy procedure (VAS$_{HyFoSy}$) is presented

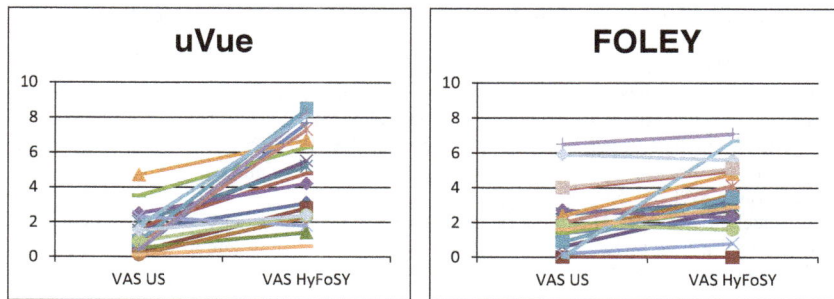

Findings

The patients' characteristics (age, parity, primary/secondary subfertility) and tubal patency for both subgroups were comparable (Table 1).

Catheter insertion failed in one patient of the uVue group (5 % failure rate) and in none of the Foley group. In the patient with failed uVue catheter insertion, a Foley was inserted successfully during the same session. Ultrasound guidance for catheter insertion was performed in 68 % of the uVue group and 20 % of the Foley group (p=0.004). The mean balloon diameter in the uVue group and the Foley group was 8.7 and 9.3 mm, respectively (p=0.22). Five women (26 %) of the uVue group reported the procedure to be really painful versus two (10 %) in the Foley group (p=0.24) (Table 2).

In the uVue group and in the Foley group, 79 and 65 %, respectively, found HyFoSy to be more painful than blood sampling (p=0.48) (Table 3), and 68 and 53 %, respectively, found HyFoSy more painful than a cervical cytology smear (p=0.33) (Table 4).

The median VAS$_{US}$ in the uVue and in the Foley group was 1.5 (0.1–4.7) and 1.9 (0–6.5), respectively (p=0.14), while the median VAS$_{HyFoSy}$ was 4.8 (0.6–8.5) and 3.5 (0–7.1), respectively (p=0.10). The median ratio (VAS$_{HyFoSy}$−VAS$_{US}$)/VAS$_{US}$ for the uVue and the Foley group was 1.82 and 0.54, respectively (p=0.005) (Fig. 2).

Conclusions

A 2-mm pediatric Foley catheter was easier to insert compared to an uVue catheter, and HyFoSy using a pediatric Foley catheter was reported by the women to be the least painful too.

The strength of this study is its strict randomized design, the blinding of the patients, and the fact that the study was performed by the same group in the same center, precluding an operators' bias. The weaknesses are the relatively small sample size and the impossible operators' blinding.

Both catheters have the same diameter (2 mm) and have a similar balloon at the tip. The main difference is the devices' rigidity, the uVue being stiffer. The latter has the advantage to allow insertion without the need of a swab forceps. Moreover,

in case of severe ante- or retroversion of the endocervical canal, it can be bent before insertion to match/fit the shape of the canal. However, in case of a tortuous or S-shaped endocervical canal, this may prove to be a disadvantage, since the catheter will keep its pre-bended shape, the tip may "scrape" the more distal part of the canal, thus causing pain. The more difficult insertion is reflected by the significantly higher proportion of patients in the uVue group necessitating ultrasound guidance. Moreover, the catheter's stiffness may cause discomfort when inserting the vaginal ultrasound probe and makes the uterus more rigid during ultrasound examination. The Foley's catheter does not have the above-mentioned disadvantages, because it has a much less rigid and removable stylet to facilitate insertion, and once the stylet has been removed, the catheter is supple.

The results of our study favor the use of the Foley's catheter over the uVue catheter in term of patients' tolerance and operators' technical preference.

Conflict of interest Dominique Van Schoubroeck, Thierry Van den Bosch, Lieveke Ameye, Thomas D'Hooghe, and Dirk Timmerman declare that they have no conflict of interest.

The author's role in the study can be summarized as follows:

D. Van Schoubroeck—participation in study design, execution, analysis, manuscript drafting, and critical discussion; corresponding author

T. Van den Bosch—participation in study design, execution, analysis, manuscript drafting, and critical discussion

L. Ameye, study design and analysis

T. D'Hooghe—critical discussion

D. Timmerman—critical discussion

Informed consent All procedures followed were in accordance with the ethical standards of the responsible committee on human experimentation (institutional and national) and with the Helsinki Declaration of 1975, as revised in 2000 (5). Informed consent was obtained from all patients for being included in the study.

References

1. Campbell S, Bourne TH, Tan SL, Collins WP (1994) Hysterosalpingo contrast sonography (HyCoSy) and its future role within the investigation of infertility in Europe. Ultrasound Obstet Gynecol 4:245–253
2. Strandell A, Bourne T, Bergh C, Granberg S, Thorburn J, Hamberger L (2000) A simplified ultrasound based infertility investigation protocol

and its implications for patient management. J Assist Reprod Genet 17: 87–92

3. Lim CP, Hasafa Z, Bhattacharya S, Maheshwari A (2011) Should a hysterosalpingogram be a first-line investigation to diagnose female tubal subfertility in the modern subfertility workup? Hum Reprod 26:967–971

4. Exalto N, Stappers C, van Raamsdonk LA, Emanuel MH (2007) Gel instillation sonohysterography: first experience with a new technique. Fertil Steril 87:152–155

5. Emanuel MH, Exalto N (2011) Hysterosalpingo-foam sonography (HyFoSy): a new technique to visualize tubal patency. Ultrasound Obstet Gynecol 37:497–499

6. Emanuel MH, van Vliet M, Weber M, Exalto N (2012) First experiences with hysterosalpingo-foam sonography (HyFoSy) for office tubal patency testing. Hum Reprod 27:114–117

7. Van Schoubroeck D, Van den Bosch T, Meuleman C, Tomassetti C, D'Hooghe T, Timmerman D (2013) The use of a new gel foam for the evaluation of tubal patency. Gynecol Obstet Investig 75: 152–156

8. Van Schoubroeck D, Van den Bosch T, Ameye L, Boes AS, D'Hooghe T, Timmerman D (2014) Pain during Fallopian tube patency testing by hysterosalpingo-foam-sonography (HyFoSy). Ultrasound Obstet Gynecol. doi:10.1002/uog.14646

7

Clinical implementation of the hysteroscopic morcellator for removal of intrauterine myomas and polyps

Tjalina Wibeke Oona Hamerlynck · Viviane Dietz · Benedictus Christiaan Schoot

Abstract The aim of this study is to report our experience with a novel technique, the hysteroscopic morcellator (HM), for removal of intrauterine myomas and polyps. We performed a retrospective study on 315 women undergoing operative hysteroscopy with the HM in our university-affiliated teaching hospital. We collected data on installation and operating times, fluid deficit, peri- and postoperative complications. In 37 patients undergoing myomectomy with the HM, mean installation time was 8.7 min, mean operating time, 18.2 min, and median fluid deficit, 440 mL. Three out of 37 HM procedures were converted to resectoscopy, related to a type 2 myoma. In 278 patients, mean installation and operating times for polypectomy with the HM were 7.3 min and 6.6 min, respectively. All procedures were uneventful. Implementation of the HM for removal of type 0 and 1 myomas ≤3 cm, and removal of polyps appears safe and effective.

Keywords Operative hysteroscopy · Hysteroscopic morcellator · Endometrial polyp · Submucous myoma

Background

The use of hysteroscopic mono- or bipolar instruments is considered the gold standard in circumstances where scissors are not successful for removal of intrauterine lesions (e.g., myomas or polyps) [1, 2]. The choice of a specific hysteroscopic instrument depends on the origin, location, as well as the size of the intrauterine lesion [1, 2]. Recently, a novel device, the hysteroscopic morcellator (HM), became commercially available, using mechanical cutting to reduce the tumor into small chips and consequently evacuating these chips out of the uterine cavity by aspiration. The HM has been reported as an effective and safe new technique to remove intrauterine lesions [3]. Furthermore, it was reported that the HM is a safe and effective alternative to conventional resectoscopy in both experienced and inexperienced hands [4]. Results with the HM in clinical practice have hardly been documented [3, 4]. In this article, we present our retrospective data on the HM for removal of intrauterine myomas and polyps.

Methods

In our university-affiliated teaching hospital (Catharina Hospital, Eindhoven, the Netherlands), the HM was introduced in 2006 for hysteroscopic removal of intrauterine lesions. Up till that year, resectoscopy had been the standard procedure. We evaluated the introduction of the HM in retrospect.

Morcellation was performed with the HM (TRUCLEAR, Smith & Nephew, Andover, USA; Fig. 1). The HM has a 4-mm blade, consisting of a rigid inner tube which rotates within an outer tube. The blade is inserted into an electrically powered control unit which connects to a handheld motor drive unit. A foot pedal activates the blade and regulates the direction of rotation of the internal blade tube. The direction can be oscillating or continuous, with the optimal number of rotations per minute being 750 or 1,100, respectively. The rotary morcellator is recommended

T. W. O. Hamerlynck (✉) · V. Dietz · B. C. Schoot
Department of Obstetrics and Gynecology,
Catharina Hospital Eindhoven,
PO Box 1350, 5602 ZA Eindhoven, The Netherlands
e-mail: tjalina.hamerlynck@ugent.be

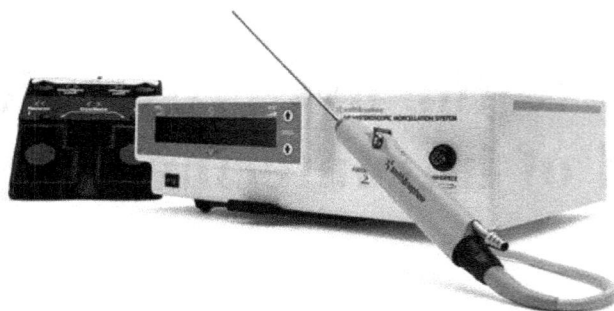

Fig. 1 The hysteroscopic morcellator

for polypectomy, and the reciprocating blade for myomectomy (Fig. 2).

The blade has a window opening at the end with cutting edges through which tissue is aspirated by means of a vacuum source. The vacuum source is connected to a regulator valve with a manometer. The optimal suction power connected to the inner tube of the HM blade is 200 mmHg. When the inner tube is not activated, the window opening is locked to prevent active suction of the distension liquid in order to avoid uterine cavity collapse. The removed tissue is discharged through the device, collected in a pouch, and made available for pathology analysis.

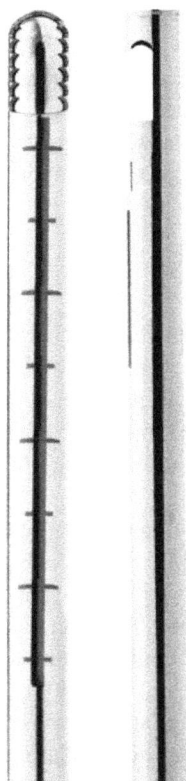

Fig. 2 The rotary and reciprocating blade of the HM

The blade of the HM was introduced into the uterine cavity through the working channel of a continuous flow 9-mm rigid hysteroscope with 0-degree optic (Smith & Nephew, Andover, USA). After dilatation of the internal os of the uterine cervix with Hegar dilators, atraumatic insertion was accomplished with the use of an obturator in the outer sheath of the hysteroscope. The working channel also acts as the inflow channel and the hysteroscope contains a separate outflow channel. Continuous flow was used for optimal distension, irrigation, and visibility. The inflow is pressurized with a peristaltic pump (Smith & Nephew, Andover, USA) with a maximum pressure setting of 120 mmHg and a maximum flow setting of 700 mL/min, similar to standard resectoscopy. The outflow is passive. Normal saline was used for distension and irrigation of the uterine cavity. All fluid was collected from the passive outflow tubing of the hysteroscope as well as from the vacuum tubing connected to the inner blade, and both measured volumes were subtracted from the measured inflow volume resulting in the fluid deficit.

First, we retrospectively describe our results with the HM—using the reciprocating blade—for removal of type 0 and 1 myomas from 2006 until 2009. We collected information on time needed to install the equipment, operating time, fluid deficit, and peri- and postoperative complications from medical records. Conversion rates to resectoscopy are mentioned.

Secondly, we report our data for removal of intrauterine polyps with the HM—using the rotary blade—between 2006 and 2009. We collected data on installation and operating time, fluid deficit, peri- and postoperative complications, and conversion rates from medical records.

For both myomas and polyps, the diameter was measured by ultrasound preoperatively. Patients were hospitalized in daycare. Procedures were performed under spinal or general anesthesia, and data on type of anesthesia are given. All patients received antibiotic prophylaxis with a single dose of metronidazole 500 mg and cefuroxime 1,500 mg. For all procedures, data on pathology analysis were available.

Findings

Myomas

Our results for removal of intrauterine myomas with the HM are summarized in Table 1. We performed this HM procedure in 37 patients aged 26 to 49 (median 45 years). The mean myoma diameter was 2.0 cm. A type 0 myoma was seen in 23 patients (62%), 11 patients had a type 1 myoma (30%), and three patients (8%) had a type 2 myoma. Since the HM can only be used for complete

Table 1 Data on hysteroscopic myomectomy and polypectomy with the HM

Tissue	N	Age (years)[a]	Diameter of tissue (cm)[b]	Installation time (min)[b]	Operating time (min)[b]	Fluid deficit (mL)[a]	Type of myoma		
							0	1	2
Myoma	37	45 (26–49)	2.0 (0.4)	8.7 (1.4)	18.2 (4.1)	440 (100–890)	23	11	3
Polyp	278	47 (23–81)	2.4 (0.7)	7.3 (2.5)	6.6 (3.3)	40 (0–300)	–	–	–

[a] Values are median (range)
[b] Values are mean (SD)

removal of type 0 and 1 myomas, in the latter three cases conversion to resectoscopy was necessary. Mean time needed to install equipment was 8.7 min, and mean operating time was 18.2 min. The limits for fluid deficit were respected. Seventy-two percent of the procedures was performed under spinal anesthesia. No complications occurred. Pathology analysis confirmed the presence of a myoma in all cases.

Polyps

We performed this HM procedure in 278 patients aged 23 to 81 (median 47 years; Table 1). The mean diameter was 2.4 cm. In 37 patients (13%), the procedure was part of an infertility treatment. Mean time to install was 7.3 min, and mean operating time was 6.6 min. Fluid deficit ranged from 0 mL to 300 mL (median 40 mL). The procedure took place under spinal anesthesia in 68% of the cases. No complications occurred. There were no conversions to resectoscopy. Pathology analysis showed 264 cases of benign intrauterine polyps, 13 cases of hyperplastic polyps, and in one patient, the intrauterine lesion appeared to be a placental site nodule.

Discussion

Few data on the use of the HM have been published so far [3, 4]. Our results with the HM over a time period of 4 years show that it's a fast technique for removal of smaller type 0 and 1 myomas, as well as larger polyps, and that no complications occurred.

The HM beholds some advantages over monopolar resectoscopy. The use of saline solution prevents hyponatremia, although meticulous measurement is indicated to prevent excessive absorption and fluid overload. When using the HM, similar to using bipolar electrosurgical systems instead of the monopolar resectoscope, there is no generation of stray currents with consequent risk of electrical burns [5]. No damage is done to the surrounding of the intrauterine lesion that needs to be removed, and we note that with the HM, no gas bubbles arise, in contrast to resectoscopy. Lethal complications have been described using hysteroscopic electrosurgery causing air bubbles and consequent gas embolism [6]. Furthermore, aspiration of the tissue fragments by the HM ensures a clear view and tissue is preserved for histological examination. In contrast, in resectoscopy, tissue fragments can block the hysteroscopic view and they need to be removed one by one, thus, making repeated in and out movements necessary, possibly causing uterine damage, and fragments might be lost.

We do acknowledge certain disadvantages of the HM. First, the inability to coagulate bleeding vessels encountered during surgery might be a disadvantage [5]. However, so far, no significant intraoperative or postoperative bleeding was documented [3]. In addition, our results show no evidence of significant bleeding during or after the HM procedure. Secondly, the HM cannot be used for the treatment of type 2 submucous fibroids [2]. Therefore, conversions to resectoscopy might occur when a type 2 myoma is misdiagnosed as a type 1 myoma preoperatively. Third, in case of larger myomas, the use of the HM can become quite time consuming. Fourth, in general, the cost of the disposables (blades and tubings) needed to perform a HM procedure is higher than that of the material needed for a hysteroscopic resection. Finally, regional or general anesthesia is mandatory for the HM procedure as it is necessary to dilate the cervix up to 8 or 9 mm. In contrast, data on successful ambulant removal of polyps, sized 2–4.5 cm [7–10], and submucous and partially intramural myomas, with a diameter up to 2 cm [7], with Versapoint (twizzle) have been published.

We report short installation and operating times for hysteroscopic myomectomy and polypectomy with the HM. Emanuel et al. report a mean operating time of 16.4 min for myomectomy and 8.7 min for polypectomy with the HM [3]. Comparing these data to other hysteroscopic techniques, the HM shows a marked reduction in the time needed to perform hysteroscopic myomectomy and polypectomy. Emanuel et al. reported a mean operating time of 42.2 min for hysteroscopic myomectomy and 30.9 min for polypectomy with the monopolar resectoscope [3]. Preutthipan et al. reported mean operating times ranging from 20.9 min to 31.9 min for polypectomy with grasping forceps, microscissors, electric probe, and resectoscope [11].

Unfortunately, data for our study were retrieved retrospectively, and in our center, no comparable control group was available for other hysteroscopic techniques. Prospective studies comparing the HM with, for example, monopolar resectoscopy are needed to confirm the possible advantages of the HM—such as the reduction of operating time—for removal of myomas and polyps. One should also retrieve more long-term follow-up data checking for persistence or recurrence of intrauterine myomas and polyps. Cost-effectiveness of the HM also needs to be evaluated.

Conclusion

We conclude that in our experience, the HM is a fast, safe, and easy method for removal of both smaller type 0 and 1 myomas, as well as polyps. Prospective data are needed to confirm these findings.

Declaration of interest   We report no conflict of interest.

References

1. Gimpelson RJ (2000) Hysteroscopic treatment of the patient with intracavitary pathology (myomectomy/polypectomy). Obstet Gyn Clin N Am 27:327–337
2. Sardo ADS, Mazzon I, Bramante S, Bettocchi S, Bifulco G, Guida M, Nappi C (2008) Hysteroscopic myomectomy: a comprehensive review of surgical techniques. Hum Reprod Update 14:101–119
3. Emanuel MH, Wamsteker K (2005) The intra uterine morcellator: a new hysteroscopic operating technique to remove intrauterine polyps and myomas. J Min Invas Gynecol 12:62–66
4. van Dongen H, Emanuel MH, Wolterbeek R, Trimbos JB, Jansen FW (2008) Hysteroscopic morcellator for removal of intrauterine polyps and myomas: a randomized controlled pilot study among residents in training. J Min Invas Gynecol 15:466–471
5. Vilos GA, Abul-Rafea B (2005) New developments in ambulatory hysteroscopic surgery. Best Pract Res Clin Obstet Gynecol 19:727–742
6. Murakami T, Tamura M, Ozawa Y, Suzuki H, Terada Y, Okamura K (2005) Safe techniques in surgery for hysteroscopic myomectomy. J Obstet Gynaecol Re 31:216–223
7. Bettocchi S, Ceci O, Di Venere R, Pansini MV, Pellegrino A, Marello F, Nappi L (2002) Advanced operative office hysteroscopy without anaesthesia: analysis of 501 cases treated with a 5 Fr. bipolar electrode. Hum Reprod 17:2435–2438
8. Garuti G, Cellani F, Colonnelli M, Grossi F, Luerti M (2004) Outpatient hysteroscopic polypectomy in 237 patients: feasibility of a one-stop "see-and-treat" procedure. J Am Assoc Gynecol Laparosc 11:500–504
9. Garuti G, Centinaio G, Luerti M (2008) Outpatient hysteroscopic polypectomy in postmenopausal women: a comparison between mechanical and electrosurgical resection. J Minim Invas Gyn L 15:595–600
10. Litta P, Cosmi E, Saccardi C, Esposito C, Rui R, Ambrosini G (2008) Outpatient operative polypectomy using a 5 mm-hysteroscope without anaesthesia and/or analgesia: advantages and limits. Eur J Obstet Gynecol Reprod Biol 139:210–214
11. Preutthipan S, Herabutya Y (2005) Hysteroscopic polypectomy in 240 premenopausal and postmenopausal women. Fertil Steril 83:705–709

8

IBS® Integrated Bigatti Shaver, an alternative approach to operative hysteroscopy

G. Bigatti

Abstract At present, conventional resectoscopy can be considered the gold standard procedure for major hysteroscopic operations [1]. Despite well-recognized advantages of resectoscopy, several problems, such as fluid overload, uterine perforation due to monopolar or bipolar current, lack of visualization resulting in a time-consuming procedure, and long learning curve, remain still unsolved. We have made, in cooperation with Karl Storz GmbH & Co., a new shaving system that, introduced through a straight operative channel of a panoramic 90° optic, allows to perform all kinds of major operative procedures such as polypectomy, G0, G1, and G2, submucosal myomectomy, and endometrial ablation. We have performed 44 operative hysteroscopy, including 24 polyps, 15 submucosal myomas, two polyps + submucosal myomas, three endometrial ablations. The polyps' size ranged from 5 to 40 mm, and all procedures were performed with the IBS®. The mean time for polyps' resection was 3'28". Ten cases of myoma's resection were performed exclusively with the IBS® of which four Type 0, two Type 1, four Type 2, the size ranged from 10 to 30 mm and the mean resection time was 14'. For five cases of myoma's resection, we started the operation with the IBS®, and we ended the procedure with the conventional monopolar resectoscope. The myomas' size ranged from 20 to 40 mm of which three Type 0, two Type 2, and the mean resection time was 32'. When the IBS® was used, the dilatation number reached 8.5 Hegar size that increased to 9.5 when we switched to conventional resectoscopy. We used sorbitol–mannitol at the beginning of the study and in all cases that we suspected the possibility of conversion to conventional monopolar resectoscope. As our learning curve improved, we switched to normal saline. No coagulation was needed when the IBS® was used. Two overload complications occurred: one was not depending on the method but to a malfunctioning of the Endomat® system. The second complication occurred during a G2—3 cm myoma's resection. This preliminary study is intended to evaluate the feasibility of this new technique that offers considerable advantages such as reduced dilatation of the cervix, better visualization during the procedure as tissue chips are removed at the same time of resection, no coagulation or cutting current is needed, the use of normal saline instead of sorbitol and mannitol, and a much faster learning curve.

Keywords Hysteroscopy · New instrumentation · Shaver

Introduction

The first resectoscope as we know today dates back 1926 and was used by Stern to remove three chips of prostatic tissue. The resectoscope Stern-McCarthy, made a few years later and that used optics with different angles 0°–30°, must be considered the precursor of the tool that we use today [2]. At present, the continuous flow monopolar or bipolar resectoscope is still considered the first-choice instrument to perform major operative hysteroscopical and urological procedures. Despite its versatility, many problems, technique-related, remain still unsolved. In case of monopolar technique, the absorption of large volumes of electrolyte-free, low viscosity fluid such as sorbitol–mannitol may result in volume overload with water intoxication [3]. Volume overload may

G. Bigatti (✉)
U.O. di Ostetricia e Ginecologia,
Ospedale Classificato San Giuseppe Via San Vittore, 12,
20123 Milan, Italy
e-mail: g.big@tiscalinet.it

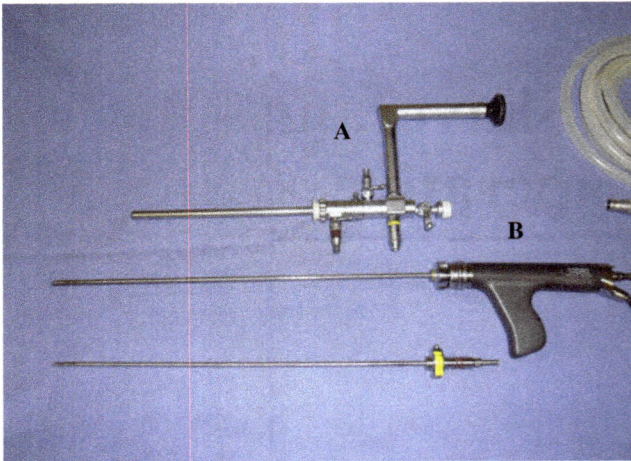

Fig. 1 IBS®: **a** 90° angulated 0°optic (Karl Storz gmbh of Tuttlingen) with a continuous flow sheath and an extra channel for the insertion of a **b** rigid shaving system

cause pulmonary edema, and water intoxication may lead to hyponatremia, hypo-osmolarity, and cerebral edema. Also, the use of bipolar technique does not prevent from these complications. If the use of isotonic solutions such as 0.9% sodium chloride prevents from dilution hyponatriemia, the risk of fluid overload is still maintained. In addition, several case reports have shown that massive fluid absorption during hysteroscopic myomectomy with normal saline solution resulted in severe hyperchloremic metabolic acidosis and dilution coagulopathy resolved with diuretic therapy [4, 5]. Another big concern is related to the use of high-frequency monopolar or bipolar current during resection. Uterine perforation with bowel injury can be caused by the loop of

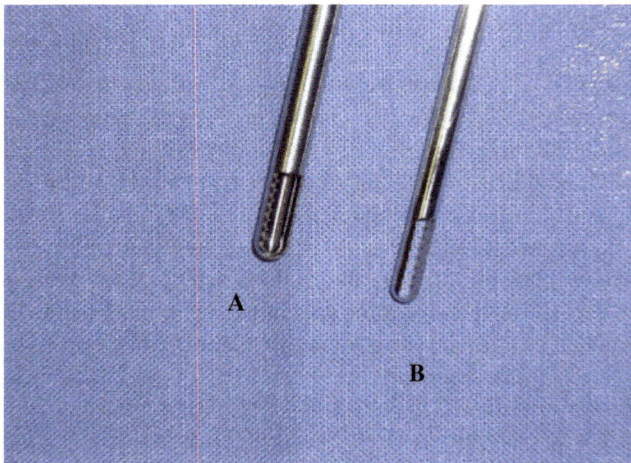

Fig. 2 a IBS® 25 mm^2 shaver tip with a **b** double window blade provided with a row of very sharp teeth

Table 1 Number of cases

	No. of cases	Percentage
Polyps	24	54.5
Myomas	15	34.1
Polyp +Myoma	2	4.5
Endometrial Hyperplasia	3	6.8
Total	44	

the resectoscope and oblige the surgeon to perform laparoscopy or laparotomy in order to repair the lesion [6]. In addition, during large polyps' or myomas' resection, the visual field of the surgeon is reduced by the tissue chips that stay inside the uterine cavity, increasing the risk of perforation. The procedure becomes time consuming, as the tissue pieces must be removed from the uterine cavity in order to continue the procedure under visual control. This tiring procedure exposes the patient to intravasation and cervical laceration. Another minor but not secondary problem is that more than half of the uterine perforations are entry related, due to the large diameter of the conventional resectoscopes [7].

All these observations explain why this technique has such a long learning curve and why only a few surgeons perform operative hysteroscopy [8].

In order to reduce the complications rate abovementioned and make this technique easier, we have made in cooperation with Karl Storz Gmbh of Tuttlingen a prototype of a new instrument.

The Integrated Bigatti Shaver (IBS®) with a double windows blade has been studied to improve the results of conventional resectoscopy. The IBS® is able to remove the tissue chips at the same time of resection so that the procedure, always done under visual control, becomes faster, and with less complications. In addition with the IBS®, there is a considerable reduction of the learning curve. The present study reports the first 44 cases made with the IBS® and debates about the feasibility of this technique.

Table 2 Polyps

No. of cases (%)	24 (54.5)
Size (mm)	5–40
IBS® Average time of resection	3′28″
Average negative fluid balance (ml)	170
Average amount of fluid used (ml)	1,195
Complications	–

Table 3 Myomas

	IBS®	IBS® + resectoscope
N° CASES (%OF MYOMAS)	10 (66,6)	5 (33.3%)
SIZE (mm)	10–30	20–40
TYPE(G)	4G0-2G1-4G2	3G0-2G2
Average Time Of Resection	14′	32′
Average negative fluid balance (ml)	540	940
Average amount of fluid used (ml)	3,910	9,300
Complications	1[a]	1[b]

[a] Malfunctioning of the Endomat® pump

[b] Rupture of the blade of the IBS®

Materials and methods

The IBS® is made of 90° angulated 0°optic (Karl Storz Gmbh of Tuttlingen) with a continuous flow sheath and an extra channel into which a rigid shaving system is introduced—Fig. 1. The continuous flow sheath is connected to a peristaltic pump (Endomat® Karl Storz gmbh of Tuttlingen) in order to maintain distension and visualization inside the uterine cavity. The outer sheath diameter is of 24 Fr (8 mm). The rigid shaving system consists of two hollow reusable metal tubes fitting to each other. The inner tube rotates within the outer tube and is connected to a handheld (Drill® cut-x Karl Storz gmbh of Tuttlingen) motor drive unit (Unidrive® eco Karl Storz gmbh of Tuttlingen) and to a roller pump (Endomat® LC Karl Storz gmbh of Tuttlingen) controlled by a foot pedal.

The foot pedal activates at the same time the movements of shaver tip and the roller pump's aspiration in order to maintain a continuous suction power on the window tip during the procedure.

The shaver tip of the IBS® has been specifically designed in order to be aggressive on any kind of tissue. The inner rotating tube has a double window blade provided with a row of very sharp teeth—Fig. 2. At the outer tube's edge there is a window, provided of teeth too, of different sizes: 10, 17, 20, and 25 mm^2.

We used a 300 to 450 oscillating rotation power per minute and a flow pressure of suction 1,000 ml/min.

After dilatation of the internal ostium of the uterine cervix up to number 8.5 of Hegar, the panoramic optic with inflow and outflow channels connected to the Endomat pump was inserted into the uterine cavity. For irrigation, we used both sorbitol–mannitol and normal physiologic saline solution according to the type of procedure. The maximal flow setting was 450 ml/min with an intrauterine pressure lower than 95 mm/Hg. Once visualized the pathological site we introduced the rigid shaving system connected to the motor drive unit and to the roller pump into the operative channel and started the procedure. Aspiration starts only when the pedal of the roller pump is pressed, this prevents from the collapse of the uterine cavity due to the massive outflow. The rotating and oscillating movement of the inner blade of the shaving system cuts the tissue and allows aspiration of specimens for histology that are collected into a glass bottle directly connected to the roller pump.

A correct fluid balance is calculated by checking the fluid aspirated by the Endomat pump and by the rollerpump connected to the shaving system plus the fluid collected into a graduated plastic bag placed under the patient.

From June 2009 to February 2010, we have performed 44 operative hysteroscopy with the IBS®. All patients underwent a diagnostic hysteroscopy before the operation.

The institutional ethical committee approved the research, and all patients gave their informed consent. All patients underwent general or regional anesthesia, and standard gynecological setup was used in the operating room.

As listed in Table 1, 24 endometrial polyps, 15 submucosal myomas, two endometrial polyps + myomas, and three endometrial abnormalities requiring endometrial ablation were included in the study. The polyps' size ranged from 5 to 40 mm, while the myomas' size was from 10 to 40 mm. All types of submucosal myomas, G0, G1, G2 classified according to the ESGE guidelines, were included in the study [9, 10]. Seven patients before myomectomy underwent a preoperative GnRH agonist

Table 4 Polyp + Myoma

N° of cases (%)	2(4,5)
Size (mm)	Polyp 10–30—Myoma 15–20(G0–G1/2)
IBS® Average time of resection	24′
Average negative fluid balance (ml)	500
Average amount of fluid used (ml)	5,750
Complications	–

therapy. Recordings were made of fluid balance, time of dilatation of the cervical canal, total operating time, time of resection, type of distension media used, and complications. For total operating time, we have considered the time of the procedure without the dilatation time. For time of resection, we have considered the time that goes from the view in the cavity of the shaver tip to the end of resection.

Results

We have analyzed the behavior of the IBS® with the different intrauterine pathologies.

The size of the polyps was between 5 mm and 4 cm with a mean time of resection of 3'28". We use an average of 1,195 ml of saline with a negative fluid loss of 170 ml. All procedures were performed exclusively with the IBS® and no complications occurred (Table 2).

Ten cases of myoma resection were performed exclusively with the IBS®, the size ranged from 10 to 30 mm of which four Type 0, two Type 1, four Type 2, and the mean resection time was 14'. We used an average of 3,910 ml of sorbitol–mannitol with a negative fluid loss of 540 ml. For five cases of myoma resection, we started the operation with the IBS®, and we ended the procedure with the conventional monopolar resectoscope. The myomas' size ranged from 20 to 40 mm of which three Type 0, two Type 2, and the mean resection time was 32' (Table 3). We used an average of 9,300 ml of sorbitol–mannitol with a negative fluid loss of 940 ml. We decided to switch to conventional resectoscopy when the negative fluid balance compared with the remaining tissue to resect was too high. Approximately with a negative fluid balance of more than 750 ml of sorbitol–mannitol, we decided to use the conventional monopolar resectoscope in order to end the procedure in one step. The average negative fluid balance increased according to the length of the operation e showed to be higher when the conventional resectoscope was used in combination with the IBS®.

Two overload complications occurred during myomectomy performed with the use of sorbitol–mannitol as distension media.

The first happened during a procedure performed exclusively with the IBS® and was due to a malfunctioning of the Endomat pump. In this case, the tubing system set was placed in the wrong position and, despite the fact that the whole procedure lasted only 20 min, we used 10,000 ml with a negative fluid loss of 1,500 ml. The second complication occurred during a G2—3 cm myoma resection done with the combination of the IBS® and the conventional resectoscope. In this case, one of the blades broke down, and we had to change it. Due to this operation,

Table 5 Endometrial hyperplasia

No. of cases (%)	3(6.8%)
Endometrial Thickness (mm)	>5
IBS® Average time of resection	12'10"
Average negative fluid balance (ml)	330
Average amount of fluid used (ml)	2,500
Complications	–

we did not properly check the fluid balance and the time of the whole operation. As a consequence, we used 12,500 ml with a negative fluid loss between 1,000 and 1,500 ml. Both cases were uneventful.

With the IBS®, we also performed two cases with the contemporary presence of a myoma and a polyp in the same patient, and the average time of resection was 24'. We used an average of 5,750 ml of sorbitol–mannitol with a negative fluid loss of 500 ml (Table 4).

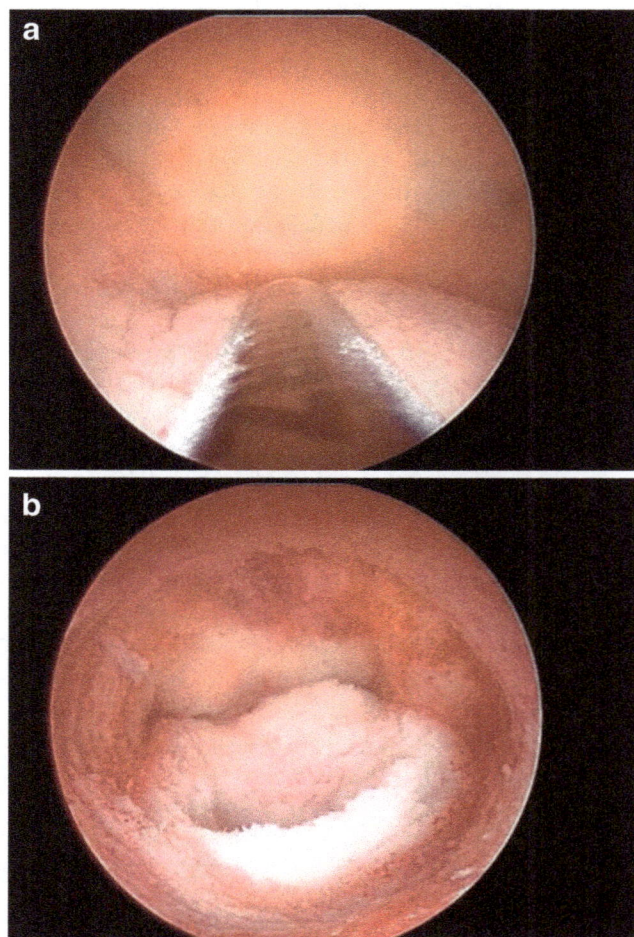

Fig. 3 IBS® resection of a G2, 2.5 cm large, submucosal myoma. **a** Before and **b** after the IBS® treatment. The Myoma is completely enucleated and the surrounding healthy endometrium is respected

We have also made three cases of endometrial ablation with an average time of resection of 12'10″. We used an average of 2,500 ml of sorbitol–mannitol with a negative fluid loss of 330 ml (Table 5). The mean dilatation time of the cervical canal was 2'.

Discussion

Polipectomy with the IBS® showed to be a very fast, clean, safe, and precise procedure. We started to remove the polyp from its top until we reached the base of the pedicle without affecting the surrounding endometrium. No bleeding was observed. Regarding myomectomy, the first remark is that we approached all types of submucosal myomas including G2 myomas. In 10 cases where the size was between 1 and 3 cm, we showed that the procedure was possible in an adequate lapse of time. When the size was approximately 4 cm, the time of the procedure became double, and conventional resectoscopy or a two-step procedure with the IBS® should be considered. What is really remarkable is that in the 10 cases done exclusively with the IBS®, the myoma was effectively enucleated, and only the intramural site of insertion of the myoma was interested by the procedure—Fig. 3. The surrounding healthy endometrium was respected without any thermal injury, compared with a less precise behavior of conventional resectoscopy. No coagulation was needed, and we had no extra bleeding problems. As our learning curve improved, only normal saline was used with less problems of fluid overload. With this paper, we want to assess the feasibility of this new technique. We believe that we should continue to work in this direction in order to reduce the time of myoma's resection that is still our major concern. To reach this goal, probably disposable and more aggressive tips are needed. At present, we have an ongoing randomized study to compare the IBS® with conventional bipolar resectoscopy. At the same time, further modifications to the IBS® are studied, in order to successfully perform all kind of hysteroscopic procedures in shorter time avoiding all major complications.

Acknowledgment This paper is dedicated to Ralph Sandler and to all members of the Roller Ball team for their enthusiasm and efforts dedicated to Hysteroscopy and for their true and long lasting friendship.

Special thanks go to H. Sonleiter, T. Weber, A. Waizenegger, H. Baher, and M Schick of Karl Storz gmbh of Tuttlingen for their technical support.

I would also like to thank my colleagues Dr. M. Rosales and Dr. C. Ferrario for their hard work in the realization of this study.

Declaration of interest The authors report no conflicts of interest. The authors alone are responsible for the content and writing of the paper.

References

1. Di Spezio SA, Mazzon I, Bramante S, Bettocchi S, Bifulco G, Guida M, Nappi C (2008) Hysteroscopic myomectomy: a comprehensive review of surgical techniques. Hum Reprod Update 14(2):101–119
2. Associazione Italiana di Endourologia - Da Lichtleiter ai Nostri Giorni - Segreteria Via Porrettana 76/2- 40033 - Casalecchio di Reno (Bo) www.ieanet.it/italiano/endourologia.php
3. Witz CA, Silverberg KM, Burns WN, Schenken RS, Olive DL (1993) Complications associated with absorption of hysteroscopic fluid media. Fertil Steril 60(5):745–756
4. Shaafer M, Von Ungern-Sternberg BS, Wight E, Schneider MC (2005) Isotonic fluid absorption during Hysteroscopy resulting in severe Hyperchloremic Acidosis. Anesthesiology 103:203–204
5. Van Kruchten PM, Vermelis JM, Herold I, Van Zundert AA (2010) Hypotonic and isotonic fluid overload as a complication of hysteroscopic procedures: two case reports. Minerva Anestesiol 76(5):373–377
6. Pasini A, Belloni C (2001) Intraoperative complications of 697 consecutive operative hysteroscopies. Minerva Ginecol 53(1):13–20
7. Jansen FW, Vredevoogd CB, Van Ulzen K, Hermans J, Trimbos JB, Trimbos-Kemper TC (2000) Complication of hysteroscopy: a prospective, multicenter study. Obstet Gynecol 96(2):266–270
8. Emanuel MH, Wamsteker K (2005) The intrauterine morcellator: a new hysteroscopic operating technique to remove intrauterine polyps and myomas. J Minim Invasive Gynecol 12(1):65–66
9. Wamsteker K, Emanuel MH, de Kruif JH (1993) Transcervical hysteroscopic resection of submucous fibroids for abnormal uterine bleeding: result regarding the degree of intramural extension. Obstet Gynecol 82:736–740
10. Salim R, Lee C, Davies A, Jolaoso B, Ofuasia E, Jurkovic D (2005) A comparative study of threedimensional saline infusion sonohysterography and diagnostic hysteroscopy for the classification of submucous fibroids. Hum Reprod 20:253–257

9

The digital operating room and the surgeon

Philippe R. Koninckx · Assia Stepanian ·
Leila Adamyan · Anastasia Ussia · Jacques Donnez ·
Arnaud Wattiez

Abstract The "word digital operating room" aims to integrate the images, information, and work flow available in the hospital and in the operating theater. In addition, it can distribute and record information while adding intelligence. The understanding of a digital operating room thus is highly variable. Whereas digital operating rooms are rapidly being incorporated in the hospitals, the clinical validation of improved quality of surgery is limited. The proven and expected usefulness of image distribution in one OR (routing and switching) or outside the OR (broadcasting), of integrating information, of image and video registration, and of intelligence, is reviewed with the perspective of quality and safety of surgery. It is expected that the digital OR will contribute to the learning and teaching and to the quality of surgery. Especially, the introduction of intelligence will be a major step forward. It remains important however that we, endoscopic surgeons, remain closely involved in shaping and orienting this future.

Keywords Digital operating room · Integrated operating room · Routing and switching · Broadcasting · Video registration · Quality of surgery

Introduction

In the last 25 years, we witnessed the explosive development of endoscopic surgery and its accompanying technological innovation. The introduction of lightweight cameras was followed by improved lens systems and better images and equipment. During the same period, diagnostic imaging such as ultrasound, MRI, and CAT scan was developed together with interventional radiology and image guidance systems. Simultaneously, the development of IT technology revolutionized communication in and between hospitals.

Philippe R. Koninckx is a professor emiritus.

P. R. Koninckx
University of KU Leuven,
Leuven, Belgium

P. R. Koninckx
University of Oxford,
Oxford, UK

P. R. Koninckx
Università Cattolica del Sacro Cuore,
Rome, Italy

L. Adamyan
Moscow State University,
Moscow, Russia

P. R. Koninckx (✉)
Vuilenbos 2,
3360 Bierbeek, Belgium
e-mail: pkoninckx@gmail.com

P. R. Koninckx
Gruppo Italo Belga, Heilig Hart,
Leuven, Belgium

A. Ussia
Villa del Rosario,
Rome, Italy

A. Stepanian
Academia of Women's Health,
Atlanta, GA, USA

J. Donnez
Université Catholique de Louvain,
Woluwe,
Brussels, Belgium

A. Wattiez
University of Strasbourg,
Strasbourg, France

The developments in these three different areas of minimal invasive surgery, imaging, and IT technology occurred simultaneously but were not or poorly coordinated, since they involved different fields of medicine and different expertise in industry. In the hospitals, this resulted in a separate development of operating theater equipment, of medical imaging systems and of digital patient records. Moreover, even within an operating theater, the development of the different equipment occurred independently, e.g., anesthesia machines, towers for endoscopic surgery, electrosurgery units, etc. The operating theaters subsequently had to change in order to accommodate orderly this various equipment and its cables into ceiling mounted booms. Operating theaters dedicated to minimal invasive surgery were developed. Radiology developed proprietary software to capture, interpret, diagnose, track, store, and recover images (the radiology information systems), and surgical information systems were developed. That these developments occurred separately is evidenced by the wide array of standards as health level 7, digital imaging and communications in medicine, picture archiving and communication system (PACS), Health Insurance Portability and Accountability Act, and clinical document architecture. Simultaneously, the individual manufacturers of operating theater equipment started the integration of their equipment. Only recently, the fast growing possibilities of integration of all these different technologies, standards, and equipment to enhance the quality and safety of surgery were realized. Introduction of intelligence will be the next step.

Digital operating room (DOR) is a much used but poorly defined word, varying from routing and switching over broadcasting, video registration, and photo documentation to integration and emerging intelligence. The usefulness of these features to improve quality and/or safety of patient care or to improve teaching and training has been poorly addressed. Indeed, a PubMed search for "digital operating room" or "integrated operating room" found a limited number of engineering articles [1–4] and two marginally relevant articles [5, 6]. Reality however is that many of us actually are already working in a digital OR whereas search engines generate numerous hits spanning advertisement by industry and hospitals, a few blogs, and one PhD on economic aspects [7]. The fast introduction of this new technology triggered this article in order to generate reflection as a basis to help with clinical validation.

The different aspects of a digital operating room

The word digital operating room aims to the integrate all images, information, and work flow available in the hospital and in the operating theater. "All information available everywhere at any moment" sounds well, but practical considerations force limitation and choices. The emphasis varies when used by hospital administration, by the IT department, or by surgeons. For the latter, quality of surgery, outcome for the patient, and teaching are the most important.

Image and video distribution in one operating theater
(also called "routing and switching")

From the beginning of endoscopic surgery, we realized for reasons of ergonomy that it was useful to have a separate screen for the surgeon and the assistant surgeon and preferably to have a third screen for the third assistant. We rapidly realized that it could be nice to display two images side by side on two screens, e.g., when placing a ureter stent under laparoscopic control or when performing simultaneously a laparoscopy and a coloscopy or ultrasound.

The basic DOR thus permits to display the images from the different image sources in the operating room to any of the available screens. This seems fairly evident for images from the endoscopic or overview camera. It is less obvious for radiology and ultrasound images and even less for the images available from PACS (with previous exams such as X-rays or MRI). In addition, versatility and integration often is an issue when plugging in a new device, e.g., a second endoscopic camera for combined laparoscopic and cystoscopic exam or for hysteroscopic resection under laparoscopic or ultrasound guidance.

Image and video distribution obviously adds versatility and makes our life easier by avoiding excessive crowding of cables around the operating theater by the additional devices. Indirect advantages for sterility, for the OR personnel, for the organization, and the work flow will result. For the quality of surgery, however, the advantage is limited, since there is little difference between the images of two endoscopic towers shown side by side and the same images shown on screens in a digital OR with image and video distribution.

Image and video distribution of images from one OR
to the outside world (often called broadcasting)

Live surgery and watching surgical interventions is widely recognized as fundamental for learning or teaching endoscopic surgery. Those having organized live surgery, however, are fully aware of the recurrent effort, cost, and technical difficulty of showing life surgery from two or three operating theaters with bidirectional audio to one meeting room in the hospital, i.e., at a reasonable distance. To distribute quality images and audio outside the hospital over longer distances requires specialized personnel and remains tricky as judged by the often imperfect images and/or failing audio. When assisting live surgery at meetings, we might have the impression that broadcasting is no longer a technical issue. We do have to realize however that broadcasting of life surgery together with audio generally has to be well planned beforehand and organized each time again. Even in the rare occasions that the infrastructure of broadcasting is structurally available, this holds true only for one or two dedicated operating rooms and still requires technicians to get it functional.

The use and the usefulness of broadcasting with bidirectional sound for training and teaching varies with its ease of use. It will be used more readily when it is as easy to be used by the surgeon as making a phone call. It moreover should be available from every operating theater. This would permit direct supervision and teaching of surgery from another operating room, from any screen in the hospital, and ideally from any computer or smartphone at distance. This would also permit to make live surgery more widely available through the Internet, eventually to selected and targeted audiences. The recent initiative of the AAGL to broadcast interventions on a regular basis is a nice example of this. Conversely, this will equally permit the surgeon to ask for advice any time he needs this even outside the hospital. This is expected to improve teaching, learning, supervision, help, and thus quality of surgery.

Important is the availability of bidirectional audio since teaching and learning is highly dependent on interactivity as is supervision and asking for advice. When considering Internet broadcast to multiple targeted audiences, other ways of asking questions will be necessary, e.g., written questions by mail or SMS to a moderator.

Empowering the surgeon

Settings of insufflation, light fountain, laser, or electro surgery are chosen before surgery or during surgery by the theater nurse or the surgeon. That the surgeon, while being sterile, can change settings himself, or can make a phone call, is nice to have. It might decrease the nursing need, but finally it will not affect much the quality of surgery performed.

The surgeon is responsible and needs to stay in control. Offering more information to the surgeon by displaying information of devices can be helpful. Sometimes, this may prevent mistakes such as "forgetting" that the initial Verres needle insufflation was done up to 25 mm for safety reasons. Additional information risks however generate information overload. The surgeon indeed is already doing surgery with two hands and with up to four pedals (for bipolar coagulation, for monopolar cutting and coagulation, and for a laser) which requires attention and information processing. In addition, he has to control the assistant, who is responsible for framing the image. Especially during live surgery, the problem of information overload is realized

since in addition the surgeon has to explain the surgery and to answer questions. The brain processing for this gets sharply worse in a nonfamiliar operating theater with a new assistant requiring increased attention. Those used to do live surgery realize that all these factors add up and that specific experience is required to manage the massive amount of information.

To give more information to the surgeon might therefore not be the right direction because of the risk of overload of information. On the contrary, what is needed is facilitating control by making the information intelligent. Examples can be very simple as preventing/warning that the irrigation bottle will be empty or that the aspiration bottle will be full. The importance of prediction is evident when these simple problems happen at the same moment a bleeding occurs. When the intraperitoneal pressure would be available to the anesthetist, he would understand immediately why ventilation is difficult when the surgeon or nurse did forget to decrease the higher insufflation pressure used for inducing the pneumoperitoneum. A nice example of intelligence enhancing safety is the indication of fluid loss during hysteroscopic surgery. The examples also emphasize the absence of communication or intelligence between different devices.

Video registration and photo documentation

Selected clips and images were shown at congresses and workshops. We all know, however, how much time and effort was spend to generate nice clips or images; even today, we often struggle to edit clips in the absence of a dedicated service to help us. What the surgeon needs is an easy way to control registration himself so that with a little training, video clips can be taken which need little or no editing afterwards.

It might be surprising that the pictures taken 20 years ago with a photo camera were of better quality than those taken today with a video camera. Indeed, the resolution of video cameras is only 640×480 pixels and even in HD only $1,920 \times 1,080$ which corresponds to 0.3 and 2 megapixels, respectively. This indeed is a low resolution in comparison with the picture of the widely available 10-megapixel photo camera. Especially when needed to be enlarged, surgical pictures of better quality would be an advantage. Photo documentation of surgery and integration of pictures in the operating report is considered a step forward since one picture tells more than 1,000 words and since it facilitates reviewing and sharing the data of surgery. Ideally, these pictures should be incorporated in a hard copy or in the electronic patient file and thus in the IT system of the hospital. Without integration in a report, isolated pictures have to be reviewed separately which is time consuming.

Video registration of entire interventions remains debated, although it might have several advantages [8]. It permits to review an intervention which can be useful when faced with a complication. It permits to debrief an operation afterwards which can improve surgery as Doyen described more than 100 years ago. Medicolegally, it can be an advantage for the surgeon, who can prove that surgery was performed meticulously without recognizable mistakes. Surgery can even be shown to have been so difficult that an error of judgment becomes understandable and that a complication does not necessarily mean a lack of precaution. Systematic video registration of complete interventions at high resolution however has the drawback of generating prohibitively large data files (some 2–5 GB/hour for a normal video camera) making registration of entire interventions impractical and expensive. Medical video registration thus has to integrate the possibilities of low quality recording for registration of entire procedures and of high quality recording which can be limited to selected clips.

Fundamental to the discussion of video registration is storage and life cycle management. A full discussion is beyond the scope of this article, but high quality recording and retrieval of all procedures is unrealistic emphasizing the need for dedicated solutions.

What is the future and what do we need?

The digital OR with video distribution in the OR is nice to have but has limited added value for the quality of surgery. The clinical value of image and video distribution in the OR and outside the OR comprises teaching, supervision of surgery, and asking for advice during surgery. The usefulness depends largely on the ease of implementation by the surgeon. When an entire operating theater complex is interconnected, several additional new applications emerge. Bringing together the videos of all ceiling cameras facilitates management of patient flow since the responsible can "see" when an operation is finished and when a room is cleaned. Showing all anesthesia monitors facilitates supervision by a senior, something similar to the central monitoring of delivery rooms. Most important is that showing the operation image to a screen in another OR greatly facilitates continuous supervision of juniors, while it permits to ask for advice without the necessity of the other surgeon to come physically to OR. It is difficult to demonstrate that this improves the quality of surgery, but it seems self-evident that with increased supervision, the risk of near accidents and accidents will decrease. Experience has demonstrated the importance of "keeping continuously an eye" on the surgery performed by a junior. The reality in surgery, however, is that most senior surgeon is not always assisting or physically present. He is called in when the junior feels the necessity, i.e., often after the accident happened or was nearly missed or more simply when a plane of cleavage was missed. When distribution of all surgical images would be made available to all monitors in the entire hospital supervision, training and quality control obviously would get a new dimension. This is even more obvious when these video images would also be available outside the hospital, e.g., to a senior surgeon at home.

In order to understand the difficulty of video distribution, we should be aware that the image quality degrades when transported over more than 12 m thus requiring intermittent amplification. Internet signals have the advantage of being transported at light speed virtually without loss of quality provided a sufficient bandwidth is available. In addition, delay of video signals can become an issue especially when used for surgery.

Photo documentation of surgery is important, especially when incorporated into the patient hospital file as an operation report with images. This indeed facilitates subsequent review and transfer of information and saves time.

The benefits and advantages of video registration of entire interventions have been discussed in detail previously [8]. It should be realized however that systematic registration of entire interventions is realistic only when a high compression limits the size of the files while keeping the quality of the image reasonable.

The real power of the digital OR will be the introduction of intelligence and of features that help the surgeon improve the quality of his surgery. The video cameras and image displayed today are similar to those used for routine filming. The following is a series of obvious examples when looking to the future. That the image on the screen no longer rotates with camera rotation will help to keep the surgeon orientated. During surgery, when looking towards the camera, the image should be flipped left–right. It would be helpful to have information of what happens outside the view of the camera. Intelligence comprises the integration of all information available in the OR. Intelligence also comprises image manipulation in real time: consider that on a separate screen side by side, or even better on the same screen, the vascularization pattern or the fluorescence of a cancer and its metastasis or of the smaller endometriotic lesions would be clearly visible. Consider what would happen to nerve sparing surgery when camera intelligence will show the difference between fibrosis and a nerve. Ureters today can be visualized with illuminated stents, but this is cumbersome and expensive; consider that the camera would recognize the ureter. All this has been summarized in Table 1 as a checklist on what a digital OR could do for you

Table 1 What a digital OR can bring to the surgeon

Distribution of image sources in 1 OR

  Video camera's (e.g., cystoscopy and laparoscopy)

  Computer screens

  PACS

  X-ray

  Ultrasound

  Is distribution plug and play or dedicated

  Maximum sources that can be handled

Broadcasting of image sources from 1 OR

  To all other theaters of the operating theater complex

  To a dedicated room of the hospital

  To each Internet connected to screens worldwide including smartphones and tablets

  With bidirectional audio

  Flexibility of display (e.g. 1 image form 12 theaters in 1 display)

  Distribution controlled by the surgeon

  Little effort and cost to setup

  What is the delay of the image

Can image "enhancement" be integrated

  Image rotation

  Fluorescence

  Spectroscopy

  Overlay of images from previous exams

Recording and reporting

  Standard quality picture

  HD quality picture

  Integrated in operation report

  Integrated in patient file

  High quality recording (>2 GB/h)

  Recording for review (<200 Mb/h)

  Adding text

  Watermark

  Rerecording

Others

  Telephone

  Display of device settings on screen

  Change of device settings by the surgeon

Discussion and conclusions

The meaning of digital operating room varies from basic image and video distribution in the OR to a tool that can improve teaching, that will help to prevent accidents, and that will improve the quality of surgery. This will be the way forward since it will benefit the patient while decreasing the cost for society.

Before discussing each item in detail, we have to realize that the needs of so-called excellent or expert surgeons which we witness during meetings are different from the needs of less experienced surgeons. We indeed demonstrated experimentally using standardized nephrectomy in rabbits that for an experienced surgeon, the quality of the image when using a 2-, 3-, 5-, or 10 -mm scope was of little importance. For the less experienced surgeon however, the quality of the surgery and the incidence of accidents [9] are strongly affected by the quality of the image which varies with the definition of detail, e.g., high definition, and the field of vision. It was suggested that experienced surgeons, while doing surgery at high magnification on a small field, have in their head at all times a 3D image of the entire pelvis. This is emphasized by the fact that all surgeons intermittently zoom out during surgery for reorientation and by the fact that often juniors have a difficulty to orient during surgery. Therefore, for training and for less expert surgeons, it is expected that the quality of image and an overview image might be an advantage. The equally valid conclusion that with experience we can do with less emphasizes the importance for training.

Manipulation of bowels often occurs outside the field of vision of the camera. Lesions therefore can occur unnoticed, as we described with small bowel perforations diagnosed after a couple of days only. Obviously, a direct image and/or a registration permitting subsequent review would be helpful. Review of the video recordings of intervention is helpful for the early diagnosis of complications, as we observed at several occasions, while a thorough analysis of a complication is the best guide to prevention in the future [10]. A more widely use of debriefing surgery would permit to identify and prevent near missers, as demonstrated for aviation.

We are at the beginning of the introduction of intelligence and of features that help the surgeon to improve the quality of his surgery. This however obviously requires that computing power is brought to the operating theater. Local computing might do; drawing in the computing power of data centers will be better. The same holds true for video registration which obviously requires dedicated recording tools. Central recording, storage, and retrieval are likely to be superior to the individual CD. The wide introduction however will require debate and consensus on ownership of the tape and of other medicolegal issues of recording.

That image and video distribution in and outside the hospital is useful for training and education and for the quality of surgery will become clear when this will be always and everywhere available when decided by the surgeon. Live surgery as evidenced by the large audiences at meetings indirectly confirms the importance. When image and video distribution would always be available, without necessitating a setup for transmission, it is expected to be used widely for training students and registrars, for supervision, and for giving advice. The lower the effort to implement image and video distribution to any video screen in or even outside the hospital, the more it will be used for direct supervision and advice. When the supervisor has to come physically to the OR, he will be asked less readily if not slightly too late. The same holds true when advice can be asked easily at a greater distance, e.g., to a senior surgeon at home during the night or to experts anywhere in the world.

In conclusion, the word digital OR is used for varying implementations, some of which are expected to improve training, prevent accidents, and improve quality of surgery. This is expected to happen when image and video distribution will become always available and as easy as making a phone call in the entire hospital and to selected targeted audiences through the Internet. Anything (any format) from anywhere (all image sources) to everywhere (also outside the hospital even on smart phones) is a reality in the near future. Systematic video recording (at high compression) with central storage and retrieval together with photo documentation in the patient record is a reality. We begin to witness the development of tools that further improve image quality. Especially when experience is less, this can compensate for our lack of 3D vision. This will bring computing power to the operating theater to improve or modify images in order to visualize and recognize structures that today are difficult to identify, such as nerves and ureters. The digital operating theater with its integration and distribution of intelligent information thus is expected to improve the quality of surgery and indirectly lower the cost for society.

Acknowledgments We do thank Dr. Karina Mailova from Moscow for reviewing this manuscript.

Disclosures PK is the chief medical officer at eSATURNUS NV, Romeinse straat, Haasrode, Belgium.

Conflict of interest The authors report no conflicts of interest. The authors alone are responsible for the content and writing of the paper.

References

1. Voruganti AK, Mayoral R, Vazquez A, Burgert O (2010) A modular video streaming method for surgical assistance in operating room networks. Int J Comput Assist Radiol Surg 5(5):489–499
2. Inamura K, Lemke HU (2007) Technology and its clinical application in the field of computer-assisted radiology and surgery. Biomed Imaging Intervent J 3(3):e41
3. Korb W, Bohn S, Burgert O, Dietz A, Jacobs S, Falk V et al (2006) Surgical PACS for the digital operating room. Systems engineering and specification of user requirements. Stud Health Technol Informatics 119:267–272
4. Ratib OM, Horii SC (eds) (2005) Workflow in the operating room: review of arrowhead 2004 seminar on imaging and informatics. 05 Feb 15; San Diego, CA
5. Buzink SN, van Lier L, de Hingh IH, Jakimowicz JJ (2010) Risk-sensitive events during laparoscopic cholecystectomy: the influence of the integrated operating room and a preoperative checklist tool. Surg Endosc 24(8):1990–1995
6. Chiu JC, Maziad AM, Rappard G, Thacker JT, Liu B, Documet J (2010) Evolving minimally invasive spine surgery: a surgeon's perspective on technological convergence and digital OR control system. Surg Technol Int 19:211–222
7. Anderson T, Tranzén R, Odén M (2006) Valuation of a digital operating room in the public health care sector. Gotheborg University, School of economics
8. Koninckx PR (2008) Videoregistration of surgery should be used as a quality control. J Minim Invasive Gynecol 15(2):248–253
9. Molinas CR, Cabral CR, Koninckx PR (1999) Effect of the diameter of the endoscope and of surgeon training on the duration and quality of laparoscopic surgery in a rabbit model. J Am Assoc Gynecol Laparosc 6(4):447–452
10. Schonman R, De CC, Corona R, Soriano D, Koninckx PR (2008) Accident analysis: factors contributing to a ureteric injury during deep endometriosis surgery. BJOG 115(13):1611–1615

10

Clinical approach for the classification of congenital uterine malformations

Grigoris F. Grimbizis · Rudi Campo ·
On behalf of the Scientific Committee of the Congenital
Uterine Malformations (CONUTA) common ESHRE/
ESGE working group: Stephan Gordts, Sara Brucker,
Marco Gergolet, Vasilios Tanos, T.-C. Li, Carlo De
Angelis, Attilio Di Spiezio Sardo

Abstract A more objective, accurate and non-invasive estimation of uterine morphology is nowadays feasible based on the use of modern imaging techniques. The validity of the current classification systems in effective categorization of the female genital malformations has been already challenged. A new clinical approach for the classification of uterine anomalies is proposed. Deviation from normal uterine anatomy is the basic characteristic used in analogy to the American Fertility Society classification. The embryological origin of the anomalies is used as a secondary parameter. Uterine anomalies are classified into the following classes: 0, normal uterus; I, dysmorphic uterus; II, septate uterus (absorption defect); III, dysfused uterus (fusion defect); IV, unilateral formed uterus (formation defect); V, aplastic or dysplastic uterus (formation defect); VI, for still unclassified cases. A subdivision of these main classes to further anatomical varieties with clinical significance is also presented. The new proposal has been designed taking into account the experience gained from the use of the currently available classification systems and intending to be as simple as possible, clear enough and accurate as well as open for further development. This proposal could be used as a starting point for a working group of experts in the field.

Keywords Uterine anomalies · Mullerian anomalies · Classification · Septate uterus

G. F. Grimbizis · R. Campo
European Academy for Gynecological Surgery,
Scientific project on Female Genital Tract Congenital Anomalies,
Diestsevest 43/0001,
3000 Leuven, Belgium

G. F. Grimbizis (✉)
First Department of Obstetrics and Gynecology,
Aristotle University of Thessaloniki,
Tsimiski 51 Street,
54623 Thessaloniki, Greece
e-mail: grigoris.grimbizis@gmail.com

G. F. Grimbizis
e-mail: grimbi@med.auth.gr

Introduction

Female genital tract anomalies are common deviations from normal anatomy with an estimated prevalence of 4–7% in the general population and even higher in selected populations such as recurrent aborters [1–3]. Their occurrence could be associated with a variety of clinical presentations ranging between life threatening complications, severe health problems in the adolescence, reproductive problems although in most of them they are asymptomatic [1, 4–16].

Due to their high prevalence and possible impact on the reproductive health of women, congenital uterine malformations of the female genital tract are a challenge for the therapeutic decision-making process. An efficient planning of the therapeutic strategy is based on their effective diagnosis and clear categorization, in view also of the numerous treatment options available for their management. The need for a reliable classification system is more than obvious [4].

The first attempt to classify female congenital anomalies goes back to the beginning of the 19th century; Strassmann described septate and bicornuate uterus and some subgroups of the disorders in 1907. However, the first classification system for categorization of congenital uterine malformations was that of the American Fertility Society (AFS) published in 1988, mostly based on the previous work of Buttram and Gibbons [17, 18]. Almost 15 years later, Acien et al. [19] proposed another option for the classification of congenital female malformations using the embryological origin as the basis of the system. A newer version of this classification has been published recently [20]. Furthermore, Oppelt et al. [21] published a very detailed classification system based on the Tumor Nodes Metastases (TNM) principle in oncology and known as vagina, cervix, uterus, adnexae and associated malformations (VCUAM) classification system. It is also interesting that, apart from these alternatives for the classification of the female genital malformations in general, some other subdivisions for certain categories of anomalies have been published [22–27].

Although the AFS classification received wide acceptance and it is still the most broadly used system, it is associated with various limitations in effective categorization of the anomalies. It is also interesting that until now none of the other available options was able to effectively replace the AFS system [4].

The European Academy for Gynaecological Surgery (EAGS), recognizing the need for an evidence-based updated classification of female genital tract malformations, has established a scientific project on that issue. As the *first step* of this project, a systematic re-evaluation of the current proposals has been done and, based on their criticism, the characteristics of the new classification system have been clarified [4]. The *second and final step* of the EAGS scientific project was to prepare a proposal for the new updated clinical classification of uterine anomalies to be used as the scientific background for a working group of experts in the field. This proposal, after extensive discussion, has been also adopted as the scientific basis for the development of a new classification system by the common working group meanwhile established by the European Society of Human Reproduction and Embryology (ESHRE) and European Society for Gynaecological Endoscopy (ESGE) under the working name CONUTA (CONgenital UTerine Anomalies). The development of the new system will run using the DELPHI procedure of consensus.

The updated new proposal for the classification of uterine congenital anomalies is designed having mainly clinical orientation and based on a critical review of the available data on female genital tract malformations with their extensive interpretation. Further subdivisions based on the cervical and vaginal anatomy, incorporating all the possible co-existent anomalies and their combinations, are feasible but they are not in the goals of the present article. Thus, the system is open for further development in order to be more comprehensive.

Design of the new system: main concepts

The first and fundamental starting point in the design of the new proposal for a classification system was, initially, *to select the basic characteristic* for patients' grouping. Thus, anatomy of the female genital tract is thought to be the most appropriate basic characteristic for the systematic categorization of the women with congenital anomalies in a new classification system for the following reasons: (1) by definition, congenital anomalies of the female genital tract are miscellaneous deviations from normal anatomy [4], (2) clinical presentation and prognosis of the patients seems to be correlated with the type and the degree of anatomical deformity of the genital tract [2, 4–16, 28–32] (3) anatomy is the basis of the AFS classification system which is successfully adopted as the main classification system for more than two decades, indicating the real value of the anatomy in that respect [4, 17].

The second point in the design of the new proposal is to decide if there is a "key" organ in the anatomy of the female genital tract that could be used by priority to build up the main groups of the system. Thus, uterine anatomy was selected as the key characteristic for the main groups of the system for the following reasons: (1) frequency should be taken into account in the design of the system and the vast majority of the congenital malformations of the female genital tract are, no doubt, uterine ones [1–3, 33, 34]; (2) uterine anatomy is the basis in the design of the AFS classification system and it is thought to be one of the advantages of this system explaining, also, its wide acceptability; the adoption of the same characteristic by the new system will facilitate the clinicians to smoothly move from the old to the new system [4, 17].

Although uterine anatomy has been selected as the main characteristic in the design of the new classification system *another crucial point was to choose if there is another supplementary characteristic* that could be used in the design of the patients' grouping. Uterine congenital malformations are the result of very discrete disturbances in the embryologic development of the Müllerian (or para-mesonephric) ducts during fetal life thus explaining their pathogenesis [9, 35, 36]. Due to its independent importance, embryological origin of uterine anomalies has been adopted as a secondary basic characteristic in the design of the main groups of the new proposal. The incorporation of embryology as an additional basic characteristic helps to create (1) more uniform classes avoiding transitional unclassified or cases with unclear classification and, (2) more "clear" classes since each class has a common pathogenesis due to the fact that, usually, very discrete embryological disturbances underlie to each patients' group.

Proposed uterine classification: key concepts

The new proposed system has the following general characteristics: (a) the main classes are based on the uterine anatomy and embryology and express main anatomical variations of uterine anatomy coming from the same embryological origin; (b) the main sub-classes are further anatomical variations of the main classes expressing different degrees of uterine deformity.

In general, two options are available for the classification of uterine anomalies: the first is to go from the normal uterus (as class 0 or I) to the more deformed types, e.g., uterine aplasia/dysplasia (as class VI), and the other one is to go from the more severe forms (uterine aplasia/dysplasia as class I) to the normal uterus (as class VI), an approach followed in the ASRM classification system. In the new system, the first way of classification is adopted, with normal uterus being class 0, since: (1) it seems to be more reasonable to start from less affected to more affected cases and (2) the scientific society is familiar mainly with this practice followed also in the categorization of cancer, endometriosis, etc.

As already mentioned, each main class is further divided into sub-classes. The mode of classification adopted in sub-classes is to go from the less severe forms to the more severe ones and the numbers are the alphabet of the Latin language (a, b, c). It should be noted that, for the needs of simplicity, an extremely detailed further sub-classification is avoided in order to stay away from too many sub-divisions, which seems not to be very functional. Thus, sub-classes include variations of the same embryological anatomical entity with clinical different significance.

The main classes and the subclasses of the new system are presented in Table 1 and are as follows (Fig. 1):

Class 0 — normal uterus
Class I — dysmorphic uterus; *Ia* T-shaped uterus and *Ib* uterus infantilis
Class II — septate uterus; *IIa* partial septate uterus and *IIb* complete septate uterus
Class III — dysfused uterus, *IIIa* partial disfused uterus and *IIIb* complete dysfused uterus
Class IV — unilaterally formed uterus (formerly unicornuate uterus); *IVa* horn with cavity (communicating or not), *IVb* horn without cavity or aplasia

Class V — aplastic/dysplastic uterus; *Va* bilateral or unilateral horn with cavity and *Ib* bilateral or unilateral horn without cavity or aplasia of both parts
Class VI — for still unclassified cases

Definitions

(a) *Class 0* incorporates all cases with normal uterus giving the opportunity to classify congenital malformations of the other parts of female genital tract apart from the uterus in the fully developed classification system [25, 26, 37–53].

(b) *Class I* incorporates all cases having a uterus with *normal outline but with an abnormal lateral wall's shape of the uterine cavity.* The Greek term "dysmorphia" is used to describe the cavity with this abnormal morphology. Class I is further subdivided into two categories: (a) T-shaped uterus characterized by a correlation of 2/3 uterine corpus and 1/3 cervix and (b) uterus infantilis characterized by an inverse correlation of 1/3 uterine body and 2/3 cervix. It should be noted, however, that both subclasses have almost the same appearance in hysterosalpingography (HSG) and magnetic resonance imaging (MRI) and differential diagnosis could be done mainly by hysteroscopy and biopsy of the endocervix and endometrium.

(c) *Class II* incorporates all cases with normal fusion and abnormal absorption of the midline septum. Thus, *septate uterus* is characterized as any uterus with a normal outline and with an inner indentation at the midline level (septum) that divides the cavity. A septum is defined any indentation at the midline level exceeding at least by 50% (half) the uterine wall thickness and reaching up to the full division of the cavity and/or the

Table 1 Classification of uterine anomalies

Main class	Uterine anomaly	Main sub-classes
Class 0	Normal uterus	
Class I	Dysmorphic uterus	a. T-shaped
		b. Infantilis
Class II	Septate uterus	a. Partial
		b. Complete
Class III	Dysfused uterus	a. Partial
		b. Complete
Class IV	Unilateral formed uterus	a. Rudimentary horn with cavity (Communicating or not)
		b. Rudimentary horn without cavity/Aplasia (no horn)
Class V	Aplastic/dysplastic uterus	a. Rudimendary horn with cavity (bi- or unilateral)
		b. Rudimentary horn without cavity (bi- or unilateral)/Aplasia
Class VI	Unclassified malformations	

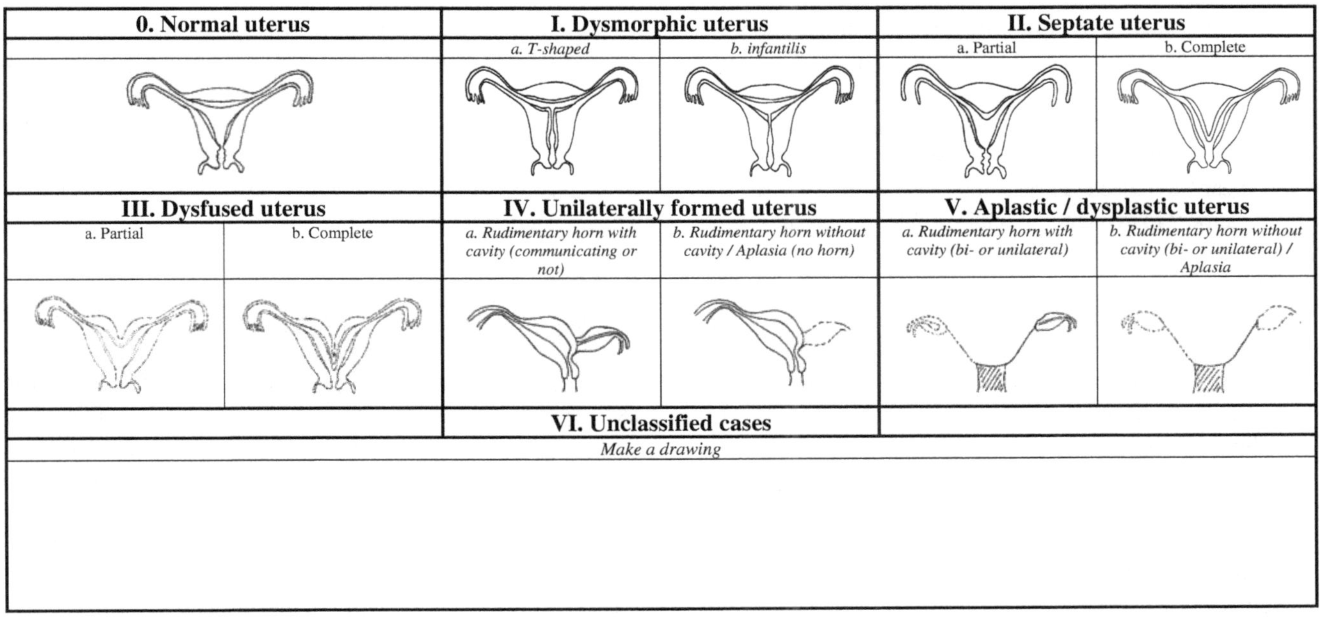

0. Normal uterus		I. Dysmorphic uterus		II. Septate uterus	
		a. T-shaped	b. infantilis	a. Partial	b. Complete
III. Dysfused uterus		IV. Unilaterally formed uterus		V. Aplastic / dysplastic uterus	
a. Partial	b. Complete	a. Rudimentary horn with cavity (communicating or not)	b. Rudimentary horn without cavity / Aplasia (no horn)	a. Rudimentary horn with cavity (bi- or unilateral)	b. Rudimentary horn without cavity (bi- or unilateral) / Aplasia
		VI. Unclassified cases			
		Make a drawing			

Fig. 1 Schematic representation of uterine anomalies' classification

cervix and/or the vagina into two distinct parts. It should be noted that in definitions, the use of absolute numbers (e.g., indentation of 5 mm) is avoided since the "normal" uterine dimensions as well as uterine wall thickness are not known and they could be different from one patient to another. Thus, it seems more justified to define uterine deformity as proportions of each patient's uterine anatomical condition [54].

Class II is further divided into two sub-classes according to the *degree of the uterine cavity deformity* (uterine corpus, including or not the cervix): (a) partial septate uterus is characterized by the presence of any septum partially dividing the uterine cavity above the level of the internal cervical oss; (b) complete septate uterus is characterized by the presence of a septum fully dividing the uterine cavity up to the level of the internal cervical oss. Cases with cervical (e.g., bicervical septate uterus) and/or vaginal defects [55–61] can be further sub-classified with the addition of cervical and/or vaginal congenital anomalies in the fully developed system.

(d) *Class III* incorporate all cases of fusion defects. The term dysfusion comes from the addition of the Greek origin "dys" to the English "fusion" to describe the abnormal fusion of the two uterine sides during embryologic development. In this main class all cases of formerly described didelphys and bicornuate uterus are included. This enables us to create a more embryological clear category without "transitional" cases [62].

Thus, a *dysfused uterus* is characterized as any uterus with an *abnormal outline* at the level of uterine midline.

As can easily be imagined, it is also associated with an inner indentation at the midline level (septum) that divides the cavity. An abnormal uterine outline is defined as any fundal indentation exceeding half of the uterine wall thickness at the midline level and reaching up to the full separation of the uterus into two distinct hemi-uterus (formerly didelphys uterus).

Class III is further divided into two subclasses according to the *degree of the uterine body deformity* (uterine corpus, including or not the cervix): (a) partial dysfused uterus is characterized by an outer form indentation at the level of uterine midline partially dividing uterine corpus above the level the cervix; (b) complete dysfused uterus is characterized by an outer form indentation at the level of uterine midline fully dividing uterine corpus up to the level of the cervix. Cases with cervical (double cervix/ formerly didelphys uterus) and/or vaginal defects (e.g., didelphys uterus with obstructing or not vaginal septum) [22, 63–72] could be sub-classified in the fully developed system with the addition of cervical and/or vaginal congenital anomalies.

A general subcategory of Class III is dysfused "septate" uterus. In these cases, fusion defects come together with absorption defects. A dysfused "septate" uterus is defined as any dysfused uterus in which the width at the midline uterine fundus' level exceeds by 50% that of the uterine wall thickness (e.g., if the uterine wall thickness is by mean 10 mm as dysfused "septate" uterus is characterized as any thickness in the midline indentation >15 mm). The necessity of creating this distinct subcategory comes from the fact that these cases can be partially treated by hysteroscopic septum resection. Furthermore, this subcategory is included in the class of dysfused uterus since: (1) by definition, any abnormal outline defect is included in this category (accuracy of definition); (2) the result of hysteroscopic treatment is a "clear" dysfused uterus; and (3) during hysteroscopic treatment to avoid complications (uterine rupture), underlining of the abnormal external outline is clinically important.

(e) *Class IV* incorporates all cases of *unilateral formed uterus* with aplasia or dysplasia of the other uterine half. It is a formation defect, but the necessity of classifying it separately from full aplasia comes from the presence of a fully developed functional uterine hemicavity, which does not exist in cases of aplasia.

A more simple subdivision is also chosen for Class IV compared to that in the ASRM classification system; it is divided into two sub-classes based on the *presence/absence of a cavity in an existing rudimentary horn*, since the presence of the cavity is the most important factor for certain complications such as ectopic pregnancy in the rudimentary horn or hematocavity [73–78]. Furthermore, treatment is only indicated in cases of patients having a rudimentary horn with cavity (laparoscopic removal) [79, 80].

It should be noted that the name of this class is derived from the normally developed horn, whereas the name of the subclasses are attributed to the characteristics of the abnormally developed horn.

(f) *Class V* incorporates only cases of *uterine aplasia/dysplasia* (formation defect) and is thus designed as a "clear" category [21, 50, 81–92]. As already mentioned, cases with cervical, vaginal or adnexal aplasia/dysplasia (having different embryological origin, clinical presentation, prognosis and treatment) can be classified in separate categories or sub-categories of the fully developed new classification system. The term "dysplasia" has a Greek origin, and it means abnormally developed uterus, which fits in cases with non-functional developed parts of the uterus. As a synonym, the term "dysgenesis" can be used; this also means abnormal formation.

Class V is further divided into two subclasses based on the *presence/absence of a cavity in an existing rudimentary horn*, avoiding an extremely detailed subdivision [21, 45, 85, 91, 93, 94]. This criterion is chosen because this seems to be a clinically significant parameter for patient's management: the presence of a cavity could be combined with complications such as "hemato-cavity" [37, 95] and gives the possibility to restore anatomical continuity after neovagina formation with isthmo-neovagina anastomosis [37, 85, 94].

(g) Finally, *Class VI* is reserved for still unclassified cases. Modern imaging technology (ultrasound and/or magnetic resonance imaging) can provide objective estimation of uterine anatomy for the needs of differential diagnosis between the six groups. However, rare anomalies, subtle changes or combined pathology may likely not to be allocated correctly to one of the six groups [96]; for these cases, in order to keep the groups "clear", a sixth class is created.

Comments on the proposed classification of uterine anomalies

In the presented classification system, arcuate uterus is deleted as a separate entity, since by definition (ASRM classification) it has no clinical significance [17]. Furthermore, all these years a great confusion has existed between arcuate and septate uteri (which are the anatomical borders), and some terms such as small septae have been also used to describe cases of arcuate (?) uterus with clinical significance in prognosis [23, 97, 98]. Hence, for the needs of clarity of the new system, only septate uterus has been included as a different class coming from an absorption defect.

An effort has been made to have clear and accurate definitions based on uterine anatomy. The degree of uterine cavity deformity has been chosen for the sub-classification of dysfused and septate uterus; any deformity reaching up to the cervix is defined as complete and any other as partial. However, another important criterion, which could be taken into account, is patient's prognosis. Thus, it is extremely important in the fore coming studies to have a clear reference to the uterus anatomical situation in order to decide what is clinically important and what not.

Imaging techniques for the diagnosis of uterine anomalies

Anatomy is the basis of the new system. Thus, diagnosis of uterine anomalies should be based on diagnostic modalities that could determine the anatomical status of the female genital tract on a more objective way [99]. The ideal diagnostic method should provide objective and measurable information on the anatomical status of the uterus in a non-invasive way

The available diagnostic methods that can be used in the investigation of the patient are as follows:

1. *Gynecological examination (GE)*. It should be noticed that gynaecological examination is very important in the diagnostic work-up of the patients with congenital malformations. Vaginal malformations (aplasia, septum) and some cervical malformations could be diagnosed objectively mainly with inspection. Furthermore, palpation through the vagina and/or the rectum (in cases of

vaginal aplasia) could provide useful but not always objective information.

2. *Two-dimensional ultrasound (2D US)*. This mainly transvaginal approach provides objective and, importantly, measurable information for the cervix, the uterine cavity, the uterine wall and the external contour of the uterus. It is very popular and accessible, non-invasive, but its accuracy highly depends on the experience of the examiner and on the examination methodology followed [100–102].

3. *Sonohysterography (SHG)*. Compared to 2D US, this method has the additional advantage of offering a better imaging of the uterine cavity, thus enhancing the accuracy in identifying the anatomy of the female genital tract and especially that of the uterus [103–110].

4. *Hysteroscopy (Hys)* is the gold standard for the examination of the cervical canal and the uterine cavity. However, as it does not provide information on the myometrial layer, hysteroscopy alone could not be used for the differential diagnosis between different groups. Nowadays, with the use of normal saline as distension medium and the miniaturization of the rigid scopes, hysteroscopy has become a minimally invasive screening tool, well tolerated by the patients and feasible for gynaecologists [34, 111, 112].

The combination of 2D US, SHG and hysteroscopy is proposed as the current standard, one "stop", evaluation protocol for the screening and diagnosis of uterine anomalies.

1. *Three-dimensional ultrasound (3D US)* provides an ideal, objective and measurable representation of the examined organs [113–120]. It provides information on the cervix, the uterine cavity, the uterine wall, the external contour of the uterus and the other structures with the exception of tubes. Theoretically, it seems to be an ideal method for the diagnostic approach of the uterus.

2. *Magnetic resonance imaging* seems to be a very useful diagnostic tool, since it can provide detailed information on the anatomical status of the female genital tract [114, 121–124]. Contrary to the visualization in ultrasound, in MRI myometrium is not seen as a homogeneous smooth muscle mass but is divided into two different structural and functional entities: the internal myometrium or junctional zone (JZ), ontogenetically related to endometrium and functionally important for reproduction, and the outer myometrium which is seen as a larger hypodense zone [125–128]. It should be noted that MRI is expensive, and its validity in the diagnosis of congenital malformations is under investigation. Until now, it has not been used as a primary diagnostic tool but was applied mainly for the investigation of complex anomalies [117, 129–132].

3. *Hysterosalpingography* has been and is still frequently the primary and only non-invasive diagnostic tool used for the diagnosis of uterine's cavity deformations. It cannot provide any information on the uterine wall and the external contour of the uterus [3, 133–135]. In order to overcome this serious limitation, Ott et al. [136] proposed the use of the angle formed by the hemicavities for the needs of differential diagnosis. It should also be noted that the quality of HSG is highly dependent on the examiner: both the examination performance and image interpretation have to be done preferably by a gynaecologist, which is not always feasible in daily practice: for example, in cases of double cervices to catheterize both of them and during the examination to pull the uterus for the best imaging of the uterine cavity [137]. Obviously, ultrasound provides superior quality information than HSG.

4. *Laparoscopy and Hysteroscopy (Lap/Hys)*. The combined application of these endoscopic techniques is thought to be the gold standard in the investigation of women with congenital malformations and especially the *uterine ones* [138]. However, the diagnosis is mainly based on the subjective impression of the clinician performing them, and this is thought to be a limitation in the objective estimation of the anomaly [15].

The specificity and sensitivity of the above-mentioned methods in the investigation of patients with *uterine malformations* have been recently reviewed [3]. Based on their diagnostic accuracy, the diagnostic methods have been categorized into four categories:

Class Ia — Those that are capable of identifying congenital uterine anomalies and classifying them into appropriate sub-types with an accuracy of >90%. Hysteroscopy plus laparoscopy, SHG and 3D US belong to this class,
Class Ib — Those that are capable of identifying congenital uterine anomalies with an accuracy of >90% without being able to classify them into appropriate sub-types. Hysteroscopy alone belongs to this class.
Class II — Those that are capable of identifying congenital uterine anomalies with an accuracy of <90%. According to the available data, HSG and 2D US belong to this class.
Class III — This includes the investigations whose diagnostic accuracy in identifying congenital uterine anomalies is still not exactly known. MRI belongs to this class.

It seems, therefore, that a wide variety of diagnostic tests are available for the interpretation of the female genital tract anatomy with different diagnostic properties as well as variable diagnostic accuracy. Thus, based on the clinical presentation of the patient, the clinician should start with gynaecological examination. HSG cannot be considered as a first line diagnostic tool, and should be used under specific conditions only. Nowadays, transvaginal 2D US seems to be the basic imaging method: it is simple, available in almost every outpatient clinic, and can give reliable, reproducible and measurable information on uterine anatomy for exact diagnosis and differential diagnosis between the different categories. Enlargement of the examination with SHG and ambulatory mini-hysteroscopy seems reasonable since they can provide additional information; they are office procedures with low risk and high patient satisfaction rates.

Further detailed information on uterine anatomy can be obtained with the use of 3D US. A disadvantage for its widespread use is that it is not available everywhere, is more expensive and can be used only by experienced personnel. MRI has comparable diagnostic accuracy with that of 3D US and provides supplementary information on the two structurally and functionally different zones of the myometrium. At the moment, its use is limited depending on the safety regulations of each country, and should be kept for research, especially for cases of complex anomalies or for cases where 3D US is necessary but unavailable or has failed to give an objective estimation of the female genital tract anatomy.

However, for the needs of patients' grouping according to the new system, a clear and exact representation of the female's genital tract anatomy is the desired result of a successful diagnostic work-up. Nowadays, endoscopic techniques (laparoscopy and hysteroscopy) should be kept mainly for the patient's treatment or for the elucidation of extremely rare and unclassified cases [139].

Conclusion

Congenital malformations of the female genital tract are a common entity with an estimated prevalence of 4–7%. The need for a new updated classification has been already underlined since currently available systems are associated with various limitations in effective categorization of the anomalies. The EAGS has established a scientific project on this issue, aiming to critically evaluate the current situation and to prepare the scientific basis for a new system. This initiative has been adopted by the recently established common ESHRE/ESGE working group of experts (CONUTA group). Consensus for the development of a new classification system should be reached using the Delphi procedure.

A new clinical approach for the classification of uterine anomalies is proposed. Uterine anatomy is the basis of the new system. Embryological origin has been adopted as the secondary basic characteristic in the design of the main classes. The system is open for further development including further subdivisions based on cervical and vaginal anatomical varieties in order to be more comprehensive. The new proposed system takes into account the experience gained from the currently available classification systems mainly that of the AFS. It is simple, clear and accurate in its definitions. It could be used as the starting point for the working group of experts in the field.

Declaration of interest The authors report no conflicts of interest. The authors alone are responsible for the content and writing of the paper.

References

1. Chan YY, Jayaprakasan K, Zamora J, Thornton JG, Raine-Fenning N, Coomarasamy A (2011) The prevalence of congenital uterine anomalies in unselected and high-risk populations: a systematic review. Hum Reprod Update 17:761–771
2. Grimbizis GF, Camus M, Tarlatzis BC, Bontis JN, Devroey P (2001) Clinical implications of uterine malformations and hysteroscopic treatment results. Hum Reprod Update 7:161–164
3. Saravelos SH, Cocksedge KA, Li T-C (2008) Prevalence and diagnosis of congenital uterine anomalies in womwn with reproductive failure: a critical appraisal. Hum Reprod Update 14:415–419
4. Grimbizis GF, Campo R (2010) Congenital malformations of the female genital tract: the need for a new classification system. Fertil Steril 94:401–407
5. Acien P (1993) Reproductive performance of women with uterine malformations. Hum Reprod 8:122–126
6. Heller-Boersma JG, Schmidt UH, Edmonds DK (2007) A randomized controlled trial of a cognitive–behavioural group intervention versus waiting-list control for women with uterovaginal agenesis (Mayer–Rokitansky–Kuster–Hauser syndrome: MRKH). Hum Reprod 22:2296–2301
7. Heinonen PK, Saarikoski S, Pystynen P (1982) Reproductive performance of women with uterine anomalies. An evaluation of 182 cases. Acta Obstet Gynecol Scand 61:157–162
8. Giannesi A, Marchiole P, Benchaib M, Chevret-Measson M, Mathevet P, Dargent D (2005) Sexuality after laparoscopic Davydov in patients affected by congenital complete vaginal agenesis associated with uterine agenesis or hypoplasia. Hum Reprod 10:2954–2957
9. Lin PC, Bhatnagar KP, Nettleton GS, Nakajima ST (2002) Female genital anomalies affecting reproduction. Fertil Steril 78:899–915
10. Mollo A, De Franciscis P, Colacurci N, Cobellis L, Perino A, Venezia R, Alviggi C, De Placido G (2009) Hysteroscopic resection of the septum improves the pregnancy rate of women with unexplained infertility: a prospective controlled trial. Fertil Steril 91:2628–2631
11. Morgan EM, Quint EH (2006) Assessment of sexual functioning, mental health and life goals in women with vaginal agenesis. Arch Sex Behav 35:607–618
12. Rackow BW, Arici A (2007) Reproductive performance of women with Mullerian anomalies. Curr Opin Obstet Gynecol 19:229–237
13. Raga F, Bauset C, Remohi J, Bonilla-Musoles F, Simon C, Pellicer A (1997) Reproductive impact of congenital Mullerian anomalies. Hum Reprod 12:2277–2281
14. Sonmezer M, Taskin S, Atabekoglou C, Gungor M, Unlu C (2006) Laparoscopic management of rudimentary uterine horn pregnancy: case report and literature review. JSLS 10:396–399

15. Woelfer B, Salim R, Banerjee S, Elson J, Regan L, Jurkovic D (2001) Reproductive outcomes in women with congenital uterine anomalies detected by three-dimensional ultrasound screening. Obstet Gynecol 98:1099–1103

16. Zlopasa G, Skrablin S, Kalafatic D, Banovic V, Lesin J (2007) Uterine anomalies and pregnancy outcome following resectoscope metroplasty. Int J Gynecol Obstet 98:129–133

17. American Fertility Society (1988) The AFS classification of adnexal aghesions, distul tubal occlusion, tubal occlusion secondary to tubal ligation, tubal pregnancies, Mullerian anomalies and intrauterine adhesions. Fertil Steril 49:944–955

18. Buttram VC, Gibbons WE (1979) Mullerian anomalies: a proposed classification (an analysis of 144 cases). Fertil Steril 32:40–46

19. Acien P, Acien M, Sanchez-Ferrer M (2004) Complex malformations of the female genital tract. New types and revision of classification. Hum Reprod 19:2377–2384

20. Acien P, Acien MI (2011) The history of female genital tract malformation classifications and proposal of an updated system. Hum Reprod Update 17:693–705

21. Oppelt P, Renner SP, Brucker S, Strissel PL, Strick R, Oppelt PG, Doerr HG, Schott GE, Hucke J, Wallwiener D, Beckmann MW (2005) The VCUAM (Vagina Cervix Uterus Adnex Associated Malformation) classification: a new classification for genital malformations. Fertl Steril 84:1493–1497

22. Burgis J (2001) Obstructive Mullerian anomalies: case report, diagnosis and management. Am J Obstet Gynecol 185:338–344

23. Gubbini G, Di Spiezio SA, Nascetti D, Marra E, Spinelli M, Greco E, Casadio P, Nappi C (2009) New outpatient subclassification system for American Fertility Society classes V and VI uterine anomalies. J Minim Invasive Gynecol 16:554–561

24. Joki-Erkkilä MM, Heinonen PK (2003) Presenting and long-term clinical implications and fecundity in females with obstructing vaginal malformations. J Pediatr Adolesc Gynecol 16:307–312

25. Rock JA, Carpenter SE, Wheeless CR, Jones HWJ (1995) The clinical management of maldevelopment of the uterine cervix. J Pelvic Surg 1:129–133

26. Rock JA, Roberts CP and Jones HW (2010) Congenital anomalies of the uterine cervix: lessons from 30 cases managed clinically by a common protocol. Fertil Steril 94:1858–1863

27. Strawbrigde LC, Crough NS, Cutner AS, Creighton SM (2007) Obstructive Mullerian anomalies and modern laparoscopic management. J Pediatr Adolesc Gynecol 20:195–200

28. Akar ME, Bayar D, Yildiz S, Ozel M, Gilmaz Z (2005) Reproductive outcome of women with unicornuate uterus. Aus N Z J Obstet Gynecol 54:148–150

29. Colacursi N, De Franciscis P, Mollo A, Litta P, Perino A, Cobellis L, De Placido G (2007) Small-diameter hysteroscopy with Versapoint versus resectoscopy with unipolar knife for the treatment of septate uterus: a prospective randomized study. J Minim Invasive Gynecol 14:622–627

30. Garcia-Enguidanos A, Calle ME, Valero J, Luna S, Dominguez-Rojas V (2002) Risk factors in miscarriage: a review. Eur J Obstet Gynecol Reprod Biol 102:111–119

31. Grimbizis G, Camus M, Clasen K, De Munck L, Devroey P (1998) Hysteroscopic septum resection in patients with recurrent abortions or infertility. Hum Reprod 13:1188–1193

32. Pabuccu R, Gomel V (2004) Reproductive outcome after hysteroscopic metroplasty in women with septate uterus and otherwise unexplained infertility. Fertil Steril 81:1675–1678

33. Aittomaki K, Eroila H, Kajanoja P (2001) A population-based study of the incidence of Müllerian aplasia in Finland. Fertil Steril 76:624–625

34. Campo R, Van Belle Y, Rombauts L, Brosens I, Gordts S (1999) Office mini-hysteroscopy. Hum Reprod Update 5:73–81

35. Acien P (1992) Embryological observations on the female genital tract. Hum Reprod 7:437–445

36. Ashton D, Amin HK, Richard RM, Neuwirth RS (1988) The incidence of asymptomatic uterine anomalies in women undergoing transcervical tubal sterilization. Obstet Gynecol 72:28–30

37. Acien P, Acien MI, Quereda F, Santoyo T (2008) Cervicovaginal agenesis: spontaneous gestation at term after previous re-implantation of the uterine corpus in a neovagina: case report. Hum Reprod 23:548–553

38. Alborzi S, Momtahan M, Parsanezhad ME, Yazdani M (2008) Successful treatment of cervical aplasia using a peritoneal graft. Int J Gynecol Obstet 88:299–302

39. Bedner R, Rzepka-Gorska I, Blogowska A, Malecha J, Kosmider M (2004) Effects of a surgical treatment of congenital cervicovaginal agenesia. J Pediatr Adolesc Gynecol 17:327–330

40. Bugmann P, Amaudruz M, Hanquinet S, La Scala G, Birraux J, Le Coultre C (2002) Uterocervicoplasty with a bladder mucosa layer for the treatment of complete cervical agenesis. Fertil Steril 77:831–835

41. Connolly G, Devaney D, McKenna P (2004) A case of cervical dysgenesis. J Obstet Gynecol 24:322–333

42. Creighton SM, Davies MC, Cutner A (2006) Laparoscopic management of cervical agenesis. Fertil Steril 85:1510.e13–15

43. Deffarges JV, Haddad B, Musset R, Paniel BJ (2001) Uterovaginal anastomosis in women with uterine cervix atresia: long-term follow-up and reproductive performance. A study of 18 cases. Hum Reprod 16:1722–1725

44. Ding D-C, Hsu S, Liu J-Y (2005) Vaginal agenesis in a girl with normal uterus and cervix reconstructed with vulvar skin graft. Eur J Obstet Gynecol Reprod Biol 123:257–258

45. Fedele L, Bianchi S, Frontino G, Berlanda N, Montefusco S, Borruto F (2008) Laparoscopically assisted uterovesticular anastomosis in patients with uterine cervix atresia and vaginal aplasia. Fertil Steril 89:212–216

46. Fujimoto VY, Miller JH, Klein NA, Soules (1997) Congenital cervical atresia: report of seven cases and review of the literature. Am J Obstet Gynecol 177:1419–1425

47. Grimbizis GF, Tsalikis T, Mikos T, Papadopoulos N, Tarlatzis BC, Bontis JN (2004) Successful end-to-end cervico-cervical anastomosis in a patient with congenital cervical fragmentation: case report. Hum Reprod 19:1204–1210

48. Jasonni VM, La Marca A, Matonti G (2007) Utero-vaginal anastomosis in the treatment of cervical atresia. Acta Obstet Gynecol Scand 86:1517–1518

49. Kresowik J, Ryan GL, Austin C, Van Voorhis BJ (2007) Ultrasound-assisted repair of a unique case of distal vaginal agenesis. Fertil Steril 87:976.e9–12

50. Miller RJ, Breech LL (2008) Surgical correction of vaginal anomalies. Clin Obstet Gynecol 51:223–236

51. Selvaggi G, Monstrey S, Depypere H, Blondeel P, Van Landuyt K, Hamdi M, Dhont M (2003) Creation of a neovagina with the use of a pudendal thigh fasciocutaneous flap and restoration of uterovaginal continuity. Fertil Steril 80:607–611

52. Shirota K, Fukuoka M, Hiroshi Tsujioka H, Inoue Y, Kawarabayashi T (2009) A normal uterus communicating with a double cervix and the vagina: a Mullerian anomaly without any present classification. Fertil Steril 91:935.e1–e3

53. Sparac V, Stilinovic K, Ilijas M, barcot Z, Kupesic S, Prka M, Bauman R, Kurjak A (2004) Vaginal aplasia associated with anatomically and functionally normal uterus. Eur J Obstet Gynecol Reprod Biol 115:110–112

54. Troiano RN, McCarthy SM (2004) Müllerian duct anomalies: imaging and clinical issues. Radiology 233:19–34

55. Chang AS, Siegel CL, Moley KH, Ratts VS, Odem RR (2004) Septate uterus with cervical duplication and longitudinal vaginal septum: a report of five new cases. Fertil Steril 81:1133–1136

56. Duffy DA, Nulsen J, Maier D, Schmidt D, Benadiva C (2004) Septate uterus with cervical duplication: a full-term delivery after resection of a vaginal septum. Fertil Steril 81:1125–1126

57. Heinonen PK (2006) Complete septate uterus with longitudinal vaginal septum. Fertil Steril 85:700–705

58. Hur J-Y, Shin J-H, Lee J-K, Oh M-J, Saw H-S, Park Y-K, Lee KW (2007) Septate uterus with double cervices, unilaterally obstructed vaginal septum and ipsilateral renal agenesis: a rare combination of Mullerian and Wolffian anomalies complicated by severe endometriosis in an adolescent. J Minim Invasive Gynecol 14:128–131

59. Patton PE, Novy MJ, Lee DM, Hickok LR (2004) The diagnosis and reproductive outcome after surgical treatment of the complete septate uterus, duplicated cervix and vaginal septum. Am J Obstet Gynecol 190:1669–1678

60. Parsanezhad ME, Alborzi S, Zarei A, Dehbashi S, Shirazi LG, Rajaeefard A, Schmidt EH (2006) Hysteroscopic metroplasty of the complete uterine septum, duplicate cervix and vaginal septum. Fertil Steril 85:1473–1477

61. Pavone ME, King JA, Vlahos N (2006) Septate uterus with cervical duplication and a longitudinal vaginal septum: a Mullerian anomaly without a classification. Fertil Steril 85:494.e9–10

62. Acien P, Acien M and Sanchez-Ferrer ML (2008) Mullerian anomalies "without a classification": from the didelphys-unicollis uterus to the bicervical uterus with or without septate vagina. Fertil Steril 91:2369–2375

63. Acien P, Sanchez-Ferrer M, Mayol-Belda M-J (2004) Unilateral cervico-vaginal atresia with ipsilateral renal agenesis. Eur J Obstet Gynecol Reprod Biol 117:249–251

64. Ballesio L, Andreoli C, De Cicco ML, Angeli ML, Manganaro L (2003) Hematocolpos in double vagina associated with uterus didelphys: US and MRI findings. Eur J Radiol 45:150–153

65. Coskun A, Okur N, Ozdemir O, Kiran G and Arykan DC (2008) Uterus didelphys with an obstructed unilateral vagina by a transverse vaginal septum associated with ipsilateral renal agenesis, duplication of inferior vena cava, high-riding aortic bifurcation and intestinal malrotation a case report. Fertil Steril 90:2006.e9–11

66. Growdon WB, Laufer MR (2008) Uterine didelphys with duplicated upper vagina and bilateral lower vaginal agenesis: a novel Müllerian anomaly with options for surgical management. Fertil Steril 89:693–698

67. Kumar S, Singh SK, Mavuduru R, Naveen A, Agarwal MM, Vanita J, Mandal AK (2008) Bicornuate uterine horns with complete cervico-vaginal agenesis and congenital vesicouterine fistula. Int Urogynecol J 19:739–741

68. Levsky MJ, Mondshine RT (2006) Hematometrocolpos due to imperforate hymen in a patient with bicornuate uterus. AJR 186:1469–1470

69. Madureira AJ, Mariz CM, Bernardes JC, Ramos IM (2006) Uterus didelphys with obstructing hemivaginal septum and ipsilateral renal agenesis. Radiology 239:602–606

70. Tsai C-H, Chen C-P, Chang MD-T, Chang S-J, Chien S-C (2007) Hematometrocolpos secondary to didelphys uterus and unilateral imperforated double vagina as an unusual cause of acute abdomen. Taiwan J Obstet Gynecol 46:448–452

71. Vercellini P, Daguati R, Somigliana E, Vigano P, Lanzani A, Fedele L (2007) Asymmetric lateral distribution of obstructed hemivagina and renal agenesis in women with uterus didelphys: institutional case series and a systematic literature review. Fertil Steril 87:719–724

72. Zurawin RK, Dietrich JE, Heard MJ, Edwards CL (2004) Didelphic uterus and obstructed hemivagina with renal agenesis: case report and review of the literature. J Pediatr Adolesc Gynecol 17:137–141

73. Arshad Z, Mohan S (2005) Pregnancy in a non-communicating uterine horn. Acta Obstet Gynecol Scand 84:1023

74. Arslan T, Bilgic E, Senturk B, Yusel N (2009) Rudimentary uterine horn pregnancy: a mystery diagnosis. Fertil Steril 92:2037.e1–e3

75. Cutner A, Saridogan E, Hart R, Pandya P, Creighton S (2004) Laparoscopic management of pregnancies occurring in non-communicating accessory uterine horns. Eur J Obstet Gynecol Reprod Biol 113:106–109

76. Heinonen PK (1997) Unicornuate uterus and rudimentary horn. Fertil Steril 68:224–230

77. Khanapure A, Aravind S, Lawley R, Verwood G (2005) Rupture of a pregnancy in the rudimentary communicating horn of the uterus. J Obstet Gynecol 25:310–311

78. Tang R, Sheng Y, Chen ZJ (2004) Rupture of pregnancy in a communicating rudimentary uterine horn after in vitro fertilization and embryo transfer. Int J Gynecol Obstet 86:394–395

79. Fedele L, Bianchi S, Zanconato G, Berlanda N, Bergamini V (2005) Laparoscopic removal of the cavitated noncommunicating rudimentary uterine horn: surgical aspects in 10 cases. Fertil Steril 83:432–436

80. Theodoridis TD, Saravelos H, Chatzigeorgiou KN, Zepiridis L, Grimbizis GF, Vavilis D, Loufopoulos A, Bontis JN (2006) Laparoscopic management of unicornuate uterus with non-communicating rudimentary horn (three cases). RBM Online 12:126–128

81. Brun J-L, Belleannee G, Grafeille N, Aslan A-F, Brun GH (2002) Long-term results after neovagina creation in Mayer–Rokitansky–Kuster–Hauser syndrome by Vecchietti's operation. Eur J Obstet Gynecol Reprod Biol 103:168–172

82. Cai B, Zhang JR, Xi XW, Yan Q, Wan XP (2007) Laparoscopically assisted sigmoid colon vaginoplasty in women with Mayer–Rokitansky–Kuster–Hauser syndrome: feasibility and short-term results. BJOG 114:1486–1492

83. Darai E, Toullalan O, Besse O, Potiron L, Delga P (2003) Anatomic and functional results of laparoscopic–perineal neovagina construction by sigmoid colpoplasty in women with Rokitansky's syndrome. Hum Reprod 11:2454–2459

84. Darwish AM (2007) A simplified novel laparoscopic formation of neovagina for cases of Mayer–Rokitansky–Kuster–Hauser syndrome. Fertil Steril 88:1427–1430

85. Fedele L, Bianchi S, Berlanda N, Bulfoni A, Fontana E (2006) Laparoscopic creation of a neovagina and recovery of menstrual function in a patient with Rokitansky syndrome: a case report. Hum Reprod 21:3287–3289

86. Fedele L, Bianchi S, Berlanda N, Fontana E, Raffaelli R, Bulfoni A, Braidotti P (2006) Neovaginal mucosa after Vecchietti's laparoscopic operation for Rokitansky syndrome: structural and ultrastructural study. Am J Obstet Gynecol 195:56–61

87. Fedele L, Bianchi S, Frontino G, Ciappina N, Fontana E, Borruto F (2007) Laparoscopic findings and pelvic anatomy in Mayer–Rokitansky–Kuste–Hauser syndrome. Obstet Gynecol 109:1111–1115

88. Fedele L, Frontino G, Restelli E, Giappina N, Motta F, Bianchi S (2010) Creation of a neovagina by Davydov's laparoscopic modified technique in patients with Rokitansky syndrome. Am J Obstet Gynecol 202:33.e1–e6

89. Guerrier D, Mouchel T, Pasquier L, Pellerin I (2006) The Mayer–Rokitansky–Kuster–Hauser syndrome (congenital absence of uterus and vagina) – phenotypic manifestations and genetic approaches. J Nedat Results Biomed 5:1–8

90. O'Connor JL, DeMarco RT, Pope JC, Adams MC, Brock JW (2004) Bowel vaginoplasty in children: a retrospective review. J Pediatr Surg 39:1205–1208

91. Oppelt P, Renner SP, Kellermann A, Brucker S, Hauser GA, Ludwig KS, Strissel PL, Strick R, Wallwiener D, Beckmann MW (2006) Clinical aspects of Mayer–Rokitansky–Kuester–Hauser syndrome: recommendations for clinical diagnosis and staging. Hum Reprod 21:792–797

92. Seccia A, Salgarello M, Sturla M, Latorre S, Farallo E (2002) Neovaginal reconstruction with the modified McIndoe technique: a review of 32 cases. Ann Plast Surg 49:379–384

93. Goluda M, Gabrys MSt, Ujec M, Jedryka M, Goluda C (2006) Bicornuate rudimentary uterine horns with functioning endometrium and complete cervical–vaginal agenesis coexisting with ovarian endometriosis: a case report. Fertil Steril 86:462.e9–e11

94. Grimbizis GF, Papanicolaou A, Papadopoulos N, Theodoridis Th, Papadopoulos M, Tarlatzis BC (2010) The chance for a successful isthmo-neovagina anastomosis after Davydov's neovagina formation. Gynaecol Surg 7(Suppl 1):S80

95. Takeuchi H, Sato Y, Shimanuki H, Kikuchi J, Kitase M, Kinoshita K (2006) Accurate preoperative diagnosis and laparoscopic removal of the cavitated non-communicated uterine horn for obstructive Mullerian anomalies. J Obstet Gynecol Res 32:74–79

96. Sadik S, Taskin O, Sehirali S, Mendilcioglu I, Onoglu AS, Kursun S, Wheeler J (2002) Complex Mullerian malformations: report of a case with hypoplastic non-cavitated uterus and two rudimentary horns. Hum Reprod 17:1343–1344

97. Mucowski SJ, Herndon CN, Rosen MP (2010) The arcuate anomaly: a critical appraisal of its diagnostic and clinical relevance. Obstet Gynecol Surv 65:449–454

98. Tomazevic T, Ban-Frangez H, Ribic-Pucelj M, Premru-Srsen T, Verderik I (2007) Small uterine septum is an important risk variable for preterm birth. Eur J Obstet Gynecol Reprod Biol 135:154–157

99. Dee Olpin J, Heilbrun M (2009) Imaging of Mullerian duct anomalies. Clin Obstet Gynecol 52:40–56

100. Kupesic S (2001) Clinical implications of sonographic detection of uterine anomalies for reproductive outcome. Ultrasound Obstet Gynecol 18:387–400

101. Lindheim SR, Adsuar N, Kushner DM, Pritts EA, Olive DL (2003) Sonohysterography: a valuable tool in evaluating the female pelvis. Obstet Gynecol Surv 58:770–784

102. Mazouni C, Girard G, Deter R, Haumonte J-B, Blanc B, Bretelle F (2008) Diagnosis of Mullerian anomalies in adults: evaluation of practice. Fertil Steril 89:219–222

103. Alborzi S, Dehbashi S, Parsanezhad ME (2002) Differential diagnosis of septate and bicornuate uterus by sonohysterography eliminates the need for laparoscopy. Fertil Steril 78:176–178

104. Cepni I, Ocal P, Erkan S, Saricalli FS, Akbas H, Demirkiran F, Idil M, Bese T (2005) Comparison of transvaginal sonography, saline infusion sonography and hysteroscopy in the evaluation of uterine cavity pathologies. ANZJ Obstet Gynecol 45:30–35

105. Grimbizis GF, Tsolakidis D, Mikos T, Anagnostou E, Asimakopoulos E, Stamatopoulos P, Tarlatzis BC (2010) A prospective comparison of transvaginal ultrasound, saline infusion sonohysterography, and diagnostic hysteroscopy in the evaluation of endometrial pathology. Fertil Steril 94:2720–2795

106. Guimarães Filho HA, Mattar R, Pires CR, Araujo Junior E, Moron AF, Nardozza LMM (2006) Comparison of hysterosalpingography, hysterosonography and hysteroscopy in evaluation of the uterine cavty in patients with recurrent pregnancy losses. Arch Gynecol Obstet 274:284–288

107. Guven MA, Bese T, Demirkiran F, Idil M, Mgoyi L (2004) Hydrosonography in screening for intracavitary pathology in infertile women. Int J Gynecol Obstet 86:377–383

108. Shokeir S, Abdelshaheed M (2009) Sonohysterography as a first-line evaluation for uterine abnormalities in women with recurrent failed in vitro fertilization-embryo transfer. Fertil Steril 91(suppl 4):1321–1322

109. Tur-Kaspa I, Gal M, Hartman M, Hartman J, Hartman A (2006) A prospective evaluation of uterine abnormalities by saline infusion sonohysterography in 1009 women with infertility or abnormal uterine bleeding. Fertil Steril 86:1731–1735

110. Valenzano MM, Mistrangelo E, Lijoi D, Fortunato T, Lantieri PB, Risso D, Costantini S, Ragni N (2006) Transvaginal sonohysterographic evaluation of uterine malformations. Eur J Obstet Gynecol Reprod Biol 124:246–249

111. Bettocchi S, Ceci O, Nappi L, Pontrelli G, Pinto L, Vicino M (2007) Office hysteroscopic motroplasty: three "diagnostic criteria" to differentiate between septate and bicornuate uteri. J Minim Invasive Gynecol 14:324–328

112. Gordts S, Campo R, Puttemans P, Verhoven H, Gianaroli L, Brosens J, Brosens I (2002) Investigation of the infertile couple: a one stop outpatient endoscopy-based approach. Hum Reprod 17:1684–1687

113. Ayoubi J-M, Fanchin R, Ferretti G, Pons J-C, Bricault I (2002) Three-dimensional ultrasonographic reconstruction of the uterine cavity: toward virtual hysteroscopy? Eur Radiol 12:2030–2033

114. Bermejo C, Ten Martinez P, Cantarero R, Diaz D, Perez Pedregosa J, Barro E, Labrador E, Ruiz Lopez L (2010) Three-dimensional ultrasound in the diagnosis of Mullerian duct anomalies and concordance with magnetic resonance imaging. Ultrasound Obstet Gynecol 35:593–601

115. Caliskan E, Ozkan S, Cakiroglu Y, Sarisoy HT, Corakci A, Ozeren S (2010) Diagnostic accuracy of real-time 3D sonography in the diagnosis of congenital Mullerian anomalies in high-risk patients with respect to the phase of the menstrual cycle. J Clin Ultrasound 38:123–127

116. Ghi T, Casadio P, Kuleva M, Perrone AM, Savelli L, Giunchi S, Meriggiola C, Gubbini G, Pilu G, Pelusi C, Pelusi G (2009) Accuracy of three-dimensional ultrasound in diagnosis and classification of congenital uterine anomalies. Fertil Steril 92:808–813

117. Imai A, Takagi H, Matsunami K (2004) Double uterus associated with renal aplasia; magnetic resonance appearance and three-dimensional computed tomographic urogram. Int J Gynecol Obstet 87:169–171

118. Jurkovic D (2002) Three-dimensional ultrasound in gynecology: a critical evaluation. Ultrasound Obstet Gynecol 19:109–117

119. Raine-Fenning N, Fleischer AC (2005) Clarifying the role of three-dimensional transvaginal sonography in reproductive medicine: an evidence-based appraisal. J Exper Clin Ass Reprod 2:10

120. Salim R, Woelfer B, Backos M, Regan L, Jurkovic D (2003) Reproducibility of three-dimensional ultrasound diagnosis of congenital uterine anomalies. Ultrasound Obstet Gynecol 21:578–582

121. Church DG, Vancil JM, Vasanawala SS (2009) Magnetic resonance imaging for uterine and vaginal anomalies. Curr Opin Obstet Gynecol 21:379–389

122. Marten K, Vosshenrich R, Funke M, Obenauer S, Baum F, Grabbe E (2003) MRI in the evaluation of Müllerian duct anomalies. J Clin Imaging 27:346–350

123. Orazi C, Lucchetti C, Schingo PMS, Marchetti P, Ferro F (2007) Herlyn–Werner–Wunderlich syndrome: uterus didelphys, blind hemivagina and ipsilateral renal agenesis. Sonographic and MRI findings in 11 cases. Pediatr Radiol 37:657–665

124. Pui MH (2004) Imaging diagnosis of congenital uterine malformation. Comput Med Imag Graph 28:425–433

125. Brosens JJ, Barker FG, deSouza NM (1998) Myometrial zonal differentiation and uterine junctional zone hyperplasia in the non-pregnant uterus. Hum Reprod Update 4(5):496–502

126. Brosens JJ, de Souza NM, Barker FG (1995) Uterine junctional zone: function and disease. Lancet 346:558–560

127. Fusi L, Cloke B, Brosens JJ (2006) The uterine junctional zone. Best Pract Res Clin Obstet Gynaecol 20(4):479–491

128. Gordts S, Brosens JJ, Fusi L, Benagiano G, Brosens I (2008) Uterine adenomyosis: a need for uniform terminology and consensus classification. RBM Online 17:244–248

129. Minto CL, Hollings N, Hall-Craggs M, Creighton S (2001) Magnetic resonance imaging in the assessment of complex Mullerian anomalies. Br J Obstet Gynecol 108:791–797

130. Mirkovic L, Ljubic A, Mirkovic D (2006) Magnetic resonance imaging in the evaluation of uterus didelphys with obstructed hemivagina and renal agenesis: a case report. Arch Gynecol Obstet 274:246–247

131. Scarsbrook AF, Moore NR (2003) MRI appearances of Mullerian duct abnormalities. Clin Radiol 58:747–754

132. Takagi H, Matsunami K, Noda K, Furui T, Imai A (2003) Magnetic resonance imaging in the evaluation double uterus and associated urinary tract anomalies: a report of five cases. J Obstet Gynaecol 23:525–527

133. Braun P, Grau FV, Pons RM, Enguix DP (2005) Is hysterosalpingography able to diagnose all uterine malformations correctly? A retrospective study. Eur J Radiol 53:274–279

134. Roma Dalfo A, Ubeda B, Ubeda A, Monzoni M, Rotger R, Ramos R, Palacio A (2004) Diagnostic value of hysterosalpingography in the detection of intrauterine abnormalities: a comparison with hysteroscopy. AJR 183:1405–1409

135. Swart P, Mol BW, van der Veen F, van Beurden M, Redekop WK, Bossuyt PM et al (1995) The accuracy of hysterosalpingography in the diagnosis of tubal pathology: a meta-analysis. Fertil Steril 64:486–491

136. Ott DJ, Fayez JA, Zagoria RJ (eds) (1998) Hysterosalpingography: a text and atlas, 2nd edn. Williams & Wilkins, Baltimore, MD

137. Renbaum L, Ufberg D, Sammel M, Zhou L, Jabara S, Barnhart K (2002) Reliability of clinicians versus radiologists for detecting abnormalities on hysterosalpingogram films. Fertil Steril 78:614–618

138. Philbois O, Guye E, Richard O, Tardieu D, Seffert P, Chavrier Y, Varlet F (2004) Role of laparoscopy in vaginal malformation. An experience in 22 children. Surg Endosc 18:87–91

139. Patterson D, Mueller C, Strubel N, Rivera R, Ginsburg HB, Nadler EP (2006) Laparoscopic neo-os creation in an adolescent with uterus didelphys and obstructed hemivagina. J Pediatr Surg 41:E19–E22

11

Current practice in the removal of benign endometrial polyps

Lotte J. E. W. van Dijk · Maria C. Breijer ·
Sebastiaan Veersema · Ben W. J. Mol ·
Anne Timmermans

Abstract The purpose of this study is to evaluate the current practice of Dutch gynecologists in the removal of benign endometrial polyps and compare these results with the results of a previous study from 2003. In 2009 Dutch gynecologists were surveyed by a mailed questionnaire about polypectomy. Gynecologists answered questions about their individual performance of polypectomy: setting, form of anesthesia, method, and instrument use. The results were compared with the results from the previous survey. The response rate was 70% (585 of 837 gynecologists). Among the respondents, 455 (78%) stated to remove endometrial polyps themselves. Polyps were mostly removed in an inpatient setting (337; 74%) under general or regional anesthesia (247; 54%) and under direct hysteroscopic vision (411; 91%). Gynecologists working in a teaching hospital removed polyps more often in an outpatient setting compared with gynecologists working in a nonteaching hospital [118 (43%) vs. 35 (19%) $p<0.001$]. These results are in accordance with the results from 2003. Compared to 2003 there was an increase in the number of gynecologists performing polypectomies with local or no anesthesia [211 (46%) vs. 98 (22%), $p<0.001$]. An increase was also noted in the number of gynecologists using direct hysteroscopic vision [411 (91%) vs. 290 (64%), $p<0.001$] and 5 Fr electrosurgical instruments [181 (44%) vs. 56 (19%), $p<0.001$]. Compared to the situation in 2003, there is an increase in removal under direct hysteroscopic vision, with 5 Fr electrosurgical instruments, using local or no anesthesia. This implies there is progress in outpatient hysteroscopic polypectomy in the Netherlands.

Keywords Polypectomy · Hysteroscopy · Inpatient · Outpatient

L. J. E. W. van Dijk (✉) · M. C. Breijer
Department of Obstetrics & Gynecology, TweeSteden Hospital,
Tilburg, The Netherlands
e-mail: jew.vandijk@gmail.com

M. C. Breijer
e-mail: m.c.breijer@amc.uva.nl

M. C. Breijer · B. W. J. Mol · A. Timmermans
Department of Obstetrics & Gynecology,
Academic Medical Center,
Amsterdam, The Netherlands

B. W. J. Mol
e-mail: b.w.mol@amc.uva.nl

A. Timmermans
e-mail: a.timmermans@amc.uva.nl

S. Veersema
Department of Obstetrics & Gynecology, St. Antonius Hospital,
Nieuwegein, The Netherlands
e-mail: s.veersema@antoniusziekenhuis.nl

Background

Benign endometrial polyps are frequently associated with abnormal uterine bleeding [1–4]. Endometrial polyps have a low potential for (pre)malignancy. However age and postmenopausal bleeding are factors which are associated with malignancy [3, 5–7]. Most gynecologists (up to 93%) will remove endometrial polyps in patients with abnormal uterine bleeding symptoms [8]. Although case series, cohort studies, and retrospective studies on this subject exist, few studies address this question prospectively in a comparative cohort study or a randomized controlled trial [9, 10]. Removing endometrial polyps is thought to improve symptoms of abnormal uterine bleeding and increase satisfaction rate in women with endometrial polyps

[11, 12]. The evidence that justifies the removal of endometrial polyps however is limited.

Traditionally, endometrial polyps were removed by dilatation and curettage (D&C). However, in approximately 57% of the D&C procedures endometrial polyps are not detected and D&C fails to extract endometrial polyps in 60–87% of the cases [13, 14]. Former surveys have demonstrated that D&C for polyp removal has not been completely abandoned: 2% of gynecologists in the UK removed polyps with D&C and 56% removed polyps with D&C following hysteroscopy [8]. In 2003, in the Netherlands, 4% of the gynecologists removed polyps with D&C and 27% used D&C following hysteroscopic localization. The preferred method of Dutch gynecologists is hysteroscopic removal (69%) [15]. Moreover, hysteroscopic polypectomy is the most performed hysteroscopic procedure in the Netherlands [16].

Large prospective cohort studies and randomized controlled trials have demonstrated that outpatient hysteroscopy and polypectomy are feasible, safe, and effective with high patient satisfaction rates [17–23]. Compared to the inpatient setting, patients treated in the outpatient setting recover faster, leading to a decrease in time away from home and work [24]. Nevertheless, our previous study revealed that in 2003, outpatient hysteroscopic polypectomy in the Netherlands was not practiced on a large scale (29% of gynecologists). However, we saw that outpatient hysteroscopic polyp removal was more often practiced in teaching hospitals compared with nonteaching hospitals. We therefore hypothesized that there might be a tendency towards outpatient hysteroscopic polypectomy. To evaluate this hypothesis, we conducted the current survey.

Materials and methods

All practicing gynecologists, holding membership of the Dutch association of obstetrics and gynecology (NVOG), in 2009 were identified from the national database. Gynecologists in training were not included. All gynecologists were approached by mail and received a questionnaire with a cover letter and prepaid return envelope. Different criteria were met to achieve the best response rate: the questionnaire was brief, fitting on one page; was explicit; and had a structured format consisting of three items subdivided in closed questions. To assure a higher response rate, a reminder was sent to the nonresponders after 8 weeks and a second reminder was sent by mail and email after another 12 weeks.

The questionnaire concerned questions about the medical practice of gynecologists, when a benign polyp was suspected following ultrasound or endometrial biopsy. Recipients were asked in what type of hospital they were working: a teaching hospital, with a residency program for gynecology, or a nonteaching hospital. Subsequently, gynecologists were asked

to report whether they performed endometrial polypectomy themselves. Only those who did were then requested to report about setting (inpatient, day care, outpatient), form of anesthesia (general, regional, local or none), method of polyp removal (D&C, D&C after hysteroscopic localization or under direct hysteroscopic visualization), and type of hysteroscopic instrument used (5 Fr mechanical instruments, 5 Fr electrosurgical instruments, resectoscope, or morcellator).

Respondents were asked to report whether they performed the different modalities as a standard method, incidentally or never at all. The options that were chosen as a standard were used for further analysis. It was possible to leave questions unanswered or give multiple answers to one question (e.g., general and regional anesthesia as a standard method).

An inpatient setting was considered an operating theater with an anesthesiologist present for general or regional anesthesia and at least one night stay in the hospital. A day care setting was considered an operating theater with an anesthesiologist present, but discharge from the hospital the same day. A "walk-in-walk-out" procedure, without the presence of an anesthesiologist and without hospital admission, was considered an outpatient setting. Since the inpatient setting and day care setting both require hospital admission and use of an operating theater, they were analyzed together as one category. The same was applied to the form of anesthesia: general and regional anesthesia both require an anesthesiologist and were analyzed as one category. Local anesthesia is administered by a gynecologist and was therefore analyzed together with no anesthesia as one category. These categories enabled comparison of the current results with the results from 2003.

Statistical analysis

All data were processed anonymously. The information was collected, and descriptive statistical analyses were performed with SPSS for Windows® Release 15.0 Standard Version (Chicago, IL, USA). Answers given by gynecologists working in teaching hospitals were compared to answers given by gynecologists working in nonteaching hospitals. The data from this study were also compared to the data from our survey conducted in 2003 [15]. The chi-square test was used to compare proportions. Differences between groups were considered statistically significant at $p < 0.05$. All p values were two sided.

Findings

In 2009 a total of 837 gynecologists were registered in the Netherlands. After the first mailing, 409 questionnaires were returned. Another 87 gynecologists responded after the first reminder. A second reminder was sent, with a response of 89. In total a number of 585 (70%) gynecologists participated. Not all respondents answered all items of the questionnaire. Therefore subcalculations with different denominators were made.

Current practice

Of the 585 participating gynecologists, 455 (78%) performed polypectomy for endometrial polyps themselves. Table 1 shows the current practice of removing endometrial polyps. An inpatient or day care setting was used routinely by 337 (74%) gynecologists, with general or regional anesthesia by 247 (54%) gynecologists. Removal under direct hysteroscopic vision was the most used method of polypectomy, used by 411 (91%) respondents. Removal under direct hysteroscopic visualization was practiced routinely with 5 Fr mechanical instruments, 5 Fr electrosurgical instruments, or resectoscope by 166 (40%), 181 (44%), and 174 (42%) respondents, respectively.

Outpatient polypectomy was carried out by 153 (34%) of the respondents, and 211 (46%) used local or no anesthesia. Separating this last group, it shows that 76 gynecologists (17%) used local anesthesia vs. 145 (32%) no anesthesia ($p < 0.001$). Table 2 shows the method of polyp removal vs. form of anesthesia. In case of D&C after hysteroscopic localization, more gynecologists used general or regional anesthesia than local or no anesthesia (13% vs. 1%, $p < 0.001$).

Teaching vs. nonteaching hospitals

In teaching hospitals, gynecologists removed polyps significantly more in an outpatient setting compared with gynecologists in nonteaching hospitals (43% vs. 19%, $p < 0.001$; Table 1). Local or no anesthesia was more often used in teaching hospitals compared with nonteaching hospitals (55% vs. 33%, $p < 0.001$). Direct hysteroscopic vision was the most common method of polypectomy in both types of hospitals.

Comparison with practice in 2003

In 2003 and in 2009, an equal number of gynecologists (455) reported to remove endometrial polyps themselves. These results turned out this way by chance. In both years the majority of Dutch gynecologists performed polypectomy in an inpatient setting under general or regional anesthesia (Table 3). Though, significantly less general or regional anesthesia (54% vs. 72%, $p < 0.001$) and more local or no anesthesia (46% vs. 22%, $p < 0.001$) is used in 2009 compared with 2003. This applies both for teaching and nonteaching hospitals (numbers not shown separately). In 2009, 145 gynecologists (32%) used no anesthesia vs. 21 (5%) in 2003 ($p < 0.001$). A shift towards the removal under direct hysteroscopic vision is seen in 2009 compared with 2003 (91% vs. 64%, $p < 0.001$), with a decrease in use of D&C (9% vs. 29%, $p < 0.001$). The 5 Fr electrosurgical instruments are more frequently used in 2009 compared with 2003 (44% vs. 19%, $p < 0.001$).

Discussion

Our survey shows that the majority of gynecologists in the Netherlands remove endometrial polyps in an inpatient setting, under direct hysteroscopic vision. More gynecologists

Table 1 Current practice in 2009 concerning removal of endometrial polyps		Total	Teaching ($n=275$)	Nonteaching ($n=180$)	p value
	Setting				
	-Inpatient/day care	337 (74)	193 (70)	144 (80)	0.019
	-Outpatient	153 (34)	118 (43)	35 (19)	<0.001
	Anesthesia				
	-General/regional	247 (54)	133 (48)	114 (63)	0.002
	-Local/no	211 (46)	152 (55)	59 (33)	<0.001
	Method				
	-D&C	6 (1)	2 (1)	4 (2)	ns
	-D&C after hysteroscopy	37 (8)	15 (6)	22 (12)	0.010
	-Direct hysteroscopic vision	411 (91)	257 (94)	154 (86)	0.005
	Hysteroscopic vision	$n=411$	$n=257$	$n=154$	
Number of performing gynecologists (in percent)	Instrument				
	-5 Fr mechanical	166 (40)	102 (40)	64 (42)	ns
Teaching academic and nonacademic teaching hospitals, *D&C*	-5 Fr electrosurgical	181 (44)	122 (47)	59 (38)	ns
dilatation and curettage, *ns* not	-Resectoscope	174 (42)	106 (41)	68 (44)	ns
significant	-Morcellator	12 (3)	10 (4)	2 (1)	ns

Table 2 Method of polyp removal versus form of anesthesia

Number of gynecologists (in percent)

D&C dilatation and curettage, *ns* not significant

	General/regional anesthesia	Local/no anesthesia	*p* value
D&C	3 (1)	1 (1)	ns
D&C following hysteroscopy	32 (13)	3 (1)	<0.001
Under direct hysteroscopic vision	214 (86)	206 (98)	ns
Total	249	210	

in teaching hospitals perform polypectomy in an outpatient setting compared with nonteaching hospitals. Comparing current practice to the situation in 2003, we found an increase in hysteroscopic polyp removal with a decrease in D&C removal. Furthermore, we noted a decrease in the use of general or regional anesthesia and an increase in the number of gynecologists performing hysteroscopy with local or no anesthesia; no difference in the use of outpatient setting was noted. We also found an increase in the number of gynecologists using 5 French electrosurgical instruments.

There are two limitations that need to be addressed regarding the present study. First, our response rate is marginal. Our results should however be considered valid as a response rate of 70% is a level where the impact of nonresponse bias is negligible [25]. Moreover, the questionnaires were concise and met different criteria to achieve the best response rate. We met these criteria by using a short one-page questionnaire with return envelopes and reminders [26, 27].

The second limitation concerns the fact that we only considered the number of gynecologists removing polyps, and we did not display the number of polypectomies they performed. This could mean that few gynecologists perform polypectomies in an outpatient setting, but the major part of the number of polypectomies in the Netherlands (by a minor group of gynecologists) is performed outpatient. To get an impression of the number of uterine polypectomies per year, we sent all departments of gynecology in the Netherlands a letter and asked for the annual report of their department. However, the annual reports of the various hospitals differed in layout and classification. Some hospitals classified their therapeutic hysteroscopies in subcategories like hysteroscopic polypectomy, while others grouped them under the same denominator, without separation in numbers of polypectomies. We could therefore not include this information in our current survey.

In 2003 we hypothesized a tendency towards outpatient hysteroscopic removal of polyps for the future. Although we could not show such an increase directly in the number of gynecologists performing outpatient hysteroscopic polypectomy, our results imply that there is a tendency towards outpatient hysteroscopic polypectomy. We found an increase in the number of gynecologists performing polypectomy under direct hysteroscopic vision with local or no anesthesia

Table 3 Comparison numbers of 2009 with 2003

D&C dilatation and curettage, *ns* not significant, *na* not applicable, *Teaching* academic and nonacademic teaching hospitals

	Total 2009, *n*=455	Total 2003, *n*=455	*p* value
Setting			
-Inpatient/day care	337 (74)	321 (71)	ns
-Outpatient	153 (34)	129 (28)	ns
Anesthesia			
-General/regional	247 (54)	326 (72)	<0.001
-Local/no	211 (46)	98 (22)	<0.001
Method			
-D&C	6 (1)	17 (4)	0.03
-D&C after hysteroscopy	37 (8)	115 (25)	<0.001
-Direct hysteroscopic vision	411 (91)	290 (64)	<0.001
Hysteroscopic vision	2009, *n*=411	2003, *n*=290	
Instrument			
-5 Fr mechanical	166 (40)	197 (68)	<0.001
-5 Fr electrosurgical	181 (44)	56 (19)	<0.001
-Resectoscope	174 (42)	159 (55)	0.001
-Morcellator	12 (3)	na	na

and a decrease in D&C after hysteroscopy and the use of general or regional anesthesia. Considering the fact that an increase in local and no anesthesia was observed, it can only be concluded that more gynecologists are performing hysteroscopy as a "walk-in-walk-out" office procedure.

Hysteroscopic polypectomy seems to be integrated in the daily practice of most hospitals in the Netherlands [16]. Possible explanations for the shift towards outpatient hysteroscopic polypectomy can be mentioned on a speculative basis. First, the Dutch obstetrics and gynecology residency curriculum requires hysteroscopic polypectomy for graduation. The curriculum includes a basic surgical skill course with additionally the possibility to attend advanced courses and congresses on hysteroscopy. Each year many residents and gynecologists participate in these courses, which enhance the implementation of basic minimally invasive surgery skills training into the residency curriculum [28, 29]. Second, in 2002 hysteroscopic sterilization was introduced in the Netherlands. This technique was set in a "see-and-treat" setting with the use of 5 Fr working channel instruments. The use of this technique has probably had a positive influence on implementation of outpatient hysteroscopy for other indications. Third, literature shows that outpatient hysteroscopy is the most cost-effective method of hysteroscopy [24].

This progress in outpatient hysteroscopic polypectomy in the Netherlands is an advantage in medical practice. Literature shows that the best method of pain control for women undergoing traditional hysteroscopy is local anesthesia [30, 31]. However, a recent systematic review reported less pain during hysteroscopy in case of vaginoscopic approach (no anesthesia) compared with traditional hysteroscopic techniques, even with use of local anesthesia [32]. We showed a significant increase in the number of gynecologists using no anesthesia in 2009 compared with 2003. This makes the vaginoscopic approach of hysteroscopy more favorable.

Conclusion

In conclusion, this study shows that although hysteroscopy without anesthesia [32] and outpatient hysteroscopic polypectomy [19, 21–23] have been described in the literature to be highly successful, it is still not practiced on a large scale in the Netherlands. However, there is progress in outpatient hysteroscopic polypectomy. This implies that daily practice is catching up with the situation described in the literature.

Acknowledgment We thank all gynecologists, who completed the questionnaire, for their cooperation.

Declaration of interest The authors report no conflicts of interest. The authors alone are responsible for the content and writing of the paper.

References

1. Karlsson B, Granberg S, Wikland M, Ylostalo P, Torvid K, Marsal K, Valentin L (1995) Transvaginal ultrasonography of the endometrium in women with postmenopausal bleeding—a Nordic multicenter study. Am J Obstet Gynecol 172(5):1488–1494

2. O'Connell LP, Fries MH, Zeringue E, Brehm W (1998) Triage of abnormal postmenopausal bleeding: a comparison of endometrial biopsy and transvaginal sonohysterography versus fractional curettage with hysteroscopy. Am J Obstet Gynecol 178(5):956–961

3. Domingues AP, Lopes H, Dias I, Oliveira CF (2009) Endometrial polyps in postmenopausal women. Acta Obstet Gynecol Scand 88(5):618–620

4. Gale A, Dey P (2009) Postmenopausal bleeding. Menopause Int 15(4):160–164

5. Kassab A, Trotter P, Fox R (2008) Risk of cancer in symptomatic postmenopausal women with endometrial polyps at scan. J Obstet Gynaecol 28(5):522–525

6. Ferrazzi E, Zupi E, Leone FP, Savelli L, Omodei U, Moscarini M, Barbieri M, Cammareri G, Capobianco G, Cicinelli E, Coccia ME, Donarini G, Fiore S, Litta P, Sideri M, Solima E, Spazzini D, Testa AC, Vignali M (2009) How often are endometrial polyps malignant in asymptomatic postmenopausal women? A multicenter study. Am J Obstet Gynecol 200(3):235–236

7. Golan A, Cohen-Sahar B, Keidar R, Condrea A, Ginath S, Sagiv R (2010) Endometrial polyps: symptomatology, menopausal status and malignancy. Gynecol Obstet Invest 70(2):107–112

8. Clark TJ, Khan KS, Gupta JK (2002) Current practice for the treatment of benign intrauterine polyps: a national questionnaire survey of consultant gynaecologists in UK. Eur J Obstet Gynecol Reprod Biol 103(1):65–67

9. Timmermans A, Veersema S, van Kerkvoorde TC, van der Voet LF, Opmeer BC, Bongers MY, Mol BW (2009) Should endometrial polyps be removed in patients with postmenopausal bleeding?—an assessment of study designs and report of a failed randomised controlled trial (ISRCTN73825127). BJOG 116(10):1391–1395

10. Lieng M, Istre O, Sandvik L, Engh V, Qvigstad E (2010) Clinical effectiveness of transcervical polyp resection in women with endometrial polyps: randomized controlled trial. J Minim Invasive Gynecol 17(3):351–357

11. Nathani F, Clark TJ (2006) Uterine polypectomy in the management of abnormal uterine bleeding: a systematic review. J Minim Invasive Gynecol 13(4):260–268

12. Lieng M, Istre O, Qvigstad E (2010) Treatment of endometrial polyps: a systematic review. Acta Obstet Gynecol Scand 89(8):992–1002

13. Epstein E, Ramirez A, Skoog L, Valentin L (2001) Dilatation and curettage fails to detect most focal lesions in the uterine cavity in women with postmenopausal bleeding. Acta Obstet Gynecol Scand 80(12):1131–1136

14. Gebauer G, Hafner A, Siebzehnrubl E, Lang N (2001) Role of hysteroscopy in detection and extraction of endometrial polyps: results of a prospective study. Am J Obstet Gynecol 184(2):59–63

15. Timmermans A, van Dongen H, Mol BW, Veersema S, Jansen FW (2008) Hysteroscopy and removal of endometrial polyps: a Dutch survey. Eur J Obstet Gynecol Reprod Biol 138(1):76–79

16. van Dongen H, Kolkman W, Jansen FW (2007) Implementation of hysteroscopic surgery in The Netherlands. Eur J Obstet Gynecol Reprod Biol 132(2):232–236

17. Bettocchi S, Nappi L, Ceci O, Selvaggi L (2004) Office hysteroscopy. Obstet Gynecol Clin N Am 31(3):641–654, xi

18. Garuti G, Cellani F, Colonnelli M, Grossi F, Luerti M (2004) Outpatient hysteroscopic polypectomy in 237 patients: feasibility of a one-stop "see-and-treat" procedure. J Am Assoc Gynecol Laparosc 11(4):500–504

19. Marsh FA, Rogerson LJ, Duffy SR (2006) A randomised controlled trial comparing outpatient versus daycase endometrial polypectomy. BJOG 113(8):896–901

20. Ghaly S, de Abreu LR, Abbott JA (2008) Audit of endometrial biopsy at outpatient hysteroscopy. Aust N Z J Obstet Gynaecol 48(2):202–206

21. Litta P, Cosmi E, Saccardi C, Esposito C, Rui R, Ambrosini G (2008) Outpatient operative polypectomy using a 5 mm-hysteroscope without anaesthesia and/or analgesia: advantages and limits. Eur J Obstet Gynecol Reprod Biol 139(2):210–214

22. Siristatidis C, Chrelias C (2010) Feasibility of office hysteroscopy through the "see and treat technique" in private practice: a prospective observational study. Arch Gynecol Obstet 283(4):819–823

23. Di Spiezio SA, Bettocchi S, Spinelli M, Guida M, Nappi L, Angioni S, Sosa Fernandez LM, Nappi C (2010) Review of new office-based hysteroscopic procedures 2003–2009. J Minim Invasive Gynecol 17(4):436–448

24. Saridogan E, Tilden D, Sykes D, Davis N, Subramanian D (2010) Cost-analysis comparison of outpatient see-and-treat hysteroscopy service with other hysteroscopy service models. J Minim Invasive Gynecol 17(4):518–525

25. Lydeards S (1996) Commentary: avoid surveys masquerading as research. BMJ 313:733–734

26. Edwards P, Roberts I, Clarke M, DiGuiseppi C, Pratap S, Wentz R, Kwan I, Cooper R (2007) Methods to increase response rates to postal questionnaires. Cochrane Database Syst Rev 2:MR000008

27. VanGeest JB, Johnson TP, Welch VL (2007) Methodologies for improving response rates in surveys of physicians: a systematic review. Eval Health Prof 30(4):303–321

28. Hiemstra E, Kolkman W, Jansen FW (2008) Skills training in minimally invasive surgery in Dutch obstetrics and gynecology residency curriculum. Gynecol Surg 5(4):321–325

29. van Dongen H, Emanuel MH, Wolterbeek R, Trimbos JB, Jansen FW (2008) Hysteroscopic morcellator for removal of intrauterine polyps and myomas: a randomized controlled pilot study among residents in training. J Minim Invasive Gynecol 15(4):466–471

30. Ahmad G, Attarbashi S, O'Flynn H, Watson AJ (2011) Pain relief in office gynaecology: a systematic review and meta-analysis. Eur J Obstet Gynecol Reprod Biol 155(1):3–13

31. Cooper NA, Khan KS, Clark TJ (2010) Local anaesthesia for pain control during outpatient hysteroscopy: systematic review and meta-analysis. BMJ 340:c1130

32. Cooper NA, Smith P, Khan KS, Clark TJ (2010) Vaginoscopic approach to outpatient hysteroscopy: a systematic review of the effect on pain. BJOG 117(5):532–539

12

Luteal phase transvaginal scan examinations have better diagnostic potential for showing focal subendometrial adenomyosis

Ahmed Abdel-Gadir · Oluseye O. Oyawoye ·
Bina P. Chander

Abstract The objective of this preliminary observational study was to monitor changes in focal cystic and non-cystic subendometrial lesions reminiscent of adenomyosis seen during the luteal phase of the cycle by repeating transvaginal ultrasound scan examinations during the follicular phase. Five patients who presented with abnormal uterine bleeding with or without dysmenorrhoea showed such lesions, following luteal phase transvaginal scanning. All lesions became smaller and less conspicuous, or an indiscriminate endometrial/myometrial interface was seen in the suspected areas during the follicular phase. Midcycle scanning of one patient showed enhancement of the irregular subendometrial area, but still without reaching the same size, or attaining an echogenic pattern as seen during the initial luteal phase examination. We hypothesise that luteal phase transvaginal scan examinations of the uterus may have better potential for diagnosing focal subendometrial adenomyosis than follicular phase scanning. This is because of the echogenic characteristics of a secretory endometrium relative to the neighbouring inner myometrium. More work is needed to verify these findings and to test our hypothesis.

Keywords Focal adenomyosis · Luteal ultrasound · Endometrial myometrial junction

A. Abdel-Gadir (✉) · B. P. Chander
London Female and Male Fertility Centre, Highgate Hospital,
17-19 View Road,
London N6 4DJ, UK
e-mail: AhmedAGadir@aol.com

O. O. Oyawoye
Department of Obstetrics and Gynaecology,
Newham University Hospital,
Glen Road, Plaistow,
London E13 8SL, UK

Background

Adenomyosis is a common cause of abnormal uterine bleeding and menstrual pain. Both magnetic resonance imaging (MRI) and transvaginal ultrasound scanning (TVS) have been used for its diagnosis, and had good correlation to the histological examination results. However, MRI findings are less observer-dependent than TVS, but still rely on the experience of the MRI observer in gynaecological imaging [1]. Furthermore, findings could fluctuate in response to hormonal changes [2]. Selective hysteroscopic resection could be helpful to remove lesions up to 3-mm deep in patients presenting with excessive uterine bleeding [3]. To facilitate such resection, accurate presurgical localisation of these lesions is essential. Transabdominal uterine biopsy performed with an ultrasound-directed biopsy gun had 100% accuracy in diagnosing myometrial disease [4]. This is in contrast to blind myometrial needle biopsies, which showed very low sensitivity for the diagnosis of subendometrial adenomyosis, even with multiple biopsies as reported by Brosens and Barker [5]. Two random myometrial biopsies picked 2.3% of adenomyotic lesions within the inner third of the myometrium, and eight biopsies were only 9.0% sensitive for diagnosing similar lesions as shown by the same authors. MRI proved to be very sensitive in this respect. It could show diffuse or focal thickening of the junctional zone, punctate foci of high-signal intensity, and ill-defined areas of low-signal intensity in the myometrium on T2-weighted imaging [2]. However, MRI is not readily available in many developing countries, and when present, services are usually prioritised to deal with more urgent medical and surgical problems. Even within the independent sector, the fees for having MRI examination are usually prohibitively high. Accordingly, efforts should be

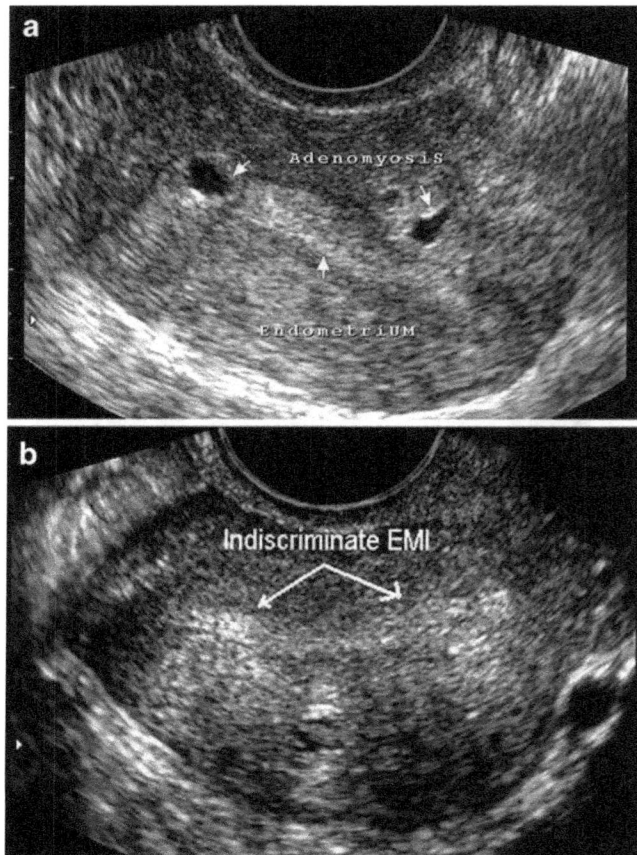

Fig. 1 **a** Shows an oblique transvaginal ultrasound scan view of a uterus during the luteal phase. Subendometrial cysts with echogenic margins are seen on the right side and in front of the left edge of a similarly echogenic endometrium. **b** Shows a similar view of the same specimen depicted in **a**. It reveals indiscriminate EMI during the early follicular phase. The cystic areas with echogenic margins seen in **a** are no longer visible

made to improve the accuracy of ultrasound scanning, which is the natural first-choice imaging technique for investigation of abnormal uterine bleeding and pelvic pain. This would also help with accurate selection of the right sites for needle biopsies, or hysteroscopic resection, when indicated. This is especially so as ultrasound machines are more readily available and cheaper to use than MRI for that purpose. The objective behind this observational study was to monitor changes in focal subendometrial lesions reminiscent of adenomyosis seen during the luteal phase of the cycle, by repeating the scan examinations during the follicular phase.

Method

Five patients who showed subendometrial focal lesions reminiscent of adenomyosis during luteal phase transvaginal ultrasound scan examinations were re-examined

during the follicular phase. Changes in the size and echotexture of the focal lesions were noted. All patients had their initial scan because of recent episodes of abnormal uterine bleeding, with or without painful menstruation. There was no evidence of endometrial polyps or intracavitary uterine fibroids.

Findings

Luteal phase transvaginal ultrasound scan examination showed echogenic endometrium in all five cases, with subendometrial cysts with echogenic margins or non-cystic echogenic lesions reminiscent of focal adenomyosis. This picture was represented by Figs. 1a, 2a, 3a and 4a in four different patients. Follow-up scans during the follicular phase showed diminution in the size or loss of these subendometrial lesions in all cases. Instead, the lesions were represented by indiscriminate EMI or by small

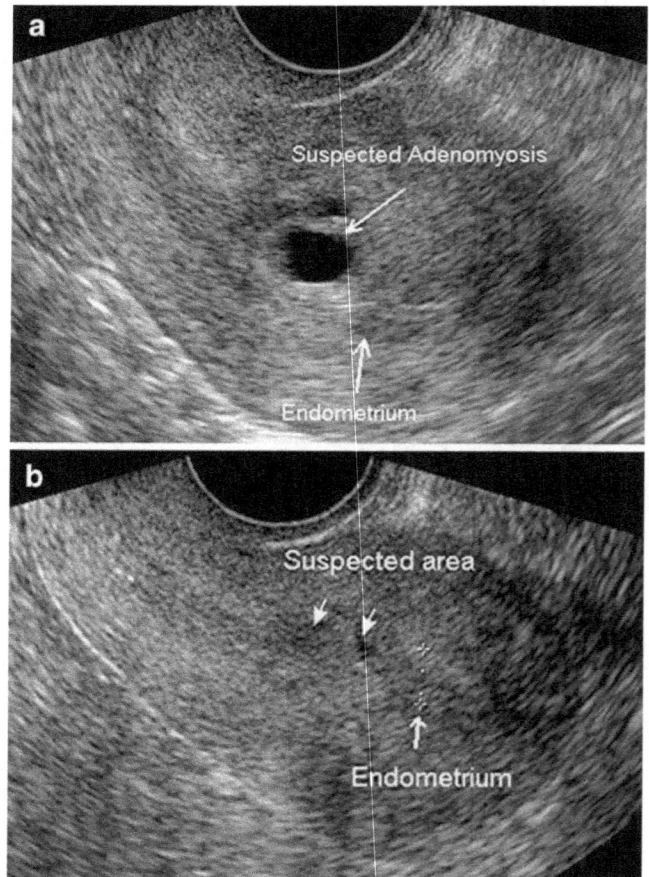

Fig. 2 **a** Shows an anterior/posterior transvaginal ultrasound view of a uterus with a large hypoechoic cyst with an echogenic margin in front of the endometrial echo. Examination was done during the late luteal phase of the cycle. **b** Shows an early follicular phase ultrasound picture of the same specimen depicted in **a**. The abnormal cystic area is represented by indiscriminate EMI marked by two arrows

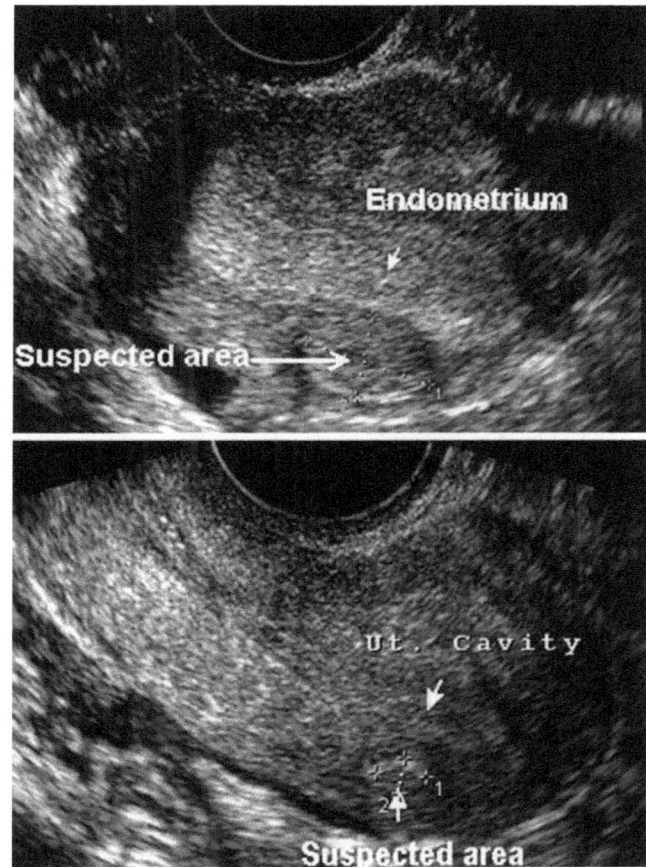

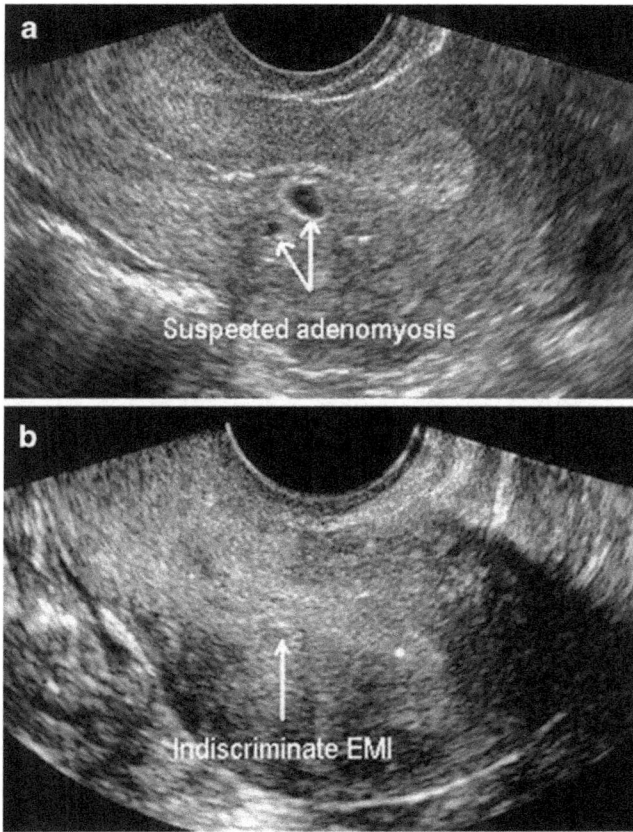

Fig. 3 **a** Image is an anterior/posterior view of a uterus showing subendometrial cysts with echogenic margin in the posterior uterine wall during the luteal phase of the cycle. **b** Image is a similar ultrasound view to the one shown in **a**. It shows early follicular phase indiscriminate EMI and disappearance of the cystic subendometrial lesions depicted in **a**

Fig. 4 **a** Shows an oblique view of a uterus during the luteal phase with 14.8×8.6 mm circumscribed area of similar texture and echogenicity to the overlying and adjacent endometrium, reminiscent of adenomyosis. **b** Shows early follicular phase anterior/posterior ultrasound picture of the same uterus depicted in **a**. The size of the suspected adenomyotic area shown in **a** is reduced to 5.3×3.8 mm

irregular areas, as seen in Figs. 1b, 2b, 3b and 4b respectively. Midcycle scanning of one patient showed enhancement of the irregular subendometrial area, but still without reaching the same size, or attaining an echogenic pattern as seen during the initial luteal phase examination. 3D rendering of the uterus during the luteal phase in the fifth patient revealed fundal adenomyotic striations which were not shown by the 2D sagittal or axial views, as shown in Fig. 5.

Discussion

In a histologically verified ultrasound study, Kepkep et al. 2007 [6] found subendometrial linear striations, myometrial cysts and globular appearance of the uterus had very high accuracy for the diagnosis of adenomyosis. Subendometrial linear striations were the most specific sonographic feature (95.5%), and had the highest positive predictive value (80.0%). However, they stressed the point that transvaginal scan examination was more useful in excluding than

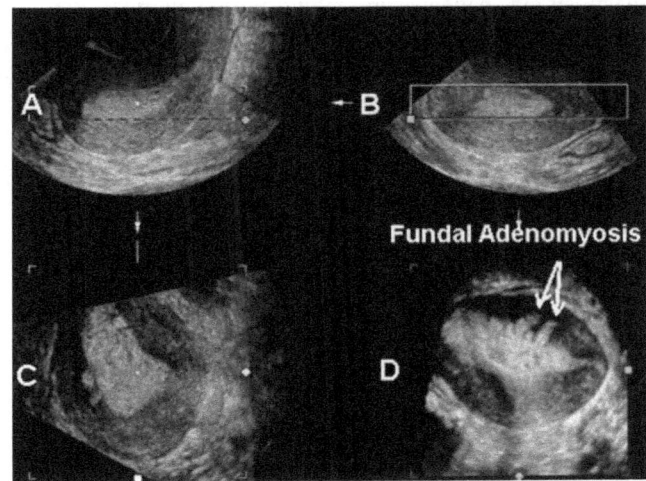

Fig. 5 Shows multiplanar views of a uterus with luteal phase echogenic endometrium. Sections *A* and *B* represent sagittal and axial views of the uterus, respectively and show no evidence of endometrial incursions into the myometrium. Fundal adenomyotic lesions are shown in section *D*, which is a rendered 3D view of the same uterus

confirming the diagnosis, as the negative and positive predictive values were 84.4% and 55.3% respectively. A higher negative predictive value of 96% for transvaginal scan examination was reported previously by Reinhold et al. in 1996 [7]. These authors found 2–6 mm myometrial cysts in 46% of the patients with histologically diagnosed adenomyosis. More important, none of the patients who proved histologically free from adenomyosis showed any myometrial cysts on presurgical transvaginal scan examination.

In this preliminary study, we used a reversed strategy, by following well-defined subendometrial cystic lesions with echogenic margins and non-cystic echogenic lesions seen during the luteal phase, to ascertain their echotexture and size during the follicular phase of the cycle. All lesions became less conspicuous, or an indiscriminate EMI was seen instead in the affected area. Since an echogenic endometrium is a luteal phase ultrasound characteristic, it is expected that luteal phase scanning would be more sensitive to reveal areas of intramural echogenic endometrial growth or cystic areas with echogenic margins, against the non-echogenic inner myometrium, compared to examinations performed at other times of the cycle. Variations in the echotexture of these subendometrial lesions during the different phases of the cycle could be a factor in explaining the differences in the quoted statistical accuracy of ultrasound scanning in diagnosing adenomyosis, depending when the scans were preformed. When available, 3D ultrasonography could help in making the diagnosis especially with fundal lesions which were not shown by routine 2D scanning, as shown in Fig. 5. With all this in mind, we put forward a hypothesis that scanning the uterus during the luteal phase might reveal focal subendometrial lesions reminiscent of adenomyosis and help with the diagnosis in patients presenting with abnormal uterine bleeding and inconclusive follicular phase ultrasound results. This could add to the diagnostic value of ultrasonography taking into account the very high specificity of both cystic and non-cystic lesions, and the high negative predictive value of ultrasound scanning [6, 7]. Alternative methods to help with the diagnosis in such cases are either too expensive (MRI), insensitive (hysteroscopy) or unavailable in certain areas. In agreement with a statement made by Margit and Erik in 2007 [1], MRI would be needed only when transvaginal ultrasound scan examination gives indefinite findings and in difficult cases with coexisting other uterine abnormalities. .

Conclusion

Focal cystic and non-cystic subendometrial lesions reminiscent of adenomyosis were detected more readily during luteal rather than follicular phase transvaginal ultrasound scanning in this small study. More work is needed to verify this finding and to test our hypothesis regarding the value of luteal phase transvaginal scanning of the uterus in the diagnosis of focal subendometrial adenomyosis. Positive findings would improve the accuracy of needle biopsies for histological diagnosis, and facilitate hysteroscopic resection when indicated. This is especially important in countries where MRI is not readily available or too expensive to afford.

Declaration of interest   The authors report no conflicts of interest.

References

1. Margit D, Erik L (2007) Transvaginal ultrasound or MRI for diagnosis of adenomyosis. Curr Opin Obstet Gynecol 19(6):505–512
2. Tamai K, Koyama T, Umeoka S, Saga T, Fujii S, Togashi K (2006) Spectrum of MR features in adenomyosis. Best Pract Res Clin Obstet Gynaecol 20(4):583–602
3. Levgur M (2007) Therapeutic options for adenomyosis: a review. Arch Gynecol Obstet 276(1):1–15
4. Wood C, Hurley VA, Fortune DW, Leoni M (1993) Percutaneous ultrasound guided uterine needle biopsy. Med J Aust 158(7):458–460
5. Brosens JJ, Barker FG (1995) The role of myometrial biopsies in the diagnosis of adenomyosis. Fertil Steril 63(6):1347–1349
6. Kepkep K, Tuncay YA, Tutal GE (2007) Transvaginal sonography in the diagnosis of adenomyosis: which findings are most accurate? Ultrasound Obstet Gynecol 30(3):341–345
7. Reinhold C, McCarthy S, Bret PM, Mehio A, Atri M, Zakarian R, Glaude Y, Liang L, Seymour R (1996) Diffuse adenomyosis: comparison of endovaginal US and MR imaging with histopathological correlation. Radiology 199:151–158

13

Minimally invasive surgical management of symptomatic uterine cysts

Atef M. Darwish · Kamal M. Zahran ·
Mohammad A. Bedaiwi · Mahmoud S. Zakherah

Abstract This study aims to evaluate the feasibility of a minimally invasive access-integrated protocol for aspiration or drainage of symptomatic uterine cysts. The design of the study is a prospective cohort study. The study setting is a tertiary care referral facility and university hospital. Twenty seven women with objective evidence of uterine cysts diagnosed by ultrasonography. The patients underwent transvaginal sonographic diagnosis of uterine cysts at different sites. Cyst aspiration was performed using interventional 2D ultrasonography, hysteroscopy and/or laparoscopy. Follow-up was performed for a maximum of 1 year to assess relief of symptoms and the recurrence rate. The main outcome measures of the study are success of aspiration tool, relief of symptoms, and persistence or recurrence rates. Cervical and corporeal uterine cysts were diagnosed in 19 and eight cases respectively. The mean size of the cervical cyst was 2.9 ± 1.21 (1.8–3.7) cm, while that of the uterine cysts was 4.8 ± 1.89 (3.4–6.1) cm. Improved health-related quality of life in the form of relief of deep dyspareunia and excessive vaginal discharge were reported in eight of 12 (66.6%) and 11/14 (78.5%) cases, respectively. Aspiration of symptomatic uterine cysts is technically feasible and achieves acceptable results. Uterine cysts may not be ignored as a potential cause of gynecologic symptoms, however, their precise pathogenesis and related co morbidities including impact on fertility should be substantiated by an adequately powered prospective randomized controlled study.

Keywords Uterine cysts · Ultrasonography · Laparoscopy · Hysteroscopy

A. M. Darwish (✉) · K. M. Zahran · M. A. Bedaiwi ·
M. S. Zakherah
Department of Obstetrics & Gynecology,
Woman's Health University Hospital,
71111 Assiut P.O. Box: (1) Assiut, Egypt
e-mail: atef_darwish@yahoo.com

Background

Intrauterine adhesions, submucous myoma, adenomyosis uterii or sometimes uterine septa are the most frequently diagnosed uterine abnormalities in gynecologic practice. Most of these abnormalities can be easily diagnosed utilizing conventional 2D transvaginal ultrasonography with or without saline infusion [1]. On the other hand, uterine cysts are rarely seen with no reported incidence in medical literature and usually accidentally detected by ultrasonography. Commonly, they are cervical due to retention of Nabothian cysts. However, they may be cystic degeneration of uterine leiomyoma, cystic adenomyosis (adenomyotic cysts), congenital uterine cysts such as mesonephric and paramesonephric cysts, hydrosalpinx densely adherent to the myometrium, and echinococcal cysts [2]. Various kinds of congenital cysts cannot be differentiated from cystic adenomatoid tumors [3] which are relatively rare benign neoplasms that usually arise in the genital tract [4–7]. Intramyometrial abscess [8] or hydatid cyst [9] are other rare possibilities. Cervical cysts may be cysts of embryonic tissues, endometriotic, or endocervicotic cysts [10]. So far, there are no published studies on the imaging of uterine cysts, their impact on health-related quality of life or the optimal line of management of such cysts. This study aims to estimate the feasibility and efficacy of a minimally access-integrated protocol for aspiration or drainage of symptomatizing sonographically diagnosed uterine cysts.

Patients and methods

This study was conducted at the Gynecologic outpatient clinic of the Woman's Health University Center, Assiut University, Assiut, Egypt between April 2001 and August 2008 and comprised 27 women with different gynecologic complaints and a transvaginal sonographic diagnosis of uterine cysts more than 2 cm in diameter at different sites.

Patients were counseled about participating in the study. A written informed consent was taken. Patients had the right to refuse to participate and/or withdraw from the study at any time without being denied their regular full clinical care. Personal information as well as data collected was subjected to confidentiality. The Institutional Review Board of the Assiut Faculty of Medicine approved this study.

Clinical work-up of the patients included entry history taking and thorough examination with stress on patients' complaints including type and duration of pelvic pain, coital-related pain, or abnormal vaginal discharge or backache. Infertile women were clearly informed that this study is not designed to help fertility. Patients with a clear potential cause of their complaints were excluded from this study, e.g., pelvic endometriosis, adenomyosis uteri, ovarian cysts, uterine fibroids, adnexal masses, pelvic inflammatory disease, or genital prolapsed. With the aid of transvaginal ultrasonography (TVS), uterine cysts appeared as a well defined hypoechogenic area not associated with uterine myomata or adenomyosis uterii. Uterine cysts more than 2 cm in diameter were included in this study. The relationship of the uterine cyst to the endometrial cavity or the cervical canal was meticulously defined. Comment on its size, fluid content, and borders were also reported. In case of suspicion, saline infusion sonohysterography (SIS) was performed in the same manner as previously described [1]. The couple was counseled for interventional 2D transvaginal sonographic aspiration of the cyst aiming at relief of the symptoms. Patients with corporeal cysts gave a written consent for laparoscopy in case of failed sonographic aspiration in the same operative setting. All procedures were done immediately postmenstrual. Under general anesthesia, TVS was performed. Sonographically guided aspiration of the cyst was done utilizing a 16-gauge aspiration needle principally designed for egg retrieval for assisted reproductive technique but used under higher pressure of the ordinary operating room suction unit at maximal power (−0.8 to −1 bar) since the cyst content is usually different from the watery follicular fluid. The

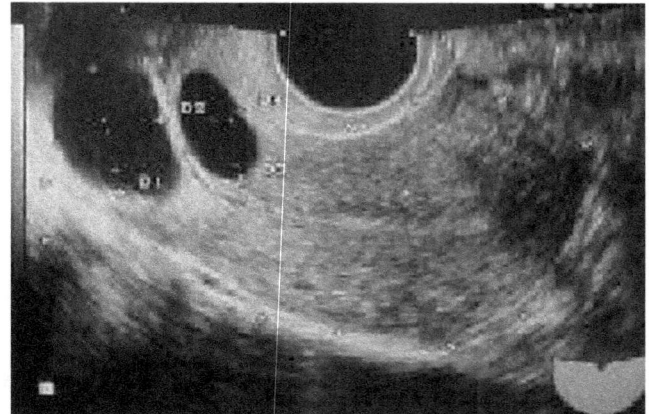

Fig. 1 Intracervical retention cysts compressing cervical canal

needle was loaded into an adaptor fitted to the vaginal probe. The procedure was considered completed once the cyst is seen entirely collapsed. The fluid content was subjected to cytologic examination after proper fixation with 95% alcohol. Failed access or aspiration of the viscid thick fluid content of corporeal cysts despite increased pressure of the suction unit were indication for operative laparoscopy in the same setting guided by the preoperative sonographic localization. Using a fine monopolar microneedle, a small incision was made over the cyst followed by drainage of its contents. The edges of the incision were coagulated with spray coagulation. The cyst content was aspirated for cytologic examination. On the other hand, if a part of the corporeal or cervical cyst is seen bulging into the endometrial or endocervical cavity respectively, a decision of hysteroscopic drainage was made. If an endocervical cyst was diagnosed, a sharp microscissors loaded into the side channel of the 7-mm operative hysteroscopy was used to puncture the cyst. If not accessible, a hook electrode of

Table 1 Basic data of the studied patients

Item	Result
Age [years] [means±SD] (range)	23.16±1.19 (18–31)
Parity	0.5±3.0 (0–2)
BMI (kg/m2) (range)	22.1±3.0 (15–30)
Menstrual disturbances (oligo or hypomenorrhea)	4 (14.8%)
Deep dyspareunia	12 (44.4%)
Excessive vaginal discharge	14 (51.8%)

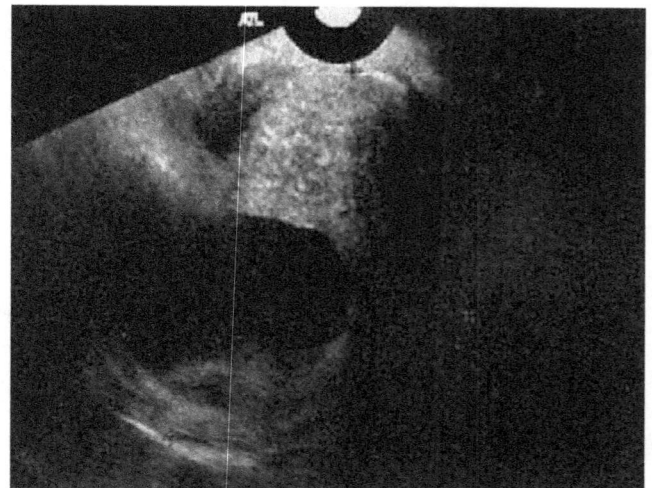

Fig. 2 A fundal corporeal cyst diagnosed by transvaginal ultrasonography

Table 2 Sonographic findings

	Cervical cysts 19 cases	Corporeal cysts eight cases	Significance p value
Cyst size (cm) (mean±SD)	2.9±1.21 2.0–3.7	4.8±1.89 (3.4–6.1)	NS
Cyst near to the cavity	11(57.8%)	1(12.5%)	0.03
accessibility	16 (48.2%)	5(62.5%)	NS
Successful sonographic aspiration	13 (68.4%)	5 (62.5%)	NS

NS non significant

monopolar resectoscope was utilized for puncture and drainage. The same instrument was used to drain any cyst bulging into the endometrial cavity. Transabdominal sonographic monitoring may be required in some difficult cases.

At the end of the operation in all cases, a broad spectrum antibiotic was prescribed and the patient was discharged few hours postoperatively. One month later, all patients were examined with TVS to comment on the site of the cyst and any evidence of recollection.

Follow-up of all cases was continued for 1 year to assess for the improvement of deep dyspareunia, abnormal vaginal discharge, or other symptoms. Data were collected and analyzed with SPSS version 11 (SPSS, Inc., Chicago, IL, USA) and expressed as mean±standard deviation (SD). Statistical methods were applied including descriptive statistics (frequency, percentage, mean, and SD) and tests of significance (X^2 and Fisher exact tests for categorical variables and Student t test and Mann–Whitney tests for continuous variables). A p value≤0.05 was considered statistically significant.

Findings

This study comprised 27 women with sonographic diagnosis of uterine cysts. Their basic data are demonstrated in Table 1. Cervical uterine cysts (Fig. 1) were diagnosed in

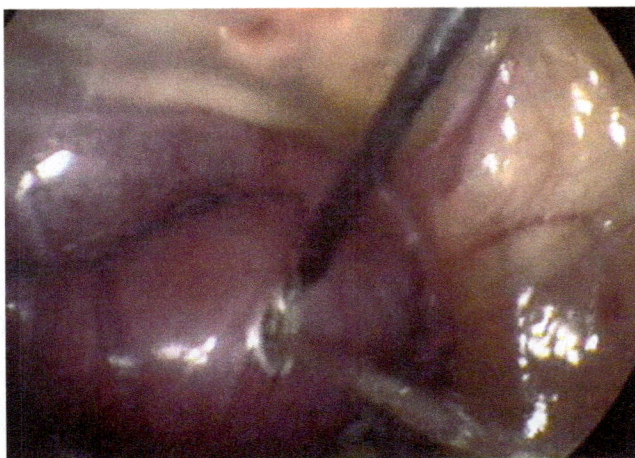

Fig. 3 Laparoscopic drainage of a fundal uterine cyst

19 cases, while corporeal cysts (Fig. 2) were diagnosed in eight cases. The mean size of the cervical cyst was 2.3± 0.9 cm, while that of the uterine cysts was 3.6±1.2 cm. Details of transvaginal aspiration are demonstrated in Table 2. Failed sonographic access or aspiration of the corporeal cysts (two cases) was managed laparoscopically guided by the previous sonographic localization without complications (Fig. 3 and Table 3). Hysteroscopic approach was tried in 16 cases with cervical and one case with corporeal cysts (Table 3). Cytologic evaluation of the cyst aspirate revealed no malignant cells in all cases. On follow-up, patients reported subjective improvement of health-related quality of life in the form of relief of deep dyspareunia and abnormal vaginal discharge in eight of 12 (66.6%) and 11/14 (78.5%) cases, respectively; this difference was statistically significant (Table 4). We did not report cyst reformation in any case on follow-up for 1 year.

Discussion

Despite being not infrequently sonographically diagnosed, uterine cysts are frequently ignored as a potential cause of gynecologic symptoms. Others may miss the diagnosis of uterine cysts particularly cervical or fundal due to lack of orientation or awareness with uterine cyst(s). The most frequently seen uterine cysts are cervical cysts. A lot of gynecologists diagnose cervical cysts but consider them insignificant follicular cervicitis. Posterior cervical cysts can be easily mistaken with follicles in the Douglas pouch during sonographic folliculometry. Many case reports on rare types of uterine cysts were published [11]. Cystic adenomyosis is a rare form of adenomyosis of the uterine myometrium that has been described in adolescents and

Table 3 Results of aspiration

	Cervical cysts 19 cases		Corporeal cysts eight cases	
	Successful	Failed	Successful	Failed
Ultrasonography	8	3	4	2
Laparoscopy	0	0	3	1
Hysteroscopy	11	5	1	0

Table 4 Persistence of the symptoms after 1 year of follow-up in the studied cases (27 cases)

	Before procedures	After procedures	Significance p value[a]
dyspareunia	12	4	0.017[a]
abnormal vaginal discharge	14	3	0.001[a]

[a] Statistically significant

adults [12]. There are some reports on primary echinococcal cysts of the uterus [13]. Commonly, non-fibroid swellings are erroneously diagnosed as adnexal enlargements and their true origin only becomes evident during surgery [14]. Others reported a case of florid cystic endosalpingiosis in the subserosa of the uterine fundus which was clinically considered to be an ovarian tumor [11]. In this study, all cases of uterine cysts were easily diagnosed utilizing conventional high resolution 2D ultrasonography with clear demarcation from adnexa masses. Moreover, the use of SIS in doubtful cases would help detect uterine cysts after proper delineation of the external uterine surface by excessive fluid in the pouch of Douglas. By this way, MRI requested for such an indication [11] can be omitted.

Some published human studies managed uterine cysts with hysterectomy [11, 14]. One case report on a complex uterine cyst demonstrated successful videohysteroscopic drainage utilizing electrocoagulation via a polypectomy snare guided by transrectal massage [15]. To the best of our knowledge, this study is the first publication in English and non-English literature that addresses the use transvaginal 2D sonographic aspiration of uterine cysts in humans. Over a 6-year period, only 29 cases were reported in one series [14]. Of these, eight corresponded to the diagnosis of a non-fibroid uterine cystic enlargement, and 21 to that of a fibroid with cystic degeneration. Histologic diagnosis showed a cystic adenomyoma in three, a congenital cyst in three, and a blind rudimentary uterine horn in two cases, respectively. In this study, just cyst aspiration was performed since these rare cysts are usually benign in nature. Moreover, cytologic examination of the aspirate in all cases in this study revealed no evidence of malignant cells. Nevertheless, cyst aspiration is not an optimal approach. Ideally, the cyst wall should be peeled off to ensure non-reformation of the cyst. Since some patients in this study were infertile, a minimally invasive procedure has been chosen and approved by the ethics committee. Moreover, many of these cysts were inaccessible for surgical removal particularly cervical retention cysts. Previously, we utilized a monopolar needle for blind puncture of these cervical cysts. However, we completely stopped this procedure due to reported cases of iatrogenic cervical atresia. Later on, we tried hysteroscopic opening of intramural cysts but unfortunately all these trials failed due to non-visualization of the cyst unless it protrudes into the cervical canal. Even after resectoscopic opening of the protruding cysts, cyst wall extraction was impossible and at the end it became just fenestration technique. In this study, hysteroscopic approach was restricted to any cyst bulging into the endocervical canal or the endometrial cavity where we achieved excellent results (11/16 and one of one

Fig. 4 Management plan of uterine cysts

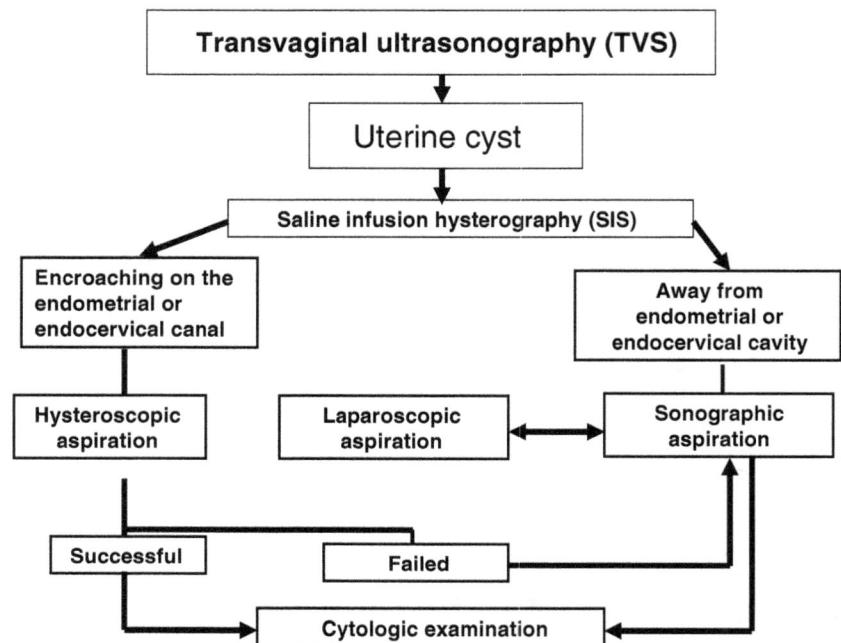

cervical and corporeal cysts, respectively). This study opens the door for a new era of hysteroscopic access to the myometrial lesions. Nevertheless, unlike hysteroscopy, sonographic approach is easier, non-invasive, available, and effective. This study addresses a laparoscopic back-up approach for treating uterine cysts. It is a simple and effective method of drainage. Moreover, those infertile women would get much more benefit of laparoscopic evaluation of their pelvis with concomitant management of any associated cause of infertility. Furthermore, we did not report cyst reformation in any case on follow-up for 1 year. This can be explained by the nature of these cysts which seems to be of embryonic origin lined by poorly developed glands in most of cases.

The impact of these cysts on fertility as well as the patient's health-related quality of life is unknown. Proposed mechanisms of impaired fertility secondary to uterine cysts would include mechanical compression of the endocervical canal or the endometrial cavity, dysrhythmic uterine contractions that interfere with proper implantation, or chronic irritation and infection. Nevertheless, we excluded fertility and pregnancy rates following cyst aspiration or drainage among infertile cases to avoid dissociation of the message of this work.

The limitations of the study

Failure to obtain cyst wall for histopathologic examination to determine the cyst nature is a clear limitation of this study. Nevertheless, we omitted this step since most of the scanty publications on uterine cysts demonstrated benign nature. Moreover, trials of cyst wall extraction or even coagulation of the whole cyst would invite adhesions for those women with unexplained infertility. Failed aspiration in some cases due to viscid nature of the fluid is another real limitation. This problem can be overcome by utilizing a larger needle caliber in the subsequent trials. Failed hysteroscopic aspiration would be minimized if concomitant sonographic guidance is used. Limited number of cases is another clear limitation of this study. Further similar studies with sufficient sample size are needed. The material of this study is quite mixed with respect to site and management options.

It is concluded that uterine cyst aspiration or drainage following an integrated protocol utilizing ultrasonography, hysteroscopy and/or laparoscopy (Fig. 4) is feasible and achieves acceptable results. While it is good to point out that uterine cysts should not be ignored, the claim that their impact on fertility and health-related quality of life is not substantiated. A randomized prospective study of large sample size would be required.

Acknowledgments We would like to thank residents and staff members of the ultrasonographic and endoscopic units of the Woman's Health University Center, Assiut University, Assiut, Egypt for their generous effort during the long study period.

Declaration of interest The authors report no conflicts of interest. The authors alone are responsible for the content and writing of the paper.

References

1. Darwish AM, Youssef AA (1999) Screening sonohysterography in infertility. Gynecol Obstet Investig 48(1):43–47
2. Kataoka ML, Togashi K, Konishi I (1998) MRI of adenomyotic cyst of the uterus. J Comput Assist Tomogr 22:555–559
3. Kim JY, Jung KJ, Sung NK, Chung DS, Kim OD, Park S (2002) Cystic adenomatoid tumor of the uterus. American Roentgen Ray Society Journal 179:1068–1070
4. Bisset DL, Morris JA, Fox H (1988) Giant cystic adenomatoid tumour (mesothelioma) of the uterus. Histopathology 12:555–558
5. Mitsumori A, Morimoto M, Matsubara S, Yamamoto M, Akamatsu N, Hiraki Y (2000) MR appearance of adenomatoid tumor of the uterus. J Comput Assist Tomogr 24:610–613
6. Livingston EG, Guis MS, Pearl ML, Stern JL, Brescia RJ (1992) Diffuse adenomatoid tumor of the uterus with a serosal papillary cystic component. Int J Gynecol Pathol 11:288–292
7. Rosa GD, Boscaino A, Terracciano LM, Giordano G (1992) Giant adenomatoid tumors of the uterus. Int J Gynecol Pathol 11:156–16
8. Erguvan R, Meydanli MM, Alkan A, Gokce MN, Kafkasli A (2003) Abscess in adenomyosis mimicking a malignancy in a 54-year-old woman. Infect Dis Obstet Gynecol 11:59–64
9. Kavak BZ, Gökaslan H, Küllü S (2002) Hydatid cyst of the uterus. Infect Dis Obstet Gynecol 10(2):67–70
10. Tindal VR (1987) Jeffcoate's principles of gynaecology, 5th edn. Butterworths, London, p 396
11. Sang Hwa Shim, Han-Seong Kim, Mee Joo, Sun Hee Chang, Ji Eun Kwak (2008) Florid cystic endosalpingiosis of the uterus—a case report. The Korean Journal of Pathology 42:189–191
12. Ho ML, Raptis C, Hulett R, McAlister WH, Moran K, Bhalla S (2008) Adenomyotic cyst of the uterus in an adolescent. Pediatr Radiol 38(11):1239–1242
13. Langley GF. Primary echinococcal cyst of the uterus British Journal of Surgery Jan1943;30,119,278-280 Online: Dec 6 2005.
14. Protopapas A, Milingos S, Markaki S, Loutradis D, Haidopoulos D, Sotiropoulou M, Antsaklis A (2008) Cystic uterine tumors. Gynecol Obstet Investig 65:275–280
15. Rambags BP, Stout TA (2005) Transcervical endoscope-guided emptying of a transmural uterine cyst in a mare. Vet Rec 156:679–682

14

Ultrasound-guided fine needle aspiration cytology in staging clinically node-negative invasive breast cancer

Daniela Huber · Cristophe Duc · Nicolas Schneider ·
Dominique Fournier

Abstract The aim of this study was to evaluate the value of ultrasound (US)-guided axillary lymph node fine needle aspiration cytology (FNAC) in staging clinically node-negative invasive breast cancer. Based on retrospective data, we analyzed sensitivity, specificity, and positive and negative predictive value and efficacy of preoperative axillary US-guided FNAC. A total of 108 consecutive female patients with histological-confirmed invasive breast cancer between January 2006 and December 2010 were included. The management decisions were based on cytological results. Twenty-two patients underwent neo-adjuvant chemotherapy and 86 remaining patients benefited of primary surgery. Patients with positive cytology or included in neoadjuvant regimens were scheduled for axillary lymph node dissection (ALND), while patient with negative or nondiagnostic cytology underwent sentinel lymph node biopsy. Axillary US-guided FNAC was compared with definitive pathology of surgically removed lymph nodes. Axillary metastases were found in 55 out of 108 patients (50.9%). In these cases we proceeded with ALND. Excluding the group benefiting from neoadjuvant chemotherapy, we could spare a second surgical intervention for 37 out of 86 patients (43%). The axillary US with FNAC has a sensitivity of 73%, a specificity of 85%, a

positive predictive value of 89%, and a negative predictive value of 66%. Without taking into account the neoadjuvant chemotherapy group, in which the statistical analyzes might be biased by the complete histological response, specificity and positive predictive value increased to 100% and negative predictive value to 71%. US combined with FNAC of axillary lymph nodes is a simple, minimally invasive, and reproducible diagnostic approach in improving the pre-operative axillary staging of invasive breast cancer patients.

Keywords Invasive breast cancer · Axillary node ultrasound · Axillary node cytology · Sentinel lymph node

Background and objective

The current goal in oncologic breast surgery is to tailor treatment options to allow optimal care without unnecessary interventions. Breast surgery has steadily evolved from an extensive to a more conservative approach. Since 2000, many clinical trials have confirmed that sentinel lymph node biopsy (SLNB) is an accurate technique that permits omitting a complete axillary lymph node dissection (ALND) in selected patients while diminishing the incidence of arm and shoulder morbidity [1, 2]. SLNB is developing in new directions (multifocal/multicentric tumors) [3]: applications with neoadjuvant chemotherapy [4–10], axillary reverse node mapping [11–13], and nanotechnology [14]. Axillary lymph node status is the single most significant predictive factor for patients with invasive breast tumors [15]. A positive sentinel lymph node (SLN) requires subsequent ALND. Sparing a second axillary surgery is a current concern that has stimulated the development of other approaches including molecular biology techniques for intraoperative assessment of SLN and preoperative detection of node metastases through the use of imaging methods. Ultrasound (US) is a simple and

D. Huber (✉) · N. Schneider
Obstetrics and Gynecology, CHCVs Sion Hospital,
Rue Champsec 80,
Sion 1950, Switzerland
e-mail: ghetudana@gmail.com

C. Duc
Pathology, ICHV Sion Hospital,
Rue Champsec 80,
Sion 1950, Switzerland

D. Fournier
Radiology, IRS Sion Radiologic Institute,
Rue du Scex 2,
Sion 1950, Switzerland

well-accepted method to examine axillary and non-axillary lymph nodes associated with breast cancer. Recent publications have reported that routine axillary US combined with cytology or core biopsy is an effective method to evaluate lymph node metastases prior to surgery [16–35]. Thus, pretreatment axillary US for early breast cancer patients and needle sampling of morphologically abnormal lymph nodes are now widely recommended [36]. The aim of our study was to establish the accuracy of US-guided fine needle aspiration cytology (FNAC) of axillary lymph nodes for the detection of clinically silent metastases and to find out how often a SLNB could be avoided.

Material and method

From January 2006 to December 2010, 144 consecutive patients with invasive breast cancer, clinical stage T1/2N0, were evaluated by axillary US with FNAC. Thirty-six patients were excluded due to a personal history of breast cancer, previous or ongoing chemotherapy or previous breast/axilla surgery, and non identifiable lymph node on axillary US. All 108 remaining patients underwent initial breast biopsy confirming invasive malignancy.

Both axillary US and node FNAC were performed by the same breast radiologist. A high-resolution probe (12 MHz electronically focused linear array transducer) of ATL HDI 500 Philips Healthcare was utilized. The suspicious ultrasound node characteristics in our study were: length/width ratio of <1.5, cortical asymmetrical thickness more than 3 mm, hypoechoic cortical nodule deforming hilum, and the absence of the fatty hilum. If at least one of these criteria was observed, the node was selected for FNAC. If more than one abnormal lymph node was found, the most suspicious one was selected. If all suspect lymph nodes were similar, the lowest one in the axilla was selected. If no suspect lymph node was detected, the lowest normal lymph node larger than 5 mm was sampled. In one case a preoperative breast NMRI identified a suspicious internal mammary lymph node that was sampled by US-guided FNAC.

All cytological samples were processed with the Thin Prep System and analyzed by a breast specialist pathologist and classified as: insufficient for diagnosis and negative or positive for malignancy. Patients with cytology that was negative or insufficient for diagnosis were referred to SLNB. Patients with positive cytologies and all patients treated with neoadjuvant chemotherapy underwent ALND. If the intraoperative imprint cytologies (Diff-Quick staining protocol) or the extemporaneous frozen sections of SLN (hematoxylin and eosine staining method) were positive for malignancy the patients underwent immediate ALND. If the SLNB were negative based on extemporaneous examination but micro or macro metastatic on final histology

(metastasis, ≥0.2 mm) the patients underwent ALND within 2 weeks. If isolated tumor cells were identified through definitive histology, no further ALND was performed.

The total number of harvested nodes, the number of positive nodes, and the size of metastasis were recorded. The tumor size and grade, histological type, lymphovascular or perinervous infiltration, the type of surgical intervention, and the neoadjuvant treatments were also included in our data. The final pathological results of harvested sentinel lymph nodes or ALND were correlated with US-guided FNAC. The sensitivity, specificity, and positive and negative predictive values were calculated.

Findings

One hundred eight patients had axillary lymph US-guided FNAC as a part of the investigation for invasive breast cancer. No immediate or late complications such as bleeding, hematoma, nerve injury, or infection were reported. Eighty-six patients underwent primary surgery and the other 22 underwent neoadjuvant chemotherapy with subsequent surgery. The median age was 58 (range 33–83) and 54 (range 33–71) years for the two groups, respectively.

The most frequent histological type of primary invasive breast tumor in our group was ductal carcinoma in 82 (76%) patients. Other described histological types were lobular carcinoma in 15 (13.9%) patients, mixed carcinoma in 9 (8.3%), and mucinous carcinoma in 2 (1.8%) cases.

As overlap of ultrasound features between reactive nodes and suspicious/metastatic ones is documented [19, 37], our breast radiologist decided to puncture also non-suspicious nodes larger than 5 mm [19, 38]. As our study is retrospective, the ultrasound reports were nonuniform and did not mention in detail the sonographic nodes description and the reasons for choosing a suspicious or a non-suspicious node. Hence, statistical analysis including the significance of each sonographic suspicious finding could not be made.

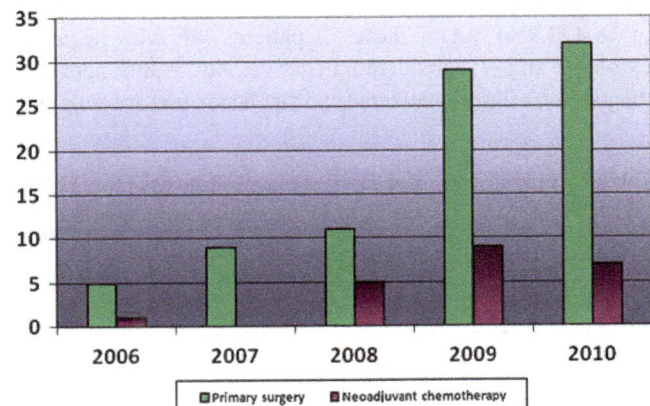

Fig. 1 Annual patient recruitment between 2006 and 2010

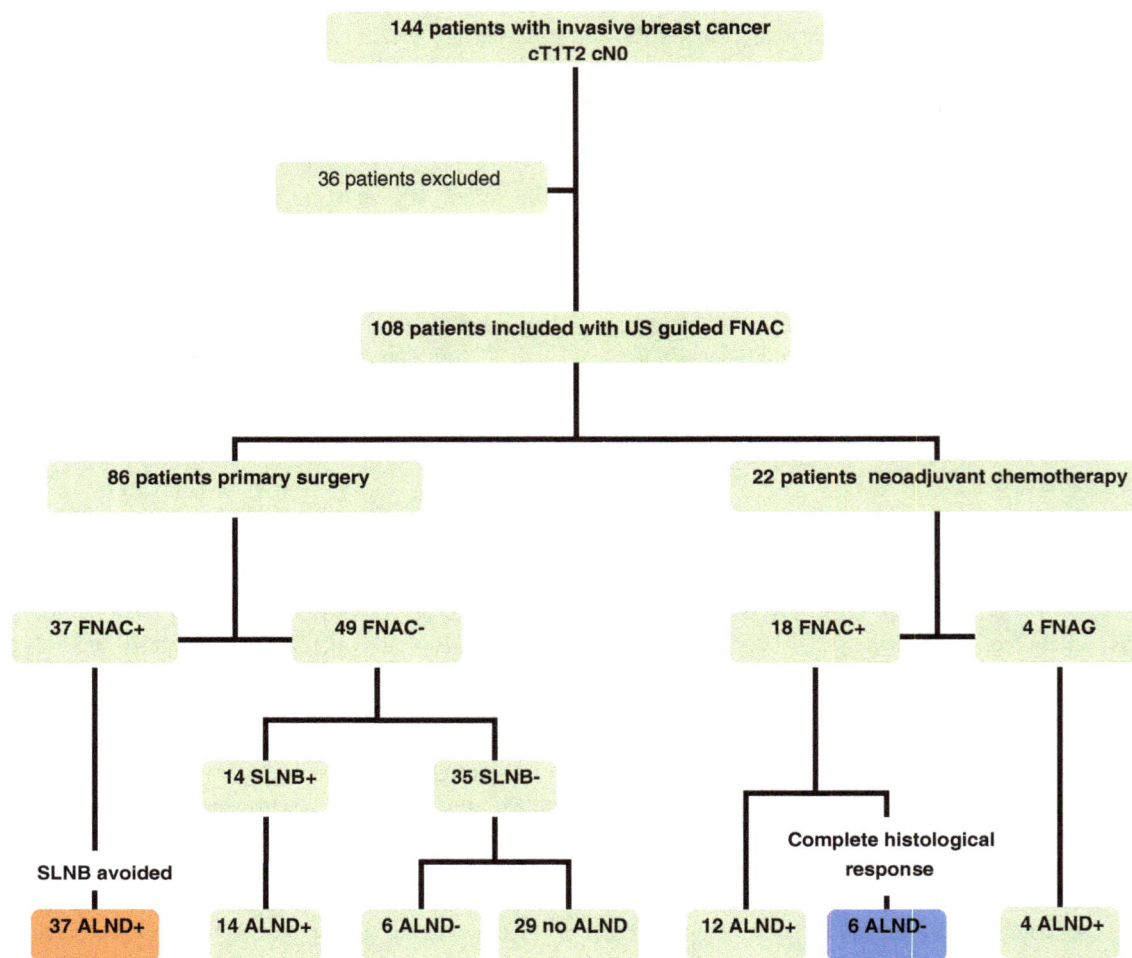

Fig. 2 Study design and results

For 55 (50.9%) patients the FNAC was positive and for 46 (42.6%) patients it was negative. In seven (6.5%) cases the FNAC was insufficient for diagnosis (in one case the FNAC sampled only necrotic cells and in six other cases there was insufficient material to reach a conclusive result). All these patients were considered to be negative for statistical analysis. False-negative results were documented in 18 (33.9%) out of these 53 patients (46 with negative cytology and 7 considered negative, but insufficient for diagnosis). Three patients had isolated tumor cells on

definitive histology despite a negative FNAC. We did not consider these results as cytohistological discordances as pathological classification remains pN0(sn) and no further ALND was performed.

For the patients in the primary surgery group, no false-positive result was documented. In the neoadjuvant chemotherapy group, 6 out of 18 patients with positive pretreatment FNAC had negative axillary lymph nodes. We have interpreted this apparent discrepancy as a complete node histological response and not as false-

Table 1 Surgical node staging compared with preoperative FNAC (108 patients)

		Surgical staging		Total
		Positive nodes	Negative nodes	
FNAC	Positive	49	6	55
	Negative	18	35	53
	Total	67	41	108

Table 2 Surgical node staging compared with preoperative FNAC in primary surgery group

		Surgical staging		Total
		Positive nodes	Negative nodes	
FNAC	Positive	37	0	37
	Negative	14	35	49
	Total	51	35	86

Table 3 Lymph node morphology by axillary ultrasound and cytological findings in the "primary surgery" group

		Lymph node morphology (US)		Total
		Normal	Suspicious	
FNAC	Positive	5	32	37
	Negative	35	14	49
	Total	40	46	86

positive results. Figure 1 shows the patients' recruitment from 2006 to 2010. Figure 2 describes our study design and the results. Table 1 reviews the final histological findings for the 86 patients treated by primary surgery. Table 2 compares the surgical node staging with FNAC for the primary surgery group. Table 3 summarizes the sonographic aspect of the punctured nodes and the cytological results in the same group. The data in Tables 4 and 5 review the clinicopathological features of invasive carcinomas and

Table 4 Clinicopathological features of invasive carcinoma primary surgery group

Pathological characteristics	N (%)
Histological type	
Invasive ductal carcinoma:	66/86 (76.7%)
Invasive lobular carcinoma	12/86 (14.0%)
Invasive mixed carcinoma	6/86 (7.0%)
Invasive mucinous carcinoma	2/86 (2.3%)
Tumor grade	
G1	10/86 (11.6%)
G2	57/86 (66.3%)
G3	19/86 (22.1%)
Pathological tumor stage	
pT1a	2/86 (2.2%)
pT1b	5/86 (5.8%)
pT1c	31/86 (36.0%)
pT2	39/86 (45.3%)
pT3	8/86 (9.6%)
pT4	1/86 (1.1%)
Lymphovascular infiltration	
Absent	65/86 (75.6%)
Present	21/86 (24.4%)
Pathological node stage	
pN0 (sn)	29/86
pN0	6/86
pN1(sn)	1/86
pN1	35/86
pN2	11/86
pN3	4/86
Total	86 (100%)

Table 5 Cytohistological discordances in primary surgery group

Histological findings	n (%)
FNAC	
Insufficient for diagnose	2 (14.3%)
Negative (false negative)	12 (85.7%)
Positive (false positive)	0%
Number of positive nodes	
1 lymph node	11 (78.5%)
2 lymph nodes	2 (14.3%)
3 lymph nodes	1 (7.2%)
Size of nodal metastasis	
Not documented	6 (42.8%)
Micrometastasis (0.2 to 2 mm)	3 (21.4%)
Macrometastasis	
2 to 4 mm	4 (28.6%)
>4 mm	1 (7.2%)
Pathological stage grouping	
IB (pT1cN1mi)	1 (7.2%)
IIA (pT1cN1a)	5 (35.7%)
IIB (pT2N1a et pT2N1b)	8 (57.1%)
Total cytohistological discordances	14 (100%)

the 14 cytohistological discordances in primary surgery group. For this group of patients, the cytohistological concordance was established in 72 (83.7%) patients (37 with positive and 35 with negative results). Consequently, for 37 patients a second axillary surgery was avoided (43.02%). Fourteen discordances were documented as either FNAC negative or insufficient for diagnosis but positive on definitive histology. In 12 patients, the FNAC was negative and in two patients the material was insufficient for cytological diagnosis. Among these 14 patients with cytohistological discordances, 11 had only one positive node, 2 patients had two positive nodes and 1 patient had three positive lymph nodes.

The internal mammary lymph node sampled by the US-guided FNAC was positive for malignancy. The patient underwent ALND (14 negative axillary lymph nodes) and the final pathological stage was pT1cN2b.

Discussion

The appropriate pretreatment evaluation enables personalized management of breast cancer patients. SLNB is widely accepted today and has led to decreased shoulder and arm morbidity. Nevertheless, this technique requires the sustained coordination of a multidisciplinary team. Some patients need a second axillary surgery if the definitive SLNB with immunostaining proves the presence of node metastases. Although there are still controversies concerning morbidity differences between immediate and delayed ALND [39–43], operating on a distorted axilla represents a surgical challenge with emotional distress for the patient as well as considerable additional medical costs [44]. Axillary ultrasound is noninvasive, reproducible, largely available, widely accepted by patients, and cost effective [35, 44]. In addition, all lymph node chains can be evaluated (intramammary, internal mammary chain, infra- and supraclavicular, or axillary nodes).

In our study, immediate assessment of the quality of FNAC was not feasible. Seven (6.5%) out of 108 FNAC specimens were insufficient for diagnosis. Immediate assessment of specimens by a pathologist might reduce the proportion of inadequate samples [45] and allow additional lymph node passes by the radiologist to improve quality [28]. For the 86 patients treated by primary surgery, the overall sensitivity was 72.55% and the specificity was 100% (Table 6) although identifiable non-suspicious nodes

were punctured and aspirated for cytological pretreatment examination. Forty-six patients of this group had sonographic suspicious nodes. Thirty-one out of these 46 nodes were positive. By puncturing normal nodes as well, a total of 37 patients with node metastasis were identified (Table 3). The major benefit of US-guided FNAC was that it spared a second surgical intervention for these 37 patients (43% of the primary surgery group). For patients with neoadjuvant treatment, this approach enables the gathering of further information about the in vivo response to chemotherapy. Patients who have a complete nodal and breast pathological response enjoy a much better outcome than those who still have residual disease after therapy [46].

Recently, the NCCN guidelines (version 2.2011) introduced prechemotherapy SLNB as an option for clinically node-negative breast cancer patients benefiting from neoadjuvant regimens. As for early breast cancer patients, we expect that FNAC will allow a better

Table 6 Sensitivity, specificity, positive predictive value and negative predictive value

Patients	n	FNAC+		FNAC−		Sensitivity	Specificity	Positive predictive value	Negative predictive value
		N+	N−	N+	N−				
All patients	108	49	6	18	35	73.13%	85.36%	89.09%	66.03%
Neoadjuvant chemotherapy group	22	12	6	4	0	66.66%		75%	
Pathological stage									
ypT0	2/22	1	1	0	0				
ypT1	6/22	2	3	1	0				
ypT2	8/22	4	2	2	0				
ypT3/T4	6/22	5	0	1	0				
Primary surgery group	86	37	0	14	35	72.55%	100%	100%	71.43%
Tumor grade									
G1	12/86	3	0	1	8	75%	100%	100%	88.88%
G2	55/86	26	0	11	18	70.27%	100%	100%	62.07%
G3	19/86	8	0	3	8	72.72%	100%	100%	72.72%
Pathological stage									
pT1	38/86	11	0	6	21	64.70%	100%	100%	77.77%
pT2	39/86	19	0	9	11	67.85%	100%	100%	55%
pT3-T4	9/86	7	0	0	2	100%	100%	100%	100%
LVI/PNI									
Present	21/86	12	0	6	3	66.66%	100%	100%	30%
Absent	65/86	25	0	9	31	73.53%	100%	100%	77.5%
Histological type									
Ductal	66/86	26	0	15	25	63.41%	100%	100%	62.5%
Lobular	12/86	6	0	2	4	75%	100%	100%	66.66%
Mixed	6/86	5	0	1	0	83.33%	100%	100%	0%
Mucinous	2/86	2	0	0	1	100%	100%	100%	100%
Type of lesion									
Unifocal	68/86	30	0	12	26	1.42%	100%	100%	68.42%
Multifocal/multicentric	18/86	7	0	3	8	70%	100%	100%	72.72%

selection of patients for prechemotherapy SLNB and will carry the same prognostic value as SLNB if complete histological response is observed.

False-positive results have seldom been reported [29, 47]. These results have been related to misinterpreting the presence of reactive lymphoid or mesothelial cells as carcinoma infiltration. The majority of cases believed to be false-positive may, in fact, be true-positive (complete histological response or failure to detect minimal residual disease in the final histology). We believe that all positive FNAC with a negative definitive histology must be treated cautiously in order to exclude a non-harvested positive node.

False-negative FNAC results probably occurred in part due to failure to target the real SLN or the most suspected region of the lymph node and perhaps to misinterpretations including failure to recognize tumor cells. As this is a retrospective study, no information about the punctured lymph node and the correlation with the SLN surgically removed was possible.

Conclusions

With a sensitivity of 73%, axillary US associated with FNAC plays an important role in preoperative lymph node staging for newly diagnosed invasive breast cancer patient. In selecting non-suspicious nodes for pretreatment lymph node cytology, we could spare a second axillary surgery for 43% of the patients. In addition, for patients included on neoadjuvant regimens, it allows a better selection for prechemotherapy SLNB and furthermore an evaluation of the histological response to treatment offering valuable information on patient prognosis and predictive factors.

Acknowledgments Many thanks go to M.E. Visher for her essential and gracious support in revising the manuscript's English.

Declaration of interest The authors report no conflicts of interest. The authors alone are responsible for the content and writing of the paper.

References

1. Veronesi U et al (2002) Twenty-year follow-up of a randomized study comparing breast conserving surgery with radical mastectomy for early breast cancer. N Engl J Med 347(16):1227–1232

2. Veronesi U et al (1997) Sentinel-node biopsy to avoid axillary dissection in breast cancer with clinically negative lymph-nodes. Lancet 349(9069):1864–1867

3. Fearmonti RM et al (2009) False negative rate of sentinel lymph node biopsy in multicentric and multifocal breast cancers may be higher in cases with large additive tumor burden. Breast J 15 (6):645–648

4. Brady EW (2002) Sentinel lymph node mapping following neoadjuvant chemotherapy for breast cancer. Breast J 8(2):97–100

5. Classe JM et al (2009) Sentinel lymph node biopsy after neoadjuvant chemotherapy for advanced breast cancer: results of Ganglion Sentinelle et Chimiotherapie Neoadjuvante, a French prospective multicentric study. J Clin Oncol 27(5):726–732

6. Hunt KK et al (2009) Sentinel lymph node surgery after neoadjuvant chemotherapy is accurate and reduces the need for axillary dissection in breast cancer patients. Ann Surg 250 (4):558–566

7. Iwase H et al (2009) Advantage of sentinel lymph node biopsy before neoadjuvant chemotherapy in breast cancer treatment. Surg Today 39(5):374–380

8. Medina-Franco H, Salgado-Nesme N, Zeron-Medina-Cuairan J (2008) Sentinel lymph node biopsy after neoadjuvant systemic chemotherapy in patients with breast cancer: a prospective pilot trial. Rev Invest Clin 60(5):390–394

9. Menard JP et al (2009) Sentinel lymphadenectomy for the staging of clinical axillary node-negative breast cancer before neoadjuvant chemotherapy. Eur J Surg Oncol 35(9):916–920

10. van Deurzen CH et al (2009) Accuracy of sentinel node biopsy after neoadjuvant chemotherapy in breast cancer patients: a systematic review. Eur J Cancer 45(18):3124–3130

11. Casabona F et al (2008) Axillary reverse mapping in breast cancer: a new microsurgical lymphaticvenous procedure in the prevention of arm lymphedema. Ann Surg Oncol 15(11):3318–3319

12. Casabona F et al (2009) Feasibility of axillary reverse mapping during sentinel lymph node biopsy in breast cancer patients. Ann Surg Oncol 16(9):2459–2463

13. Khan SA (2009) Axillary reverse mapping to prevent lymphedema after breast cancer surgery: defining the limits of the concept. J Clin Oncol 27(33):5494–5496

14. Johnson L, Charles-Edwards G, Douek M (2010) Nanoparticles in sentinel lymph node assessment in breast cancer. Cancers 2:1884–1894

15. Mainiero MB (2010) Regional lymph node staging in breast cancer: the increasing role of imaging and ultrasound-guided axillary lymph node fine needle aspiration. Radiol Clin North Am 48(5):989–997

16. Park S et al (2011) Impact of preoperative ultrasonography and fine-needle aspiration of axillary lymph nodes on surgical management of primary breast cancer. Ann Surg Oncol 18 (3):738–744

17. Abe H et al (2009) Axillary lymph nodes suspicious for breast cancer metastasis: sampling with US-guided 14-gauge core-needle biopsy—clinical experience in 100 patients. Radiology 250 (1):41–49

18. Baruah BP et al (2010) Axillary node staging by ultrasonography and fine-needle aspiration cytology in patients with breast cancer. Br J Surg 97(5):680–683

19. Bonnema J et al (1997) Ultrasound-guided aspiration biopsy for detection of nonpalpable axillary node metastases in breast cancer patients: new diagnostic method. World J Surg 21 (3):270–274

20. Britton PD et al (2009) Use of ultrasound-guided axillary node core biopsy in staging of early breast cancer. Eur Radiol 19 (3):561–569

21. Cowher MS et al (2008) Correlation of the use of axillary ultrasound and lymph node needle biopsy with surgical lymph node pathology in patients with invasive breast cancer. Am J Surg 196(5):756–759

22. Damera A et al (2003) Diagnosis of axillary nodal metastases by ultrasound-guided core biopsy in primary operable breast cancer. Br J Cancer 89(7):1310–1313

23. Davey P et al (2011) The value of axillary ultrasound with fine needle aspiration as a preoperative staging procedure in breast cancer: Northern Irish experience. Ir J Med Sci 180 (2):509–511

24. Garcia-Ortega MJ et al (2011) Pretreatment axillary ultrasonography and core biopsy in patients with suspected breast cancer: diagnostic accuracy and impact on management. Eur J Radiol 79(1):64–72

25. Hinson JL et al (2008) The critical role of axillary ultrasound and aspiration biopsy in the management of breast cancer patients with clinically negative axilla. Ann Surg Oncol 15(1):250–255

26. Jain A et al (2008) The role of ultrasound-guided fine-needle aspiration of axillary nodes in the staging of breast cancer. Ann Surg Oncol 15(2):462–471

27. Jung J et al (2010) Accuracy of preoperative ultrasound and ultrasound-guided fine needle aspiration cytology for axillary staging in breast cancer. ANZ J Surg 80(4):271–275

28. Krishnamurthy S (2009) Current applications and future prospects of fine-needle aspiration biopsy of locoregional lymph nodes in the management of breast cancer. Cancer 117(6):451–462

29. Kuenen-Boumeester V et al (2003) Ultrasound-guided fine needle aspiration cytology of axillary lymph nodes in breast cancer patients. A preoperative staging procedure. Eur J Cancer 39 (2):170–174

30. Lemos S et al (2005) Detection of axillary metastases in breast cancer patients using ultrasound and colour Doppler combined with fine needle aspiration cytology. Eur J Gynaecol Oncol 26 (2):165–166

31. MacNeill M, Arnott I, Thomas J (2011) Fine needle aspiration cytology is a valuable adjunct to axillary ultrasound in the preoperative staging of breast cancer. J Clin Pathol 64(1):42–46

32. Oruwari JU et al (2002) Axillary staging using ultrasound-guided fine needle aspiration biopsy in locally advanced breast cancer. Am J Surg 184(4):307–309

33. Ou YT et al (2008) Role of ultrasound-guided needle biopsy of ultrasonographic abnormal axillary lymph nodes in patients with breast cancer. Zhonghua Yi Xue Za Zhi 88(2):82–84

34. Swinson C et al (2009) Ultrasound and fine needle aspiration cytology of the axilla in the preoperative identification of axillary nodal involvement in breast cancer. Eur J Surg Oncol 35 (11):1152–1157

35. Schiettecatte A et al (2011) Initial axillary staging of breast cancer using ultrasound-guided fine needle aspiration: a liquid-based cytology study. Cytopathology 22(1):30–35

36. Yarnold J (2009) Early and locally advanced breast cancer: diagnosis and treatment National Institute for Health and Clinical Excellence guideline 2009. Clin Oncol (R Coll Radiol) 21 (3):159–160

37. de Kanter AY et al (1999) Multicentre study of ultrasono-graphically guided axillary node biopsy in patients with breast cancer. Br J Surg 86(11):1459–1462

38. Alvarez S et al (2006) Role of sonography in the diagnosis of axillary lymph node metastases in breast cancer: a systematic review. AJR Am J Roentgenol 186(5):1342–1348

39. Husted-Madsen A et al (2008) Arm morbidity following sentinel lymph node biopsy or axillary lymph node dissection: a study from the Danish Breast Cancer Cooperative Group. Breast 17 (2):138–147

40. Husen M, Paaschburg B, Flyger HL (2006) Two-step axillary operation increases risk of arm morbidity in breast cancer patients. Breast 15(5):620–628

41. Olson JA Jr et al (2008) Impact of immediate versus delayed axillary node dissection on surgical outcomes in breast cancer patients with positive sentinel nodes: results from American College of Surgeons Oncology Group Trials Z0010 and Z0011. J Clin Oncol 26(21):3530–3535

42. Holwitt DM et al (2008) Scientific Presentation Award: the combination of axillary ultrasound and ultrasound-guided biopsy is an accurate predictor of axillary stage in clinically nodenegative breast cancer patients. Am J Surg 196(4):477–482

43. Liu CQ et al (2009) Late morbidity associated with a tumour-negative sentinel lymph node biopsy in primary breast cancer patients: a systematic review. Eur J Cancer 45(9):1560–1568

44. Boughey JC et al (2010) Cost modeling of preoperative axillary ultrasound and fine-needle aspiration to guide surgery for invasive breast cancer. Ann Surg Oncol 17(4):953–958

45. Ciatto S (2004) Sentinel lymph node biopsy: sentinel node technique has drawbacks. BMJ 329(7458):170

46. Chollet P et al (2002) Prognostic significance of a complete pathological response after induction chemotherapy in operable breast cancer. Br J Cancer 86(7):1041–1046

47. Tate JJ et al (1989) Ultrasound detection of axillary lymph node metastases in breast cancer. Eur J Surg Oncol 15(2):139–141

15

Prostaglandins prior to hysteroscopy

Fady M. Shawky Moiety · Amal Azzam

Abstract This prospective randomized controlled study was conducted to assess the role of misoprostol, given sublingually or rectally, on the outcome of hysteroscopic procedures. A total of 212 premenopausal patients undergoing hysteroscopic procedures were randomly allocated into three groups: group 1 ($n=71$), sublingual misoprostal given 2 h before the procedure; group 2 ($n=71$) rectal misoprostal 2 h before the procedure; group 3 ($n=70$), control group, no medications were given. Main outcome measures were ease of cervical dilatation, dilatation time to Hegar 6, complications as cervical laceration and postoperative cramps, bleeding and pyrexia. The cervical canal at the start was significantly wider misoprostol groups ($P=0.038$). Cervical dilatation was significantly easier in the rectal misoprostol group over control ($P=0.035$). Misoprostol groups showed significant reduction in the mean time needed to dilate to Hegar 6 ($P=0.021$). Postoperative pain and cramps were significantly higher in misoprostol groups ($P=0.002$). Misoprostol before hysteroscopy demonstrates a benefit in the ease of cervical dilatation, cervical width at the start and time for dilatation with low risk of cervical tears. Rectal misoprostol appears advantageous than sublingual one. However, postoperative adverse effects are more common with misoprostol groups.

Keywords Sublingual · Rectal · Misoprostol · Hysteroscopy

F. M. S. Moiety (✉) · A. Azzam
Department of Obstetrics and Gynecology, Shatby Maternity
University Hospital,
Shatby, Alexandria 21526, Egypt
e-mail: fmoeity@hotmail.com

Introduction

Advances in endoscopic instrumentations and fiber optics made hysteroscopy an important diagnostic and therapeutic tool for patients with intrauterine diseases. Hysteroscopy provides detailed observation and optional management of intrauterine lesions, thus constituting a valuable gynecologic procedure [1].Many patients require cervical dilatation prior to hysteroscopy, which might lead to considerable traumatization of tissues especially in women with firmly closed rigid cervix. Furthermore, complicated cervical dilatation is attended by the risk of lacerations caused by the tenaculum, the creation of false passages and an increased risk of uterine perforation especially in nulliparous and postmenopausal women [2–4].

Ripening or softening of the uterine cervical tissue is a complex process recommended before procedures where intrauterine manipulations either for diagnostic or therapeutic purposes are needed [5]. Cervical ripening can be achieved in various ways, mechanically and biologically with agents such as prostaglandins, antiprogestins or nitric oxide donors, although prostaglandins are the most commonly used agent for cervical ripening [6]. Misoprostol, a prostaglandin E1 analogue (PGE1) was first approved in 1988 by the US Food and Drug Administration for prevention and treatment of gastric ulcer induced by nonsteroidal anti-inflammatory drugs, and because of its cervical ripening and uterotonic activity effects, it has been used prior to hysteroscopy in order to reduce the complications occurring during the dilatation procedures [7, 8]. The routes of administration can be oral, vaginal or sublingual. However, it is still unclear which route is more effective for cervical dilatation before transcervical procedures in non pregnant premenopausal women [9]. This study evaluated the effect of misoprostol, given preoperatively sublingually or rectally, on intraoperative and postoperative outcomes during hysteroscopic procedures in premenstmal non-pregnant women.

Subjects and methods

The approval of the official ethical committee of the faculty of medicine was granted before the research commenced. From October 2009 until September 2010, 212 premeno-pausal patients scheduled for hysteroscopic procedures were recruited from the outpatient Gynecology clinic of our university hospital by two senior staff physicians. Indications for hysteroscopy were: infertility work-up ($n=98$), abnormal uterine bleeding ($n=102$) and uterine abnormality (uterine septum, $n=7$) and endometrial polyp ($n=5$). All eligible subjects were non-pregnant, who had their last menstrual period within the last 2 months. However, those with untreated genital infection, allergy to prostaglandins or ongoing pregnancy were excluded. A fully informed consent was obtained from all participants.

All participants underwent a physical examination and detailed medical obstetric and gynecologic histories were obtained. Women were randomly allocated into three groups by another senior staff researcher using the online researcher randomizer software (www.randomizer.org/form.htm]: group 1 ($n=71$), sublingual misoprostol (400 µg) (two tablets, cytotec 200 µg/tablet, a synthetic prostaglandin E_1 analog; Searle, England) was given 2 h before the procedure. In group 2 ($n=71$), rectal misoprostol 400 µg was given 2 h before the procedure. In group 3 ($n=70$; control group), no medications were given. There were no dropouts.

The primary outcome measures were the ease of cervical dilatation recorded on a 5-point Likert scale [10] by the subjective assessment of the performing surgeon and Hegar size that could be first inserted with feeling of resistance. Secondary outcome measures included the duration of cervical dilatation up to Hegar 6, potential intraoperative complications as cervical laceration and postoperative complications as pain (cramps), vomiting, diarrhea, bleed-ing and pyrexia.

Surgical procedure

All hysteroscopic procedures were performed by the first author. All patients were in the proliferative phase of the menstrual cycle. General anesthesia was used. A standard, rigid, 9-mm hysteroscope with a 30° forward-oblique lens was used (Karl Storz GmbH, Tuttlingen, Germany). Serial cervical dilatation was done starting from Hegar 1 dilator. For diagnostic purposes, if the endocervical canal was tight, the cervix was dilated to Hegar 6. If the operative sheath

was required, the cervix was dilated to Hegar 9. Normal saline solution was used as a distention medium for diagnostic procedures, whereas 1.5% Glycine was used with the monopolar energy.

Statistical methodology

Using a one-tailed test with an alpha level of 0.50 and a 90% power, the sample size was calculated to be a total of 195 patients, i.e., 65 patient per group. Data were collected, coded and entered into IBM compatible computer, using SPSS version 12 for windows. Qualitative variables were expressed as the number and percentage, while the quantitative variables were expressed as the mean and standard deviation. Comparison of means was performed using the one-way ANOVA as a parametric test or Kruskal–Wallis test as a non-parametric test. Frequency distributions between categorical variables among the three groups were compared using the χ^2 test. The 5% level of significance was chosen.

Findings

Patients' characteristics were comparable in terms of age, parity, body mass index (BMI) and the number of patients with previous cervical dilatation (Table 1). Different hysteroscopic procedures were done as indicated to the three random groups. The difference between the studied groups in terms of the primary and secondary outcome measures is shown in Table 2 and Fig. 1. The adverse effects in the present study were abdominal pain due to cramp and bleeding that were significantly greater in the misoprostol groups compared to control group ($P=0.002$ and $P=0.003$, respectively). Other adverse effects in the form of vomiting, diarrhea and pyrexia occurred only in misoprostol groups and were significant in sublingual misoprostol group compared to rectal one ($P=0.003$, $P=0.003$ and $P=0.023$, respectively; Table 3). Mean time of surgery was 32.55 ± 11.42, 32.89 ± 12.65, and 33.25 ± 15.55 min in groups 1, 2 and 3, respectively, which showed no significant difference.

Discussion

Prostaglandins had been shown to be effective for cervical ripening in non-pregnant women undergoing hysteroscopic procedures being administered orally or vaginally [11–13]. However, misoprostol use via rectal or sublingual route for the same indication was not thoroughly studied and there is scarce evidence to support or decline such role. Hence it was considered worthwhile to investigate such role in this work.

Table 1 Patients' characteristics

		GI (n=71)	G2 (n=71)	G3 (n=70)	F or χ^2	P	LSD
	Age (years)						
	Mean ± SD	29±4.3	29±4.21	29.9±5.05	F=1.03	0.22	N.S.
	Range	22–37	22–37	22–44			
	Parity						
	Mean ± SD	0.90±1.21	0.9±1.43	0.79±1.16	F=2.22	0.109	N.S.
	Range	0–4	0–5	0–5			
	BMI (kg/m^2)						
	Mean ± SD	27.35±2.76	25.7±2.91	25.6±3.14	F=2.66	0.101	N.S.
	Range	23.5–36	19–31	19–33.5			
N.S. not significant, *SD* standard deviation, *LSD* least significant difference	Previous surgery No. (%)	18 (25.35)	15 (21.27)	17 (24.29)	χ^2=1.036	0.411	N.S.

In the present study, sublingual and rectal misoprostol groups were associated with easy cervical dilatation as well as, significantly shorter time to dilate to Hegar 6. We used 400 μg misoprostol rectally or sublingually 2 h before hysteroscopy based on the studies of pregnancy termination [14, 15]. The plasma concentration of misoprostol biologically active metabolite peaks less than 30 min after oral or sublingual administration and 1 h after the vaginal one, then it gradually decreases [16]. The systemic bioavailability of sublingually administered misoprostol is significantly better than oral or vaginal routes [16]. Rectally administered misoprostol is associated with a qualitatively similar absorption curve as that vaginally administered but with lower bioavailability [17]. Also, studies have found that higher doses of misoprostol did not provide greater cervical response than lower dosages [15]. Ngai et al. [18] studied the effect of 400 μg oral misoprostol on premenopausal women undergoing hysteroscopy for infertility and demonstrated that the cumulative forces required to dilate the cervix were 61% lower in misoprostol group compared to

placebo and the mean baseline cervical width was significantly greater in the misoprostol group. The same was also observed by Batukan et al. [19]. Similarly, Preutthipan and Herabutya [20] evaluated the effectiveness of 200 μg vaginal misoprostol on cervical dilatation in non-pregnant premenopausal women undergoing hysteroscopy and found that the mean baseline cervical width was significantly greater and the mean time of cervical dilatation to Hegar 9 was significantly shorter after misoprostol compared to placebo. They also mentioned more cervical tears in the control group. Similar results were reported by Singh et al. [12] and Choksuchat et al. [13]. Only a few studies evaluated the effectiveness of sublingual misoprostol for cervical ripening in non-pregnant premenopausal women undergoing hysteroscopy. In agreement, Mulayim et al. [21] compared the effectiveness of 200 μg sublingual misoprostol vs. placebo and found that less patients needed cervical dilatation in the misoprostol group whereas, the duration of dilatation was longer in the placebo group. Also, Lee et al. [22] compared sublingual to oral/vaginal misoprostol

Table 2 Main outcome measures

		GI (n=71)	G2 (n=71)	G3 (n=70)	F or χ^2	P	LSD
	Primary outcome measures						
	Ease of cervical dilatation						
	Mean ± SD	2.63±0.95	2.03±0.74	2.97±0.81	F=4.65	0.035*	2#3
	Range	1–5	1–3	2–5			
	Baseline cervical width						
	Mean ± SD	4.25±0.98	4.27±0.79	3.22±1.03	F=4.05	0.038*	1,2#3
	Range	2.5–6.5	2–5.5	1–5			
	Secondary outcome measures						
Ease of cervical dilatation is scored from 1 to 5 on a Likert scale, with 1 being easier than normal and 5 more difficult than normal	Time to Hegar 6 (s)						
	Mean ± SD	63.77±9.69	63.24±9.03	73.24±11.15	F=6.98	0.021*	1,2#3
	Range	45–85	45–85	55–95			
SD standard deviation	Cervical lacerations						
*Significant at *P*<0.05	n (%)	3 (4.23)	1 (1.4)	9 (12.85)	χ^2=5.38	0.02*	2#3

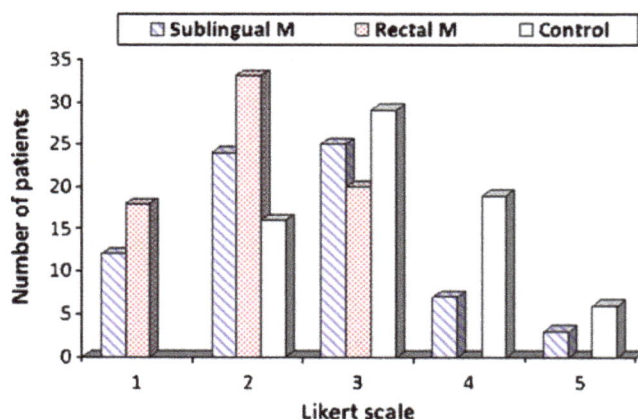

Fig. 1 Ease of cervical dilatation in the studied groups on a Likert Scale

before hysteroscopic procedures in non-pregnant premenopausal women. They concluded that the preoperative cervical width and time to Hegar 10 were comparable among the three groups. In addition, the sublingual route was effective when compared with the vaginal and the oral routes for pregnancy termination [23, 24]. However, to our knowledge, there have been no published studies comparing sublingual to other routes (including rectal) in non-pregnant premenopausal women undergoing hysteroscopy.

In the present study, rectally administered misoprostol was as effective as sublingual misoprostol in producing cervical ripening during hysteroscopy with ease cervical dilatation and shorter time to dilatation to Hegar 6. Since the rectal misoprostol has similar absorption curve as the vaginal one, therefore, it is expected to behave in a similar manner as the vaginally administered misoprostol with the added advantage of shorter time of administration before hysteroscopic procedures (2 vs. 6–12 h) and avoidance of instrument interferences with tablet residue. In contrast to the present results, Bisharah et al. [25] tested sublingual misoprostol (100 μg) 12 h before hysteroscopy against placebo in a cohort of 40 patients, they pointed no difference between the two groups in terms of cervical width and time to dilate to Hegar 9. This might be

attributed to leuprolide's hypoestrogenic effect, to which patients were subjected 4 weeks before the procedures. Also, Healey et al. [26] studied 64 premenopausal women and found no improvement in baseline cervical width and time required to dilate the cervix with oral misoprostol 12 h before diagnostic hysteroscopy compared to placebo. This might be explained by a long interval between drug intake and hysteroscopic procedure.

In the present study, the incidence of cervical lacerations was significantly lower in misoprostol groups, unlike the adverse effects, namely; pain and bleeding, which were significantly more severe with misoprostol. The occurrence of abdominal pain after misoprostol might be attributed to the uterotonic activity of prostaglandins inducing uterine contractions. The reduction in the incidence of cervical laceration after misoprostol was also confirmed by Preutthipan and Herabutya [20]. Also, some authors believed that the severity of the adverse effect after misoprostol varies considerably and are often not correlated with dosage, interval of use or route of administration [27]. Lee et al. [22] reported adverse effects in the form of cramp (10.6%), bleeding (4.3%), nausea (4.3%) and shivering (2.1%) after 400 μg sublingual misoprostol 2–4 h prior to hysteroscopy. Also, Bisharah et al. [25] found mild abdominal cramp (20%) and vaginal bleeding (20%) after 100 μg sublingual misoprostol 12 h prior to hysteroscopy.

Conclusion

In premenopausal non-pregnant women, misoprostol appears to be a promising cervical ripening agent prior to hysteroscopy, being safe, effective and cheap. Its use led to ease of cervical dilatation, with a short time of dilatation to Hegar 6 and with minimal cervical laceration. Rectal misoprostol (400 μg) was as effective as the 400 μg sublingual one when given 2 h before hysteroscopy with the added advantage over oral or vaginal misoprostol of being administered shortly before hysteroscopy and avoidance of instrument interference

Table 3 Adverse effects of sublingual and rectal misoprostol groups vs. control group

	G1		G2		G3		χ^2	P	LSD
	n	%	n	%	n	%			
Pain (cramps)	27	38.03	30	42.25	3	4.29	15.98	0.002*	1,2#3
Bleeding	10	14.08	9	12.68	2	2.86	8.98	0.003*	1,2#3
Vomiting	18	25.35	6	8.45	0	0.00	8.25	0.003*	2,3#1
									2#1
Diarrhea	18	25.35	6	8.45	0	0.00	8.25	0.003*	2,3#1
									2#1
Pyrexia	6	8.45	0	0.00	0	0.00	5.65	0.023*	1#2.3

*Significant at P<0.05 level

with tablet residue. The adverse effects after rectal misoprostol appear to be less when compared with the sublingual route. Further studies are required on a large number of women to reassess the use of sublingual and rectal misoprostol on non-pregnant premenopausal women undergoing hysteroscopy.

Acknowledgements The authors thank the University of Alexandria for funding most of the stages of this study. The study was entirely funded by Alexandria University-administered research funds, together with the Obstetrics and Gynecology Department's own funds.

Authors' contribution F. Moiety designed the study, operated on all the patients, supervised the analysis and interpreted the results. A. Azzam performed the statistical analysis and contributed to study design and interpretation. All authors have approved the final version.

Conflicts of interest The authors report no conflicts of interest. The authors alone are responsible for the content and writing of the paper.

References

1. Preutthipan S, Herabutya Y (1999) A randomized controlled trial of vaginal misoprostol for cervical priming before hysteroscopy. Obstet Gynecol 94(3):427–430
2. Loffer FD (1995) Complications of hysteroscopy: their causes, prevention and correction. J Am Assoc Gynecol laparosc 3:11–26
3. Bradely LD (2002) Complications in hysteroscopy: prevention, treatment and legal risk. Curr Opin Obstet Gynecol 14:409–415
4. Lieng M, Qvigstad E, Sandvik L, Jorgensen H, Langeorekke A, Istre O (2007) Hysteroscopic resection of symptomatic and asymptomatic endometrial polyps. J Minim Invasive Gynecol 14:189–194
5. Stjernholm-Vladic Y, Stygar D, Mansson C, Masironi B, Akerberg S, Wang H et al (2004) Factors involved in the inflammatory events of cervical ripening in humans. Reprod Biol Endocrinol 2:74–78
6. Blanchard K, Clark S, Winikoff B, Gaines G, Kabai G, Shannon C (2002) Misoprostol for women's health. Obstet Gynecol 99:316–332
7. Garris RE, Kirkwood CF (1989) Misoprostol: a prostaglandin E_1 analogue. Clin Pharm 8:627–644
8. Crane JM, Healy S (2006) Use of misoprostol before hysteroscopy: a systemic review. J Obstet Gynecol Can 28:373–479
9. Darwish AM, Ahmad AM, Mohammad AM (2004) Cervical priming prior to operative hysteroscopy: a randomized comparison of laminaria versus misoprostol. Hum Reprod 19:2391–2394
10. Likert R (1932) A Technique for the Measurement of Attitudes. Arch Psychol 140:1–55
11. Waddell G, Desindes S, Takser L, Beauchemin MC, Bessette P (2008) Cervical ripening using vaginal misoprostol before hysteroscopy: a double-blind randomized trial. J Minim Invasive Gynecol 15:739–744
12. Singh N, Ghosh B, Naha M, Mittal S (2009) Vaginal misoprostol for cervical priming prior to diagnostic hysteroscopy: efficacy, safety and patient satisfaction, a randomized controlled trial. Arch Gynecol Obstet 279:37–40
13. Choksuchat C, Cheewadhanaraks S, Getpook C, Wootipoom V, Dhanavoravibul K (2006) Misoprostol for cervical ripening in non-pregnant women: a randomized double-blind controlled trial of oral versus vaginal regimens. Hum Reprod 21:2167–2170
14. Hamoda H, Ashok PW, Flett GM, Templeton A (2004) A randomized controlled comparison of sublingual and vaginal administration of misoprostol for cervical ripening before first-trimester surgical abortion. Am J Obstet Gynecol 190:55–59
15. Saxena P, Salhan S, Sarda N (2004) Comparison between the sublingual and oral route of misoprostol for pre-abortion cervical priming in first-trimester abortions. Hum Reprod 19:77–80
16. Tang OS, Schweer H, Seyberth HW, Lee SW, Ho PC (2002) Pharmacokinetics of different routs of administration of misoprostol. Hum Reprod 17:332–336
17. Khan RU, El-Refaey H, Sharma S, Sooranna D, Stafford M (2004) Oral, rectal and vaginal pharmacokinetics of misoprostol. Obstet Gynecol 103(5):866–870
18. Ngai WN, Chan YM, Liu KL, Ho PC (1997) Oral misoprostol for cervical priming in non-pregnant women. Hum Reprod 12:2373–2375
19. Batukan C, Ozgun MT, Ozcelik B, Aygen E, Sahin Y, Turkyilmaz C (2008) Cervical ripening before operative hysteroscopy in premenopausal women: a randomized, double-blind, placebo-controlled comparison of vaginal and oral misoprostol. Fertil Steril 89:966–9673
20. Preutthipan S, Herabutya Y (2000) Vaginal misoprostol for cervical priming before operative hysteroscopy: a randomized controlled trial. Obstet Gynecol 96:890–894
21. Mulayim B, Celik NY, Onalan G, Bagis T, Zeyneloglu HB (2010) Sublingual misoprostol for cervical ripening before diagnostic hysteroscopy in premenopausal women: a randomized, double blind, placebo-controlled trial. Fertil Steril 93(7):2400–2404
22. Lee YY, Kim TJ, Kang H, Choi CH, Lee JW, Kim BG, Bae DS (2010) The use of misoprostol before hysteroscopic surgery in non-pregnant premenopausal women: a randomized comparison of sublingual, oral and vaginal administrations. Hum Reprod 25 (8):1942–1948
23. Carbonell-Esteve JL, Mari JM, Valero F, Llorente M, Salvador I, Varela K, Leal P, Candel A, Tudela A, Serrano M et al (2006) Sublingual versus vaginal misoprostol (400 microg) for cervical ripening in first-trimester abortion: a randomized trial. Contraception 74:328–323
24. Aronsson A, Helstrom L, Gemzell-Danielsson K (2004) Sublingual compared with oral misoprostol for cervical dilatation prior to vacuum aspiration: a randomized comparison. Contraception 69:165–169
25. Bisharah M, Al-Fozan H, Tulandi T (2003) A randomized trial of sublingual misoprostol for cervical priming before hysteroscopy. J Am Assoc Gynecol Laparosc 10(3):390–391
26. Healey S, Butler B, Kum FN, Dunne J, Hutchens D, Crane JM (2007) A randomized trial of oral misoprostol in premenopausal women before hysteroscopy. J Obstet Gynecol Can 29(8):648–652
27. Choksuchat C. Clinical use of misoprostol in non-pregnant women: review article. K Minim Invasive Gynecol 2010; 17(4): 449: 55

16

The relevance of endometrial polyps: a bibliometric study

Pietro Gambadauro · Rafael Torrejón

Abstract The aim of this study was to explore and describe the status and trends of scientific literature on endometrial polyps. We have conducted a systematic search for publications related to endometrial polyps from 1982 to 2012 using Scopus. The original search was refined with the additional keywords: "infertility", "bleeding", and "cancer". We have collected and analyzed quantitative data on number of publications, journals, language, and origin of each article. Descriptive statistics and charts were used to analyze data and provide information on publication trends. Out of a database of 12,125,345 articles published in the past 30 years, our systematic search retrieved 1,144 relevant publications. The amount of articles/year related to endometrial polyps has been significantly growing throughout the study period (1982–1996, 14±11.988; 1997–2012, 58.38± 11.506; $p<0.0001$). A similar positive trend is observed for relative number of yearly publications (% retrieved/indexed; 1982–1996, 0.0044 %±0.0035; 1997– 2012, 0.0127 %±0.0025; $p<0.0001$). The proportion of articles related to "infertility" and "bleeding" has been growing more than that of papers related to "cancer". English is the dominant language (79 %), and the USA is the most prolific country (19 %), followed by Italy (8 %) and the UK (7,8 %). During the last 5 years, *Gynecological Surgery* has been the journal with the highest proportion of publications on endometrial polyps (2.11 % of all its articles). In conclusion, the publications related to endometrial polyps have increased steadily during the last 30 years, particularly those related to bleeding and infertility. Not all the journals publishing regularly on "endometrial polyps" are indexed in Medline/Pubmed. Scholars interested in this field should consider comprehensive bibliographic search strategies.

Keywords Endometrial polyps · Hysteroscopy · Infertility · Abnormal uterine bleeding · Endometrial cancer · Bibliometrics

Background

Endometrial polyps are commonly described as sessile or pedunculated overgrowths of the endometrial layer. The clinical relevance of endometrial polyps is linked to abnormal uterine bleeding, infertility, and the risk of endometrial atypia and cancer [1–3]. Scientific advances during the last decades have contributed to the evidence-based establishment of reliable tools for diagnosis and treatment of endometrial polyps, such as transvaginal ultrasound and hysteroscopy [4, 5]. Nevertheless, the clinical relevance of endometrial polyps, particularly in asymptomatic and premenopausal women, is debated and expectancy has been advocated, keeping in mind that one out of four polyps can regress without treatment [6].

We have conducted this bibliometric study in order to explore, analyze, and describe the current status and past trends of scientific literature on endometrial polyps.

Methods

We have conducted a systematic, electronic search through scientific literature published between 1982 and 2012, with the aim to retrieve publications related to the topic of endometrial polyps. In order to achieve our goal, we searched the Scopus database (http://www.scopus.com) during autumn 2012 for the terms "endometrial polyps", "endometrial polyp", and "hysteroscopic polypectomy". Our search strategy was based on the following query:

P. Gambadauro (✉)
Centre for Reproduction,
Department of Obstetrics and Gynaecology,
Uppsala University Hospital, 751 85 Uppsala, Sweden
e-mail: gambadauro@gmail.com

R. Torrejón
Department of Obstetrics and Gynaecology, "Puerta del Mar"
University Hospital, University of Cádiz, Cádiz, Spain

TITLE-ABS-KEY("endometrial polyps" OR "endometrial polyp" OR "hysteroscopic polypectomy") AND SUBJAREA(medi OR nurs OR heal) AND PUBYEAR > 1981 AND (EXCLUDE(SUBJAREA, "VETE"))

This original search was then refined with the additional keywords: "infertility", "bleeding", and "cancer". Data were extracted from the original and refined searches regarding number of retrieved publications, source journals, the language, and the geographical origin of each article. The number of retrieved articles per year was also normalized to the total number of articles indexed by Scopus. We divided the retrieved articles into two different periods (1982–1996 and 1997–2012) in order to allow for comparative analysis. For source journals analysis, we focused on the period 2007–2012, in order to provide recent data.

All data were initially stored on a custom-made, online electronic database, based on Google Drive spreadsheets (http://drive.google.com). This allowed simultaneous access to both authors [7].

Descriptive statistics and charts were used to analyze data and provide information on publication trends. Student's *t* test and Fisher's exact test were used were appropriate and differences were considered statistically significant with

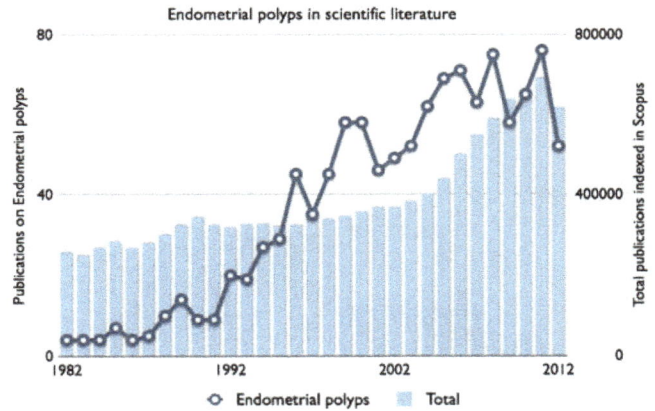

Fig. 1 Our systematic search (Autumn 2012, Scopus) shows a growing trend of publications retrieved with the keywords "endometrial polyps", "endometrial polyp", or "hysteroscopic polypectomy" throughout the last 30 years

a *p* value <0.05. The software Numbers '09 v2.2 (Apple Inc.) and SPSS v20 (IBM) for Mac OSX were respectively used for charts and statistical calculations. The global map on publications was generated on Google Drive.

Findings

Our systematic search retrieved 1,144 relevant publications out of a database of 12,125,345 articles published in the past 30 years in the subject area of interest. An overview of descriptive findings is given in Table 1.

Analysis of the yearly publication trends reveals how the absolute number of articles related to endometrial polyps has been growing since 1982 (Fig. 1). Significantly more articles per year have been published after 1997 (1982–1996, 14 ± 11.988; 1997–2012, 58.38 ± 11.506; $p<0.0001$). A similar statistically significant difference is found when normalizing the yearly amount of retrieved articles to the

Table 1 Summary of findings

	N of articles	Percent
Total	1,144	(0.009[a])
1982–1996	210	18.36
1997–2012	934	81.64
Language		
English	913	79
Other	231	21
Geographical distribution per country[b]		
United States	213	19.0
Italy	90	8.0
United Kingdom	88	7.8
Turkey	79	7.0
Spain	63	5.6
Others	589	52.6
Geographical distribution per continent[b]		
Europe	513	45.7
Asia	260	23.1
North America	236	21
South America	68	6
Africa	23	2
Oceania	22	1.9
Refined search		
"cancer"	431	37
"bleeding"	376	33
"infertility"	132	11.5

[a]Percent of articles retrieved out of the total amount of articles (*n* 12,125,345) indexed by Scopus in the same period and subject areas
[b]Calculated on 1,122 articles with retrievable information on source country

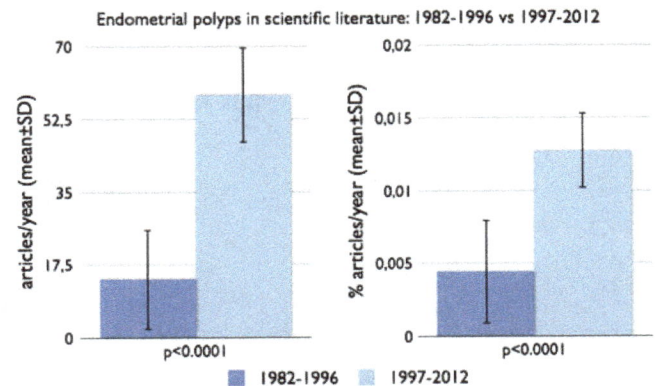

Fig. 2 This figure shows a significant increase of mean yearly publications related to endometrial polyps after 1997. The *chart on the right* shows the yearly publications normalized to the total amount of articles indexed in Scopus

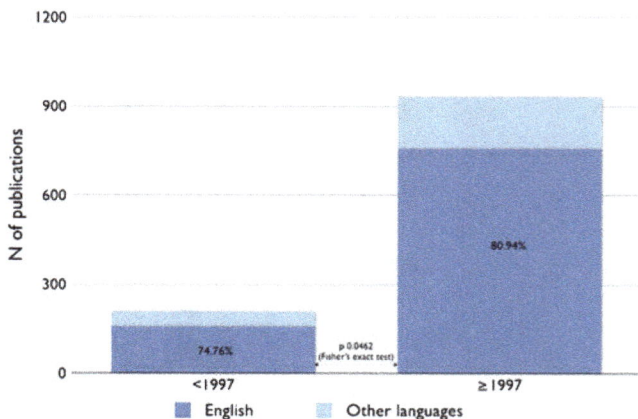

Fig. 3 English is the dominant language in this field of research

total of publications indexed by Scopus (1982–1996, 0.0044 %±0.0035; 1997–2012, 0.0127 %±0.0025; $p <$ 0.0001; Fig. 2).

English was dominant over other languages (913/1,144 publications; 79 %). The proportion of publications in English has significantly increased from 74.76 % in the period 1982–1996, to 80.94 % in the period 1997–2012 (157/210 vs 756/934; $p = 0.046$; Fig. 3).

The USA is by far the most prolific country (19 %), followed by Italy (8 %) and the UK (7,8 %). While 65 countries contributed with at least one publication, nearly half of all the retrieved articles originated from the five top countries: US, Italy, UK, Turkey, and Spain (Table 1). The global geographic distribution is shown in Fig. 4.

After refining our original search query with three additional keywords, we observed that more articles were retrieved by the keywords "cancer" and "bleeding" (respectively 37 and 33 %) respect to "infertility" (11.5 %). A publication trend analysis shows how the proportion of articles related to "infertility" and "bleeding" has been growing more than that of papers related to "cancer" during the last 30 years (Fig. 5). Interestingly, the geographical distribution of publications is more even in the case of papers dealing with "infertility", where Turkey, USA, UK, and Italy have got similar shares (respectively 17, 15, 10, and 10 %).

A total of 160 publishing sources have contributed articles included in this study. The journal mostly represented in our search results is *Obstetrics and Gynecology* with a total of 37 publications retrieved belonging to the period 1982–2012. When restricting our search to recent literature (from 2007), *Fertility and Sterility* was the journal with most publications retrieved (25/389; 6.4 %), followed by the *Journal of Minimally Invasive Gynecology* (18/389; 4.62 %) and the *European Journal of Gynaecological Oncology* (14/389; 3.59 %). After normalizing the number of retrieved publications to the total amount of articles indexed for each journal, *Gynecological Surgery* is the journal with the highest proportion of publications on endometrial polyps (2.11 % of all its articles; Table 2).

Discussion

We have conducted this study in order to explore the scientific relevance of endometrial polyps by means of a quantitative bibliometric analysis of scientific literature published from 1982 to 2012.

Our results show that both the absolute and relative number of publications related to endometrial polyps have increased steadily during the last 30 years, testifying growing interest in the

Fig. 4 Geographical distribution of publications related to endometrial polyps, by country, 1982–2012 (autumn 2012, Scopus)

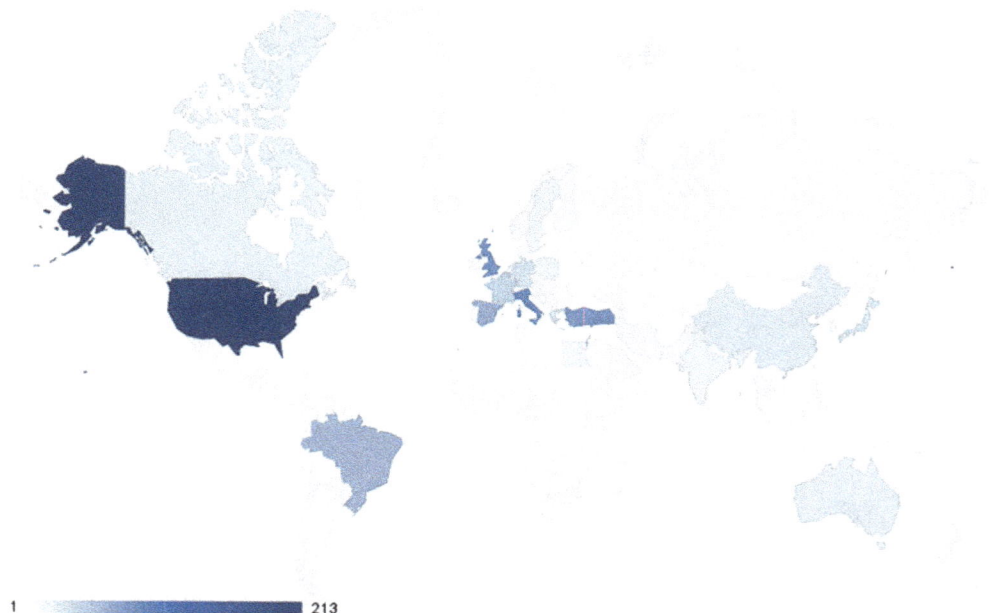

Fig. 5 We have refined our main Scopus search with the additional keywords "cancer", "bleeding", and "infertility". This graph shows the publication trends per each one of those additional keyword (autumn 2012, Scopus)

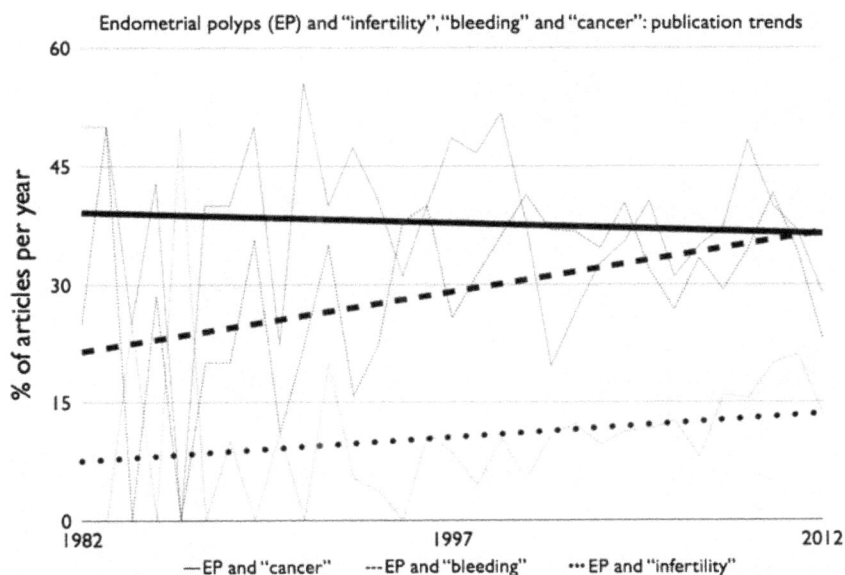

subject. During the same period great progress has occurred concerning the development of minimally invasive methods for diagnosis and treatment of intrauterine pathology [8, 9]. We are now simply better than 30 years ago at looking inside the uterus and operating effectively, and with minimal invasiveness, conditions which in the past required a hysterectomy [10–12]. Endometrial polyps represent just one example of the different abnormalities of the uterine cavity frequently related to abnormal bleeding, infertility, or cancer risk [13]. We might speculate that the increase in the clinical use of minimally invasive methods for diagnosis and treatment [14] might have played a role in the increase of scientific interest on endometrial polyps, but this should be confirmed by other studies.

Another fact emerging from our study is the uneven linguistic and geographical distribution of publications in

Table 2 The 12 top publishing journals in the field of "endometrial polyps" (2007–2012)

Journal	Retrieved	Indexed	Percent
Fertil Steril	25	5,716	0.44
J Minim Invasive Gynecol	18	1,080	1.67
Eur J Gynaecol Oncol	14	945	1.48
Arch Gynecol Obstet	13	2,445	0.53
Eur J Obstet Gynecol Reprod Biol	13	2,129	0.61
Gynecol Surgery	11	519	2.12
Menopause	10	1,275	0.78
Int J Gynec Pathol	10	569	1.76
Ultrasound Obstet Gynecol	8	1,657	0.48
Am J Obstet Gynecol	7	3,785	0.18
J Obstet Gynaecol	7	1,679	0.42
Reprod Biomed Online	7	1,576	0.44

the field of endometrial polyps. This is certainly not unexpected, but deserves a few comments.

English is the predominant language in this field of research, and its relevance has been increasing throughout the study period. This is in line with common knowledge and several other reports, and might only partially be justified by the fact that two of the five top countries in our study have English as official language (USA and UK). English is universally acknowledged as the *lingua franca* in science and the language of most medical literature. As a result, authors and researchers choose to submit the results of their research to journals published in English, since those usually have broader audience and better bibliometric indicators, such as the *impact factor* [15]. In spite of well-grounded criticism [16], the impact factor is still misused to evaluate a researcher's performance, and publishing on high impact factor journals might be as important as publishing "good" research in order to disseminate your own work and get cited by colleagues [17].

We have also analyzed the geographical distribution of research reports in the field of endometrial polyps. While as many as 65 countries, spread throughout the five continents, have contributed to scientific literature on this topic, only few of them have originated the majority of all articles. A geographical bias in publication patterns has been previously reported in other fields of research [18–20]. Such circumstance might be related to local interests in this field, or socioeconomic factors such as population, investments in research, or gross domestic product (total and per capita). We cannot speculate on those hypotheses since they fall beyond the goals of this observational study.

Endometrial polyps are commonly associated with abnormal bleeding, infertility, and risk of endometrial atypia/cancer. The relevance of those associations is reflected in scientific literature, where more than 1/3 of articles is linked to the keywords "cancer" and "bleeding". Moreover, the association with "bleeding" and "infertility" is acquiring relevance, as demonstrated by our trend analysis. Interestingly, the USA loses the predominance as source country in the specific subset of articles retrieved by the keyword "infertility".

We would like to point out that several online tools exist to assist us in the search for scientific literature for bibliometrics. The most commonly used are PubMed (by the United States National Library of Medicine, NLM; http://www.pubmed.com), Web of Science (by Thomson Reuters; http://http:// wokinfo.com/wok/products_tools/multidisciplinary/ webofscience/) and, as in our case, Scopus (by Elsevier B.V.; http://www.scopus.com). The latter was a natural choice for us since we are familiar with its system of queries that, in our opinion, facilitates searching by keywords and result retrieval. Moreover, Scopus covers a wider journal range than the other databases [21]. For instance, by searching on PubMed we would have missed the publications of *Gynecological Surgery*, journal of the European Society for Gynecological Endoscopy, which is not currently indexed on MEDLINE. This would have compromised our analysis, since we found that *Gynecological Surgery* dedicates more of its editorial space than other journals to "endometrial polyps". A logical consequence of this finding would be a strong recommendation for scholars conducting research on endometrial polyps to consider searching for references in more comprehensive databases than PubMed, as already recommended in other research fields [22].

Finally, our search strategy was meant to use only electronic queries, and its results are depending on the quality of indexing [23]. It seems reasonable to mention how hand-searching, possibly with the help of desktop search engines [24], might be the best complement of database searching in order to increase the accuracy of the results particularly when qualitative analysis is the goal.

Conclusions

The relevance of endometrial polyps as a scientific subject is growing, as shown by a positive trend in related publications during the last 30 years. This area of research is dominated by Europe, although the USA is the country publishing most articles.

Several journals contribute articles to endometrial-polyps-related research, some of them not covered by the most popular database, PubMed. Researchers in this field should adopt comprehensive search strategies in order to retrieve information also from journals not indexed by PubMed.

Acknowledgement Pietro Gambadauro had the idea and designed the study. Both author's contributed to the acquisition, analysis and interpretation of data. Pietro Gambadauro wrote all drafts of the manuscript and both author's revised it critically for important intellectual content, and gave their final approval of the version to be published.

Declaration of interest The authors report no conflicts of interest. The authors alone are responsible for the content and writing of the paper.

References

1. Lieng M, Istre O, Sandvik L, Qvigstad E (2009) Prevalence, 1-year regression rate, and clinical significance of asymptomatic endometrial polyps: cross-sectional study. J Minim Invasive Gynecol 16 (4):465–471

2. Afifi K, Anand S, Nallapeta S, Gelbaya TA (2010) Management of endometrial polyps in subfertile women: a systematic review. Eur J Obstet Gynecol Reprod Biol 151(2):117–121

3. Lee SC, Kaunitz AM, Sanchez-Ramos L, Rhatigan RM (2010) The oncogenic potential of endometrial polyps: a systematic review and meta-analysis. Obstet Gynecol 116(5):1197–1205

4. Salim S, Won H, Nesbitt-Hawes E, Campbell N, Abbott J (2011) Diagnosis and management of endometrial polyps: a critical review of the literature. J Minim Invasive Gynecol 18 (5):569–581

5. Sharma M, Taylor A, Magos A (2004) Management of endometrial polyps: a clinical review. Rev Gynaecol Pract 4(1):1–6

6. American Association of Gynecologic Laparoscopists (2012) AAGL practice report: practice guidelines for the diagnosis and management of endometrial polyps. J Minim Invasive Gynecol 19 (1):3–10

7. Gambadauro P, Magos A (2008) Office 2.0: a web 2.0 tool for international collaborative research. Lancet 371(9627):1837–1838

8. Kamel HS, Darwish AM, Mohamed SA (2000) Comparison of transvaginal ultrasonography and vaginal sonohysterography in the detection of endometrial polyps. Acta Obstet Gynecol Scand 79(1):60–64

9. Di Spiezio SA, Taylor A, Tsirkas P, Mastrogamvrakis G, Sharma M, Magos A (2008) Hysteroscopy: a technique for all? Analysis of 5,000 outpatient hysteroscopies. Fertil Steril 89(2):438–443

10. Sharma M, Taylor A, di Spiezio SA, Buck L, Mastrogamvrakis G, Kosmas I, Tsirkas P, Magos A (2005) Outpatient hysteroscopy: traditional versus the 'no-touch' technique. BJOG 112 (7):963–967

11. Gambadauro P, Magos A (2010) Pain control in hysteroscopy. Finesse, not local anaesthesia. BMJ 340:c2097

12. Papalampros P, Gambadauro P, Papadopoulos N, Polyzos D, Chapman L, Magos A (2009) The mini-resectoscope: a new instrument for office hysteroscopic surgery. Acta Obstet Gynecol Scand 88:227–230

13. Marbaix E, Brun JL (2004) Concise survey of endometrial pathologies detected at hysteroscopy. Gynecol Surg 1(3):151–157

14. van Dijk LJEW, Breijer MC, Veersema S, Mol BWJ, Timmermans A (2012) Current practice in the removal of benign endometrial polyps: a Dutch survey. Gynecol Surg 9(2):163–168

15. Lenhard MS, Johnson TR, Himsl I, Ditsch N, Rueckert S, Friese K, Untch M (2006) Obstetrical and gynecological writing and publishing in Europe. Eur J Obstet Gynecol Reprod Biol 129 (2):119–123

16. Gambadauro P, Torrejón R (2007) Impact factor and the quality of research: what is a rose defined by, its name or its scent? Eur J Obstet Gynecol Reprod Biol 134(2):269–270

17. Callaham M, Wears RL, Weber E (2002) Journal prestige, publication bias, and other characteristics associated with citation of published studies in peer-reviewed journals. JAMA 287(21):2847–2850

18. Tutarel O (2002) Geographical distribution of publications in the field of medical education. BMC Med Educ 2:3

19. Boulos MN (2005) On geography and medical journalology: a study of the geographical distribution of articles published in a leading medical informatics journal between 1999 and 2004. Int J Health Geogr 4(1):7

20. Yeung M, Bhandari M (2012) Uneven global distribution of randomized trials in hip fracture surgery. Acta Orthop 83 (4):328–333

21. Falagas ME, Pitsouni EI, Malietzis GA, Pappas G (2008) Comparison of PubMed, Scopus, Web of Science, and Google Scholar: strengths and weaknesses. FASEB J 22(2):338–342

22. Suarez-Almazor ME, Belseck E, Homik J, Dorgan M, Ramos-Remus C (2000) Identifying clinical trials in the medical literature with electronic databases: MEDLINE alone is not enough. Control Clin Trials 21:476–487

23. Dickersin K, Scherer R, Lefebvre C (1994) Identifying relevant studies for systematic reviews. BMJ 309:1286–1291

24. Magos A, Gambadauro P (2005) Desktop search engines: a modern way to hand search in full text. Lancet 366(9481):203–204

A virtual reality simulator for hysteroscopic placement of tubal sterilization micro-inserts: the face and construct validity

Juliënne A. Janse · Sebastiaan Veersema ·
Frank J. Broekmans · Henk W. R. Schreuder

Abstract This study investigated the validity of a virtual reality simulator for hysteroscopic tubal sterilization. Initially performed laparoscopically, the hysteroscopic sterilization method is becoming increasingly popular. An adequate training model could enhance one's skills prior to the start of performing the procedure on the real patient. This prospective study (Canadian Task force II-2) enrolled 69 residents and gynecologists who were divided into three groups, based on vaginoscopic hysteroscopy and Essure® experience level: novices (N=17), intermediates (N=35), and experts (N=17). Participants completed two cases on a virtual reality simulator (EssureSim™) in which four Essure® placements were performed. A questionnaire was completed to assess face validity, and reality scores were given on a 5-point Likert scale. Construct validity was represented by the ability of six simulator-derived parameters to significantly differentiate between different hysteroscopic experience levels. Reality of the sterilization procedure was scored with a median of 5.00 points on a 5-point Likert scale by all participants with prior sterilization experience. Of these participants, 95.5 % indicated the simulator as a useful preparation for real-time Essure® placement. The expert and intermediate group performed both cases significantly faster than novices (p=.001). The novices had a significantly longer path length in comparison to the other groups (p=.006). Analysis of the remaining parameters did not show a persistent ability to differentiate between experience levels. Satisfactory validity was demonstrated for the EssureSim™ by high reality scores and moderate ability to distinguish between different performance levels.

Keywords Hysteroscopy · Training · Sterilization · Essure® · Virtual reality

Background

Female sterilization is the most common method of contraception worldwide [1]. More than 600,000 tubal sterilizations are performed annually in the USA [2]. Initially performed laparoscopically, the hysteroscopic sterilization method is becoming increasingly popular [3, 4].

Hysteroscopy is generally considered as a safe procedure with a low complication rate [5, 6]. Its practice ranges from diagnostics in an outpatient setting to a surgical alternative for many gynecological problems. Teaching hysteroscopy skills traditionally has been based on a mentored model, where trainees are exposed to procedures with the guidance of an experienced teacher. However, in recent years, the surgical volume has been limited by restrictions on resident working hours and less highly skilled teachers are available [7, 8]. This results in difficulties in acquiring sufficient skills in advanced endoscopic surgery [9, 10]. Effective usage of simulation and training models is a possible solution to this problem [9–11].

Development and validation research on training models and simulators has been mainly focused on laparoscopy. Training models allow a surgeon to safely overcome the learning curve of a new technique before practicing on a patient [9, 12, 13]. Virtual reality (VR) simulators especially allow more independent instruction and objective immediate feedback for more reliable, unbiased assessment of

---

All authors contributed extensively to the work presented in this paper.

J. A. Janse (✉) · S. Veersema
Department of Gynecology and Obstetrics, Sint Antonius Hospital
Nieuwegein, Koekoekslaan 1,
3435 CM Nieuwegein, Netherlands
e-mail: julienne.janse@gmail.com

F. J. Broekmans · H. W. R. Schreuder
Division of Woman and Baby, University Medical Center Utrecht,
3508 GA Utrecht, Netherlands

psychomotor skills [9, 12, 14]. In addition, it allows for repeated practice without any risk to patients. Training on a VR system bypasses the ethical concerns associated with practice on animals or cadavers. Besides, many VR systems allow for practice at varying levels of difficulty and across a wide range of scenarios, thus accommodating trainees at many levels [14, 15].

Prior to implementation of a new training tool in a curriculum, evaluation and validation of the simulator and its parameters are mandatory [16–19]. Validity measures whether a simulator is actually teaching or measuring what it is intended to teach or measure [17]. Different aspects of validity exist. Face validity refers to whether the model resembles the task or procedure it is aiming to train for, by determining the opinion of users on realism of the simulation. Objective approaches consist of construct and predictive validity. Construct validity refers to whether the model measures the quality or ability it is supposed to measure [17]. In this regard, the simulator must be able to differentiate between the experienced and the inexperienced surgeon, or in addition, measure improvement in novices' performance by training. Predictive validity is the extent to which the simulator predicts future performance by assessing whether the skills acquired on a simulator actually result in improved skills in patients in the real-time clinical setting [17, 20].

Excellent data are available to support the validity and effectiveness of VR training of surgical skills in general surgery [21–23], urology [20] as well as in gynecology [24, 25]. VR training leads to more efficient movements and less errors, which translates into less operating time and improved patient safety.

In comparison to laparoscopy, little work has been done regarding hysteroscopy training despite its upcoming use and applicability during the last decades. Several training methods have been designed, focusing mainly on the development of physical models and box trainers [26–28]. A collaboration between gynecologists and technicians in Switzerland led to the development of the Hysteroscopic Surgery Simulator System (HystSim™)—a VR simulator for hysteroscopic interventions. Face and construct validity have been established for a diagnostic training module [29, 30]. Recently, a new procedural training module became available by which the Essure® sterilization method can be practiced (EssureSim™).

The hysteroscopic sterilization method by Essure® Permanent Birth Control system (Conceptus; Mountain View, CA, USA) was approved in 2001 by the European Health Office and in 2002 by the U.S. Food and Drug Administration. Micro-inserts placed in both the tubal ostia cause a sterile inflammatory response of the intramural and isthmic parts of the Fallopian tube, thereby occluding the tubes within 3 months. Since the introduction of this method, it is performed by gynecologists around the world and has become an accepted alternative to laparoscopic sterilization.

Initially taught with significant hands-on supervision, the EssureSim™ is developed to train gynecologists who want to start performing this procedure in a more efficient manner and without risks for the patient.

The aim of this study is to determine the face and construct validity of this VR training module for the hysteroscopic placement of tubal sterilization micro-inserts.

Methods

Participants

Between June 2010 and April 2011, 25 ob-gyn residents and 44 consultant gynecologists ($N=69$) were randomly recruited at the Annual Meeting of the Dutch Society of Obstetrics and Gynecology and from a university hospital and a major teaching hospital in the Netherlands.

Given that hysteroscopic sterilization is performed as a type of therapeutic vaginoscopic hysteroscopy, without use of a speculum and tenaculum, three groups were made. This division was based on a combination of Essure® experience level and experience level in therapeutic vaginoscopic hysteroscopy. "Novices" ($N=17$): never performed an Essure® placement nor a therapeutic vaginascopic hysteroscopy, "experts" ($N=17$): performed >25 Essure® placements and >25 therapeutic vaginascopic hysteroscopies, "intermediates" ($N=35$): any experience varying between a novice and expert. The assessment of the participants' experience was made by self-estimated numbers of both procedures.

Equipment

The EssureSim™ consists of an adapted hysteroscope (10-mm resectoscope), an Essure® simulation device, simulation hardware and software (Fig. 1). The simulation software runs on standard laptop hardware (2.40 GHz Intel® Core™ 2 DUO CPU P8600, 2 GB RAM, NVIDIA Quadro FX 2700 M graphic card). The system does not possess haptic feedback. The software contains eight different cases with varying degrees of difficulty.

Face validity

Participants completed a questionnaire immediately after completing the cases on the simulator. It included questions about participants' demographics and experience level in hysteroscopy training, several hysteroscopy procedures, and hysteroscopic sterilization. The opinion of each participant was assessed with 14 questions about the simulator and sterilization module. These questions concerned the realism of the simulation and training capacities, and were presented on a 5-point Likert scale [31]. Additionally, two statements were

Fig. 1 Set up EssureSim™ (with permission of VirtaMed AG)

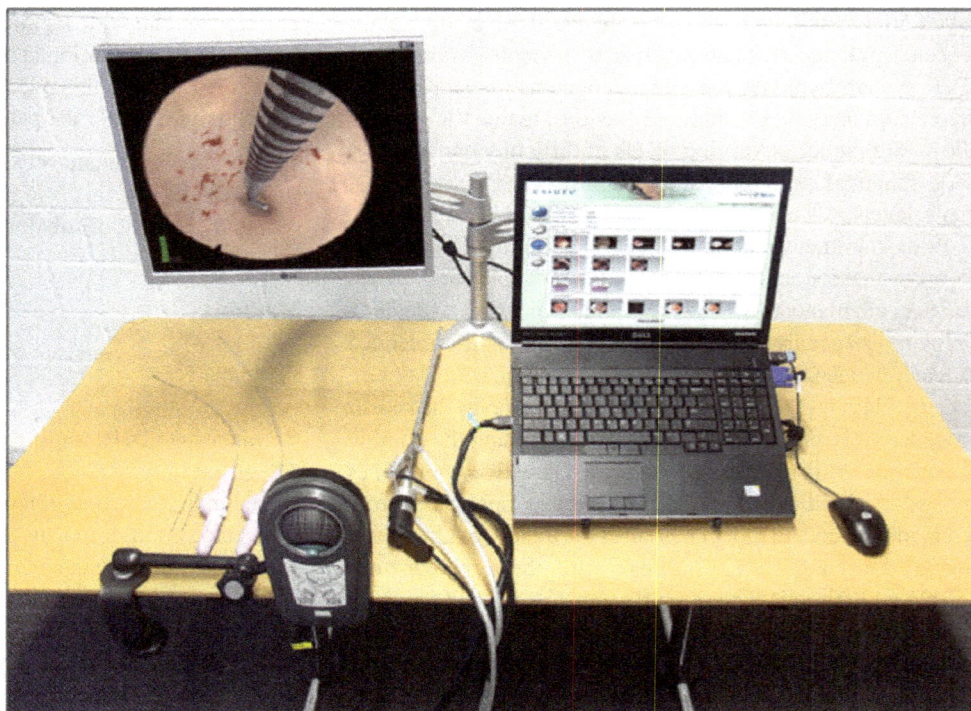

proposed for further opinion inquiry. These were answered with "agree," "disagree," or "no opinion." Face validity was determined by analyzing the opinion of the participants with prior Essure® experience. In this manner, realism and training capacity of the simulator was evaluated only by the participants who had knowledge of the real-time procedure and who could make a comparison between both environments.

Construct validity

To investigate construct validity, the participants performed tasks on the simulator. To all participants, a standard introduction of the simulator and sterilization procedure was given. A familiarization with the VR simulator was executed, consisting of one tubal micro-insert placement in a uterus with normal tubes. In the first case (case 1), the participant performed a bilateral sterilization in a uterus with normal tubes, as shown in the animation (Online Resource 1). The second case (case 2) comprised a bilateral placement in a uterus of a more difficult level, because of the thickened endometrium of this uterus, decreased visibility, and slightly more lateral insertion of the tubes (Online Resource 2). All participants were supervised by one supervisor (J.A.J.), who gave answers to questions and gave instructions if one was not able to proceed.

Case 1 and 2 were used for analysis. Parameters being measured by the simulator and used for data analysis were task time, path length, trauma, patient comfort, amount of distension fluid used, and successful placement. A description

of all parameters used is given in Table 1. These parameters were compared between the different groups for both cases separately, since they were of a different level.

Use of statistics

Data were analyzed using the statistical software package SPSS 17.0 (SPSS, Inc., Chicago, IL). Differences between the general demographics and performances between the three groups were analyzed using the Kruskal–Wallis test for nonparametric data. If the Kruskal–Wallis test resulted in

Table 1 Description of all parameters used

Parameter	Description
Task time	Time of the total procedure, from insertion of scope into cervix to removal of scope, in seconds
Path length	Path length of the tip of the hysteroscope in millimeters
Trauma	Cumulative number of contacts of the scope with the cervix and uterine wall
Patient comfort	Combination of number of trauma and the distension pressure of the fluids exerted on the uterine wall, given on a 10-point scale, 1 = extremely uncomfortable, 10 = no discomfort at all
Correct placement	1 to 8 coils of the micro-insert need to be visible after placement
Distension fluid used	The amount of distension fluid used in milliliters

a significant difference, then a comparison between two separate groups was done using the Mann–Whitney U test with post hoc Dunn's (Bonferroni) correction. To verify the minimum sample size, a power analysis was performed. A total sample of 69 subjects achieves a power of >.80 with the Kruskal–Wallis test with a target significance of .05. The average within-group standard deviation assuming the alternative distribution is 1.0 (PASS 2008 NCSS; LCC, Kayville, UT). A p value of <.05 was considered to be statistically significant. Values are presented as medians with interquartile ranges unless stated otherwise.

Findings

Table 2 shows the general demographics of the participants. A significant difference for age was seen between groups ($p<.05$), while gender and handedness did not differ significantly. Of all participants, one expert and three participants of the intermediate group had been introduced to the HystSim™ at other conference venues.

Face validity

Of the 69 participants, all completed the entire questionnaire. Table 3 summarizes the median values of the scores considering the realism and training capacity of the simulator, awarded by the participants with prior Essure® experience ($N=22$). In the questionnaire, realism of the sterilization procedure was scored with a median of 4.00 points on a 5-point Likert scale. Training capacity of the sterilization procedure was awarded a median of 5.00 points. Of all participants with prior Essure® experience, 100.0 % agreed with the statement that the hysteroscopy simulator offers procedural training of hysteroscopic skills. Furthermore, 95.5 % indicated the training module for the Essure® sterilization method as a useful preparation for real-time placement.

Construct validity

All of the 69 participants completed all cases. Median values of the assessed parameters for case 1 and 2 are shown in Table 4. The simulator was able to differentiate between

Table 2 Baseline characteristics of all participants

	All participants ($N=69$)	Novices ($N=17$)	Intermediates ($N=35$)	Experts ($N=17$)
Age, median in years (IQR)	39.0 (31.5–48.0)	26.0 (25.5–32.5)	41.0 (33.0–52.0)	43.0 (37.5–48.0)
Gender, % male/female	28.6:71.4	17.6:82.4	31.4:68.6	23.5:76.5
Handedness, % right/left	91.3:8.7	82.4:17.6	94.3:5.7	94.1:5.9
Status, % resident/ consultant	36.2:63.8	82.4:17.6	31.4:68.6	0.0:100.0
Hysteroscopy training courses, in hours (%)				
0	20 (29.0)	12 (70.6)	7 (20.0)	1 (5.9)
1–10	29 (42.0)	5 (29.4)	19 (54.3)	5 (29.4)
11–20	15 (21.7)	0	5 (14.3)	10 (58.8)
>20	5 (7.2)	0	4 (11.4)	1 (5.9)
Experience with virtual reality in general, in hours (%)				
0	38 (55.1)	13 (76.5)	15 (42.9)	10 (58.8)
1–10	21 (30.4)	4 (23.5)	12 (34.3)	5 (29.4)
11–20	7 (10.1)	0	5 (14.3)	2 (11.8)
>20	3 (4.3)	0	3 (8.6)	0
Experience with HystSim (%)	4 (5.8)	0	3 (8.6)	1 (5.9)
Number of therapeutic vaginoscopic hysteroscopies performed (%)				
0	17 (24.6)	17 (100.0)	0 (0.0)	0
1–25	17 (24.6)	0	17 (48.6)	0
26–50	10 (14.5)	0	9 (25.7)	1 (5.9)
>50	25 (36.2)	0	9 (25.7)	16 (94.1)
Number of Essure® placements performed (%)				
0	47 (68.1)	10 (100.0)	30 (85.7)	0
1–25	5 (7.2)	0	5 (14.3)	0
26–50	6 (8.7)	0	0	6 (35.3)
>50	11 (15.9)	0	0	11 (64.7)

IQR interquartile ranges

Table 3 Results face validity

	Participants with prior Essure® experience (N=22)
What is your opinion about the realism of the following items? (1=not realistic...5=very realistic)	
Instrumentation	4.00 (3.75–5.00)
Setting	4.00 (3.00–5.00)
Navigation	4.00 (4.00–5.00)
In- and outflow valves	4.00 (4.00–5.00)
Quality of images	5.00 (4.00–5.00)
Depth perception	4.00 (3.00–4.25)
Essure® procedure	4.00 (4.00–5.00)
General impression	5.00 (4.00–5.00)
What is your opinion about the training capacity of the following items? (1=very bad...5=very good)	
Camera navigation	4.50 (4.00–5.00)
Hand–eye coordination	5.00 (4.00–5.00)
Depth perception	4.00 (3.00–4.25)
Operative hysteroscopy	4.00 (4.00–5.00)
Essure® procedure	5.00 (4.00–5.00)
Training capacity in general	4.00 (4.00–5.00)

Statement 1: the HystSim™ offers procedural training of hysteroscopic skills

Agree: 100.0 % Disagree: 0.0 % No opinion: 0.0 %

Statement 2: the EssureSim™ offers a useful preparation for the real-time Essure® sterilization procedure

Agree: 95.5 % Disagree: 4.5 % No opinion: 0.0 %

Median scores (with interquartile ranges) are given for the realism and training capacity of the simulator on a 5-point Likert scale. Results are presented for those participants who have prior Essure® experience

subjects with varying hysteroscopy experience for two out of six parameters.

The parameter task time was able to differentiate significantly between all groups in both cases. The novice group performed both cases significantly slower in comparison to the other groups ($p=.001$ for both cases). In addition, all groups required more time to finish the second case, a uterus of a more difficult level, in comparison to the first case.

Similarly, the parameter path length showed significant differences between groups in both cases. The novices had a significantly longer path length in comparison to the intermediate and expert group (case 1, $p=.001$ in both groups; case 2, $p=.006$ in comparison with the intermediate group).

The results for parameter task time and path length are visualized in Fig. 2. Both parameters reflect a more efficient performance of hysteroscopy by experienced gynecologists; however, the clinical relevance of a shorter duration of 1 to 1.5 min per patient is uncertain.

In the first case, the parameter trauma displayed a significant difference between the novices and the intermediate group and a similar trend in comparison to the expert group. However, in the second case, a reversed (nonsignificant) effect is observed. The novice group achieved a median score of 8 contacts in comparison to 13 in the expert group. A similar contradictory trend in both cases is seen for the parameter patient comfort.

The analysis of the parameter distension medium did not show significant results, while the intermediate group used the largest amount of fluid in both cases. The last parameter, the number of correctly placed devices, did not differ significantly between the three groups and no specific trend could be observed. Both inexperienced and experienced

Table 4 Results of construct validity for each group

	Novices (N=17)	Intermediates (N=35)	Experts (N=17)	p value
Case 1				
Time (s)	203.40, IQR 172.65–302.65	161.90, IQR 123.00–180.40	118.70, IQR 103.80–146.60	.001
Path length (mm)	647.30, IQR 583.55–946.05	498.60, IQR 412.60–553.80	462.20, IQR 383.05–545.60	.001
Trauma (number)	11.00, IQR 5.50–17.00	7.00, IQR 2.00–9.00	6.00, IQR 3.00–8.50	.033
Patient comfort (10-point scale)	6.90, IQR 6.80–7.80	7.10, IQR 6.70–7.70	7.30, IQR 6.75–7.70	.831
Distension medium (mL)	558.90, IQR 267.15–791.40	600.20, IQR 449.95–905.55	489.60, IQR 193.08–571.15	.102
Correct placement left/right (percentage)	94.1/82.4	91.4/91.4	82.4/94.1	.481/.481
Case 2				
Time (s)	224.90, IQR 180.30–279.25	177.60, IQR 150.30–197.40	136.70, IQR 120.35–174.30	.001
Path length (mm)	665.40, IQR 586.40–837.85	538.70, IQR 504.90–626.20	561.40, IQR 495.95–677.75	.009
Trauma (number)	8.00, IQR 4.50–28.00	10.00, IQR 5.00–28.00	13.00, IQR 6.50–25.50	.791
Patient comfort (10-point scale)	7.90, IQR 6.60–8.10	7.20, IQR 6.20–8.00	7.30, IQR 7.00–8.10	.377
Distension medium (mL)	671.45, IQR 180.55–831.40	836.50, IQR 503.45–1141.63	635.55, IQR 438.48–873.38	.173
Correct placement left/right (percentage)	100.0/100.0	97.1/100.0	100.0/100.0	.615/1.00

Median values (interquartile ranges) for all analyzed parameters are given. For every parameter, a p value is stated per exercise to indicate whether a significant effect between any of the groups is observed (nonparametric, Kruskal–Wallis test)

IQR interquartile ranges

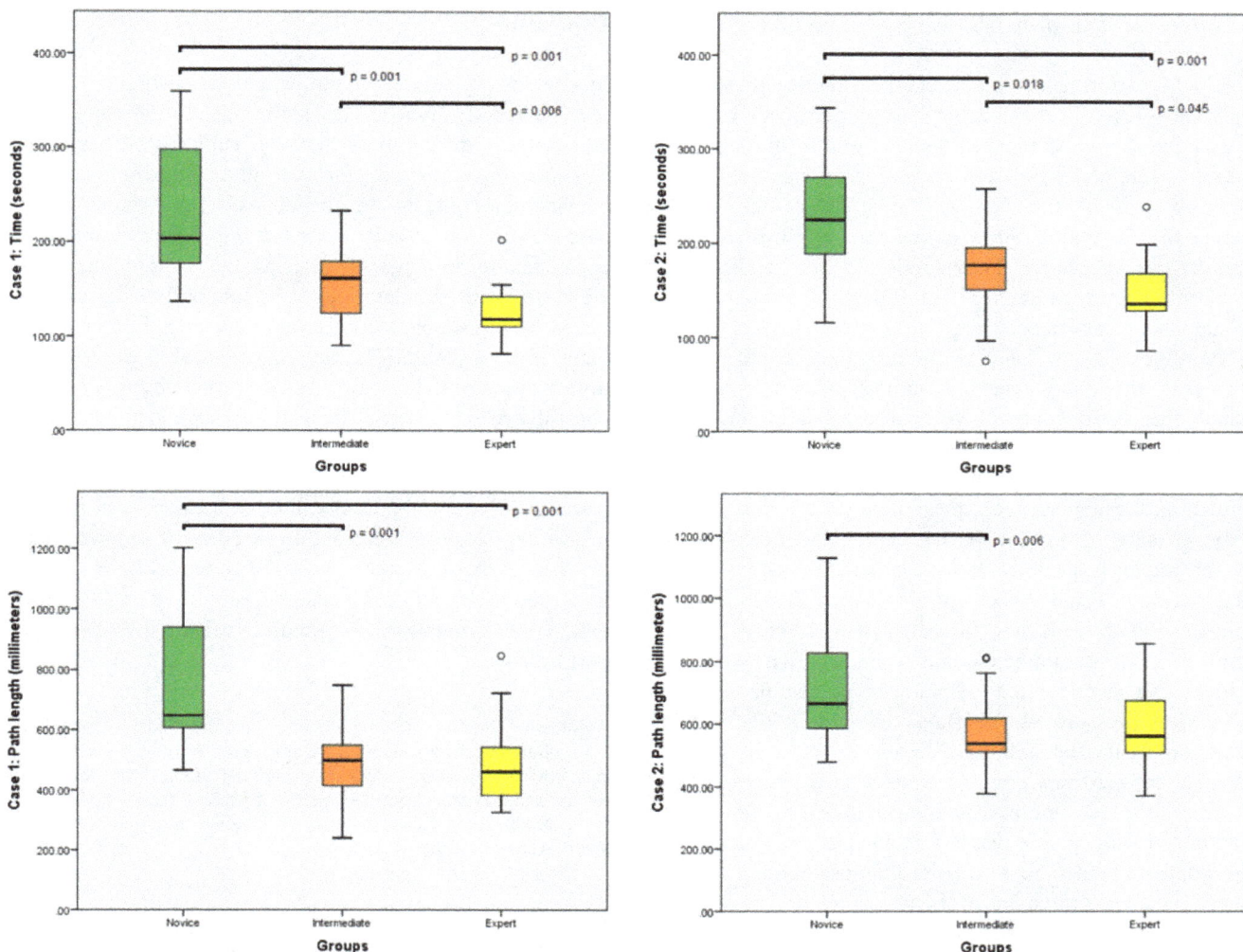

Fig. 2 Results of construct validity in *box plots*. *Box plots* for parameters task time and path length, for all groups performing case 1 and 2. *Bars* are medians, *boxes* show interquartile range, *whiskers* show range, *dots* are outliers, and *large horizontal bars* indicate statistically significant differences, specified with *p* values

participants were able to position the sterilization micro-inserts in a correct manner.

Discussion

The aim of this study was to determine the validity of a new training module by which the Essure® sterilization method can be practiced on a commercially available VR simulator. We assessed the realism of the simulator by questionnaires (face validity) and determined the capacity of the simulator to distinguish between experienced and inexperienced hysteroscopists (construct validity). Face validity was established with high scores, while construct validity showed moderate results.

The study was preceded by a power analysis and contained a sufficient number of participants. One supervisor coached all participants to limit inter-supervisor bias.

According to the fact that hysteroscopic sterilization is usually performed as a type of therapeutic vaginoscopic hysteroscopy [32, 33], participants were grouped by their experience in both procedures.

In general, gynecologists with ample experience in performing hysteroscopies are considered experts. In the absence of generally accepted criteria for the classification of experience levels, we applied the arbitrary number of 0 and 25 therapeutic procedures to form three levels. Both the novice and expert group were of similar size (*N*=17), whereas the intermediate group consisted of clearly more participants (*N*=35), indicating that the majority of our study population had some or more therapeutic vaginoscopic hysteroscopy experience. Face validity was assessed by taking into account only the opinion of those participants who had tubal sterilization experience (performed ≥1 Essure®). In this manner, realism was evaluated only by those participants who had knowledge of the real-time procedure.

Not all performance parameters measured by the simulator were able to differentiate between participants with varying hysteroscopy experience. We hereby confirm findings of previous studies by Bajka et al. [30] and Panel et al. [34], who investigated the face and construct validity of the diagnostic and sterilization module on this hysteroscopy simulator, respectively. Both studies found that less than half of all used parameters significantly correlated with hysteroscopy experience.

Possible reasons for the current study could be the fact that an active coaching strategy was adopted, by which the supervisor was easily accessible for questions and practical advice. It should be emphasized that this might have reduced possible differences between experienced and inexperienced participants. Another reason may possibly be the lack of haptic feedback, which might impair especially the experienced hysteroscopist. Not only the visual aspect but also haptic feedback gives guidance to the operator for efficient and safe hysteroscopies. Both parameters trauma and patient comfort, which is a combination of number of trauma and the distension pressure of the fluids exerted on the uterine wall, might not be able to differentiate in a consequent manner between novices and experts as a result.

Also, the parameter distension medium should be interpreted with caution due to a number of missing data, as the simulator tended not to register fluid use during all placements. Further refinement of the software and scoring systems is therefore necessary. Incorrectly placed devices were mainly caused by placing them too deeply into the tubes, whereby the coils were not visible in the uterine cavity after deployment. The fact that novices scored high percentages for correctly placed devices might be explained by the observation that those participants without any hysteroscopy experience tended to adhere more closely to any practical advice given during device placement, in contrast to the more experienced groups. In addition, one needs to realize that the assessment of the participants' experience was self-reported and therefore is subject to recall bias. Also, the division into three levels of experience could be seen as a potential source of bias since the norm of both sufficient hysteroscopy and sterilization experience must be met to be classified as an expert.

One could ask oneself in general if a slower performance with more use of distension medium is not preferred when a higher correct placement rate is achieved with better patient comfort. The parameters used by this simulator might not be the only measures of hysteroscopy performance. For procedural exercises, one could design a global rating scale (GRS), which is a scoring system that is built on certain clinically relevant performance parameters [35, 36].

Conclusion

In conclusion, this simulator received the highest scores regarding both procedure realism and training capacity. It was able to differentiate between subjects with varying hysteroscopy experience for two out of six parameters. We consider this study as an essential basic step in the validation cascade of a VR simulator for training operative hysteroscopies and for hysteroscopic sterilization in particular. Also, we believe this simulator could be suitable for future training of hysteroscopic sterilization skills, after further refinement of the software. The next important step would be the investigation of the learning curve, with concurrent use of a clinically relevant GRS. The learning curve is a vital part of construct validity and in addition addresses implementation of the simulator in hysteroscopy training curricula. The learning curve could possibly indicate the necessary number of training sessions contributing to efficient and safe daily practice. Assessing predictive validity would be a last and ideal step in the validation cascade, providing data to which extent the simulation can predict real-life hysteroscopic performance.

Acknowledgments We would like to thank the residents and consultants who voluntarily participated in this study. We would like to thank Ass. Prof. M.J.C. (René) Eijkemans from the Julius Centre for Health Sciences and Primary care, University of Utrecht, the Netherlands for his help with the statistical analysis. No funding resources or compensation disclosure is applicable.

Potential conflict of interest J.A.J. has nothing to disclose. S.V. has received honorariums for training sessions on the Essure® device for Conceptus and was involved in the development of the EssureSim™. F.J.B. has nothing to disclose. H.W.R.S. has nothing to disclose. No funding was received for this study.

References

1. Peterson HB (2008) Sterilization. Obstet Gynecol 111:189–203
2. Chan LM, Westhoff CL (2010) Tubal sterilization trends in the United States. Fertil Steril 94:1–6
3. Levie M, Chudnoff MS (2011) A comparison of novice and experienced physicians performing hysteroscopic sterilization: an analysis of an FDA-mandated trial. Fertil Steril 96:643–648
4. Shavell VI, Abdallah ME, Shade GH Jr, Diamond MP, Berman JM (2009) Trends in sterilization since the introduction of Essure hysteroscopic sterilization. J Minim Invasive Gynecol 16:22–27
5. Jansen FW, Vredevoogd CB, van Ulzen K, Hermans J, Trimbos JB, Trimbos-Kemper TC (2000) Complications of hysteroscopy: a prospective, multicenter study. Obstet Gynecol 96:266–270
6. Aydeniz B, Gruber IV, Schauf B, Kurek R, Meyer A, Wallwiener D (2002) A multicenter survey of complications associated with 21,676 operative hysteroscopies. Eur J Obstet Gynecol Reprod Biol 104:160–164
7. Blanchard MH, Amini SB, Frank TM (2004) Impact of work hour restrictions on resident case experience in an obstetrics and gynecology residency program. Am J Obstet Gynecol 191:1746–1751

8. Van Dongen H, Kolkman W, Jansen FW (2006) Hysteroscopic surgery: perspectives on skills training. J Minim Invasive Gynecol 13:121–125

9. Gallagher AG, Cates CU (2004) Virtual reality training for the operating room and cardiac catheterization laboratory. Lancet 364:1538–1540

10. Shoukrey MN, Fathulla BI, Al Samarrai T (2008) Hysteroscopy training in the UK: the trainees' perspective. Gynecol Surg 5:213–219

11. Chudnoff SG, Liu CS, Levie MD, Bernstein P, Banks EH (2010) Efficacy of a novel educational curriculum using a simulation laboratory on resident performance of hysteroscopic sterilization. Fertil Steril 94:1521–1524

12. Chou B, Handa VL (2006) Simulators and virtual reality in surgical education. Obstet Gynecol Clin North Am 33:283–296

13. Ahlberg G, Enochsson L, Gallagher AG et al (2007) Proficiency-based virtual reality significantly reduces the error rate for residents during their first 10 laparoscopic cholecystectomies. Am J Surg 193:797–804

14. Palter VN, Grantcharov T (2010) Virtual reality in surgical skills training. Surg Clin North Am 90:605–617

15. Neary PC, Boyle E, Delaney CP, Senagore AJ, Keane FB, Gallagher AG (2008) Construct validation of a novel hybrid virtual–reality simulator for training and assessing laparoscopic colectomy; results from the first course for experienced senior laparoscopic surgeons. Surg Endosc 22:2301–2309

16. Verdaasdonk EG, Stassen LP, Monteny LJ, Dankelman J (2006) Validation of a new basic virtual reality simulator for training of basic endoscopic skills: the SIMENDO. Surg Endosc 20:511–518

17. McDougall EM (2007) Validation of surgical simulators. J Endourol 21:244–247

18. Schout BM, Hendrikx AJ, Scheele F, Bemelmans BL, Scherpbier AJ (2010) Validation and implementation of surgical simulators: a critical review of present, past, and future. Surg Endosc 24:536–546

19. Gallagher AG, Ritter EM, Satava RM (2003) Fundamental principles of validation, and reliability: rigorous science for the assessment of surgical education and training. Surg Endosc 17:1525–1529

20. Schout BM, Ananias HJ, Bemelmans BL et al (2009) Transfer of cysto-urethroscopy skills from a virtual–reality simulator to the operating room: a randomized controlled trial. BJUI Int 106:226–231

21. Seymour NE, Gallagher AG, Roman SA et al (2002) Virtual reality training improves operating room performance: results of a randomized, double-blinded study. Ann Surg 236:458–463

22. Grantcharov TP, Kristiansen VB, Bendix J, Bardram L, Rosenberg J, Funch-Jensen P (2004) Randomized clinical trial of virtual reality simulation for laparoscopic skills training. Br J Surg 91:146–150

23. Van Sickle KR, Ritter EM, Baghai M et al (2008) Prospective, randomized, double-blind trial of curriculum-based training for intracorporeal suturing and knot tying. J Am Coll Surg 207:560–568

24. Larsen CR, Soerensen JL, Grantcharov TP et al (2009) Effect of virtual reality training on laparoscopic surgery: randomized controlled trial. BMJ 338:b1802. doi:10.1136/bmj.b1802

25. Schreuder HW, van Dongen KW, Roeleveld SJ, Schijven MP, Broeders IA (2009) Face and construct validity of virtual reality simulation of laparoscopic gynecologic surgery. Am J Obstet Gynecol 200:540.e1-8

26. Burchard ER, Lockrow EG, Zahn CM, Dunlow SG, Satin AJ. Simulation training improves resident performance in operative hysteroscopic resection techniques. Am J Obstet Gynecol 197:542.e1-4.

27. Kingston A, Abbott J, Lenart M, Vancaillie T (2004) Hysteroscopic training: the butternut pumpkin model. J Am Assoc Gynecol Laparosc 11:256–261

28. Wallwiener D, Rimbach S, Bastert G (1994) The HysteroTrainer, a simulator for diagnostic and operative hysteroscopy. J Am Assoc Gynecol Laparosc 2:61–63

29. Bajka M, Tuchschmid S, Streich M, Fink D, Székely G, Harders M (2009) Evaluation of a new virtual–reality training simulator for hysteroscopy. Surg Endosc 23:2026–2033

30. Bajka M, Tuchschmid S, Fink D, Székely G, Harders M (2010) Establishing construct validity of a virtual–reality training simulator for hysteroscopy via a multimetric scoring system. Surg Endosc 24:79–88

31. Mattel MS, Jacoby J (1972) Is there an optimal number of alternatives for Likert-scale items? J App Psychol 56:506–509

32. Miño M, Arjona JE, Cordón J, Pelegrin B, Povedano B, Chacon E (2007) Success rate and patient satisfaction with the Essure sterilisation in an outpatient setting: a prospective study of 857 women. BJOG 114:763–766

33. Ubeda A, Labastida R, Dexeus S (2004) Essure: a new device for hysteroscopic tubal sterilization in an outpatient setting. Fertil Steril 82:196–199

34. Panel P, Bajka M, Le Tohic A, Ghoneimi AE, Chis C, Cotin S (2012) Hysteroscopic placement of tubal sterilization implants: virtual reality simulator training. Surg Endosc. doi:10.1007/s00464-011-2139-6

35. Reznick RK (1993) Teaching and testing technical skills. Am J Surg 165:358–361

36. Martin JA, Regehr G, Reznick R et al (1997) Objective structured assessment of technical skill (OSATS) for surgical residents. Br J Surg 84:273–278

18

Asherman's syndrome after removal of placenta remnants: a serious clinical problem

A. B. Hooker · A. Thurkow

Abstract Intrauterine adhesions (IUA) or Asherman's syndrome is thought to develop after trauma to the uterine cavity by destruction of the basal layer of the endometrium. IUA can result in menstrual disorders, infertility, and complication during pregnancy and delivery. IUA formation is multifactorial, with pregnancy being an important etiologic factor. Performing a postpartum exploration/evacuation or curettage can lead to adhesion formation. We present three patients who presented with a menstrual disorder after postpartum surgical intervention on suspicion of placental remnants. Hysteroscopic evaluation revealed severe intrauterine adhesions with complete obliteration of the uterine cavity. Repeated and extensive hysteroscopic adhesiolysis is performed to acquire a cavity with a normal appearance. Besides the puerperal uterus, the time of surgical performance is crucial in the risk for adhesion formation. Performing a late surgical intervention, as from 24–48 h after delivery, leads to an increased risk for adhesion formation. Prevention of IUA can be established by an accurate indication for late postpartum surgical interventions. When performing a late surgical intervention, hysteroscopic surgery is preferable. Firstly, hysteroscopy allows the possibility for identification of placental remnants, and secondly, the possibility for selective removal, thus avoiding unnecessary trauma to the endometrium compared to blindly curettage. Caution is advised when performing a late puerperal surgical intervention. An accurate indication is essential, and when needed, hysteroscopic surgery is preferable, minimizing trauma to the endometrium.

Keywords Asherman's syndrome · Adhesion · Pregnancy · Placental remnants · Surgical intervention · Puerperium · Prevention · Curettage

Background

Intrauterine adhesion (IUA), also known as posttraumatic amenorrhea, was first described in 1894 by Fritsch [1]. In 1948, Joseph Asherman was the first to describe the frequency of this syndrome, which has borne his name ever since [2]. Asherman's syndrome, defined as adhesion in the uterine cavity, is thought to develop following trauma to the uterine cavity by destruction of the basal layer, the regenerative reservoir of the endometrium. In the healing process, fusion between the injured opposing uterine walls may arise, and as a consequence, partial or complete obliteration of the uterine cavity may occur [3, 4]. IUA can cause menstrual disturbances, infertility, and recurrent abortions. If pregnancy occurs, it is frequently complicated by miscarriage, ectopic pregnancy, abnormal placentation, fetal growth restriction, fetal anomalies, premature labor and delivery, and postpartum hemorrhage [3, 5, 6].

IUA formation is multifactorial with multiple predisposing and causal factors. The specific cause of IUA formation is difficult to determine because the true pathophysiological process that leads to IUA formation is still obscure. Pregnancy appears to be an important etiologic cause as it is one of the dominating predisposing factors in 91% of the patients with adhesions; adhesions appear in 67% after miscarriage curettage and in 22% after postpartum curettage [3]. Other studies have confirmed the predisposing condi-

A. B. Hooker (✉) · A. Thurkow
Department of Obstetrics and Gynaecology,
Sint Lucas Andreas Hospital,
Amsterdam, The Netherlands
e-mail: a.hooker@slaz.nl

tion of the gravid uterus [6–9]. Besides the gravid uterus, other determinants as surgery, infection, inflammation, and constitutional characteristics play a role in adhesion formation. There is a lack of studies/reports addressing the prevalence of adhesion formation, especially in relation to puerperal surgical interventions.

Method

The indication to perform a secondary postpartum curettage and/or digital evacuation is suspicions of placental remnants. The surgical procedure is often performed in daily practice, but there is lack of information concerning frequency and possible complications. We present three patients who developed severe adhesions and Asherman's syndrome after undergoing surgical treatment on suspicions of placental remnants after delivery. We propose treatment strategies to prevent or reduce the formation of adhesions.

Case 1

A 34-year-old primigravida was initially in primary care with an independent midwife. At 33 weeks of gestation, the membranes ruptured, and she was transferred to our teaching hospital. She was treated with steroids to enhance pulmonary maturity and calcium channel blocker (nifedipine) for tocolysis. Despite tocolytic therapy, the patient was in labor and spontaneously delivered a healthy girl, weighing 2,000 g (P50) with 1- and 5-min Apgar scores of 9 and 10, respectively. The newborn baby was admitted at the neonatal intensive care unit. The retained placenta was managed by manual removal under general anesthesia. The placenta localized at the right fundus could be easily removed. The uterine cavity was normal, in particular, no signs of congenital uterine anomalies. The estimated amount of blood loss was 2,500 ml, and blood transfusion was not necessary. After a short observation period, the patient and newborn could be discharged in good clinical condition.

Two months later, the patient still had irregular blood loss. Transvaginal ultrasonography was performed to evaluate the blood loss. A white, not well-defined structure in the uterine cavity was detected with a maximum diameter of 5.2 by 2.7 cm (Fig. 1). The structure had the echogenic appearance of placenta tissue. A puerperal curettage was performed; macroscopic placental tissue was removed. The postoperative period was unremarkable. Histological examination proved placental remnants.

Six months after delivery, the patient was referred because of secondary amenorrhea. An attempt to perform a saline infusion sonography (SIS) failed because of a cervical stenosis. Hysteroscopic adhesiolysis under general anesthesia was performed. Because of the cervical stenosis,

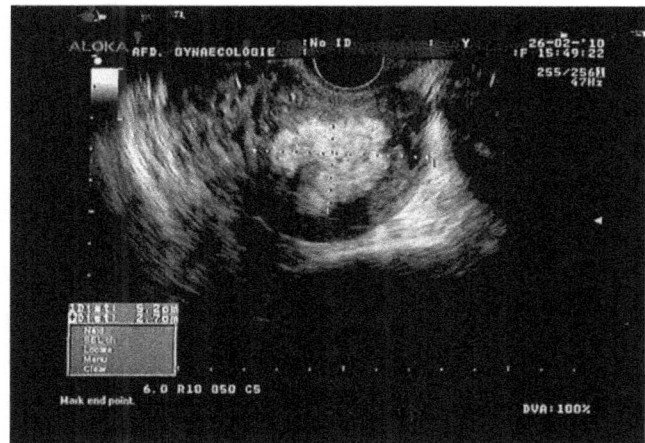

Fig. 1 Transvaginal ultrasonography performed 8 weeks after delivery. A white, not well-defined structure is seen in the uterine cavity, with a maximum diameter of 5.2×2.7 cm. The structure has the echogenic appearance of placenta tissue

introduction was difficult; the uterine cavity was reached but was unrecognizable. A small channel could be detected at the left side connected with the left tube. A hysterosalpingography performed during the operation confirmed the image (Fig. 2). At the right side, a niche was found, probably the remains of the right side of the uterine cavity. The niche could not be reached by hysteroscopy; adhesiol-

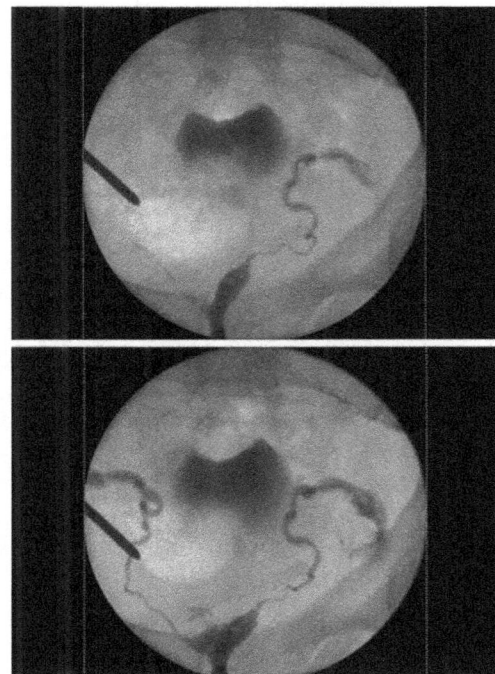

Fig. 2 Hysterosalpingography performed in case 1. *Top*: At the *left side*, a small channel is connected with the left tube. At the *right side*, no cavity can be visualized; there seems to be minimal connection with the right tube. *Bottom*: After extensive adhesiolysis, a normal uterine cavity with connection with both tubes is visible

ysis was performed. After adhesiolysis, the cavity was enlarged, but still incomplete. A second session was necessary. After extensive adhesiolysis, the uterine cavity had a normal appearance. After the procedure, the patient regained a normal menstrual cycle. One year later, the patient still has a regular menstrual cycle.

Case 2

A 34-year-old primigravida with an unremarkable medical history was initially in primary care but was transferred in late pregnancy to our teaching hospital because of pregnancy-induced hypertension. The labor was induced by amniotomy and intravenous administration of oxytocin. The patient spontaneously delivered a healthy girl, weighing 3,500 g with 1- and 5-min Apgar scores of 9 and 10, respectively. Spontaneous placental separation and delivery occurred. Because of a primary postpartum hemorrhage despite treatment with uterotonic drugs, digital exploration and evacuation under general anesthesia was performed. The uterus was atonic and filled with clots. After removal of blood clots, the uterine cavity felt normal; there were no signs of congenital uterine malformations or placental remnants. Contraction of the uterus and normalization of the blood loss occurred after additional treatment with uterotonic drugs. The estimated blood loss was 4,000 ml; the patient received 4 units of red cells and 2 units of fresh frozen plasma. After a short clinical observation, the patient was discharged in good clinical condition.

Two months later, the patient reported persistent, irregular blood loss. Ultrasonography showed a uterine cavity with a structure suspicious for placenta remnants. Curettage was performed with removal of tissue. Histological examination did not prove placental residue.

Six months after delivery, the patient was referred because of amenorrhea. The patient stopped lactation for several months; thereafter, no menstrual bleeding occurred. A SIS was attempted, but was inconclusive because of insufficient distension or enlargement of the cavity. An outpatient hysteroscopy showed exhaustive adhesions. A second procedure under general anesthesia was planned. Introduction of the hysteroscope was difficult because of a cervix stenosis; the passageway of the cervix was narrow and fibrotic. Because of the unclear picture, a hysterosalpingography was performed during operation, which shows an asymmetric uterine cavity with a remarkable wide open right tube (Fig. 3). Hysteroscopically, the cavity was reached and was unrecognizable. At the right side, a niche was visible with endometrium, which could be followed into the right, distended tube, possibly a hydrosalpinx. At the left side, no cavity could be identified, and the origin of the left tube is identified by hysterosalpingography; with the hysteroscope, the origin of the left tube was not visible.

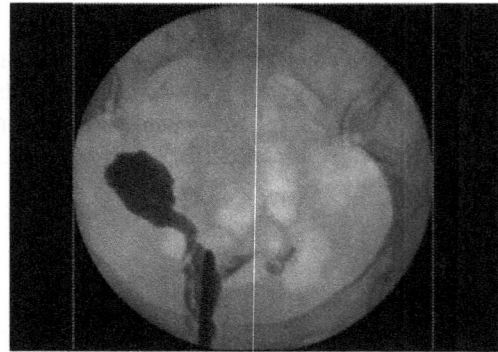

Fig. 3 Hysterosalpingography. At the *right side*, a niche is visible, which is connected to the distended right tube, possibly a hydrosalpinx. At the *left side*, no cavity or left tube could be identified, and the origin of the left tube cannot be identified

Adhesiolysis was started, but because there was difficulty in identifying the boundaries of the cavity and suspicion of intra-abdominal involvement, a new combined session with hysteroscopy, hysterosalpingography, and laparoscopy was planned.

At the third session, the uterine cavity could ultimately be reached under transrectal ultrasonographic guidance. The impression of the cavity is equal to that of the second session. With the combination of hysteroscopy and hysterosalpingography, the right tube and the right side of the cavity could be identified. At laparoscopy, the right tube ran into the uterine cavity through a perforation gap near the origin of the right tube. First, laparoscopic adhesiolysis was performed; thereafter, the right tube could be removed from the cavity. The uterine defect was closed after excision of the margins. Secondly, hysteroscopic adhesiolysis was performed with removal of the remains of the fimbriae, ultimately with a more or less normal cavity. For the prevention of adhesions, Hyalobarrier® was administered, but because of persistent blood loss, a Cook balloon was inserted. The patient was treated with an additional regimen of cyclical estrogen and progesterone for 7 days during two cycles. A fourth and last session for hysteroscopic check-up revealed a more or less normal cavity. The patient has a regular cycle.

Case 3

A 28-year-old gravida 3 para 1, with a spontaneous delivery and a miscarriage in history, was followed in primary care by an independent midwife. At 39 weeks of gestation, she spontaneously delivered a healthy boy, weighing 3,950 g with 1- and 5-min Apgar scores of 9 and 10, respectively. Because of a primary postpartum hemorrhage, the patient was transferred to secondary care. Treatment with uterotonic drugs normalized the blood loss, and the patient was discharged in good clinical condition after a short observation period.

Three weeks later, the patient was readmitted because of excessive bleeding. Ultrasonographic imaging was performed. Curettage was performed because of suspicion of placental remnants, and macroscopic placental tissue was removed. The postoperative course was uncomplicated. Because of a hemoglobin level of 4.2 mmol/l, iron therapy was started. Histological evaluation proved placental remnants.

Six months later, the patient was referred to our outpatient department because of pelvic pain and amenorrhea, despite the use of oral contraceptive. Transvaginal ultrasonography revealed a thin endometrium, and the image of the uterine cavity was not clear. A SIS could not be performed because the catheter could not be introduced in the cervical channel; cervix stenosis was suspected. A hysteroscopy was performed; an obliterated cervix was seen and could be opened after adhesiolysis under ultrasonographic guidance. After reaching the uterine cavity, widespread adhesions were encountered with an obliterated cavity. Adhesiolysis was performed under ultrasonographic guidance. The ostia of the left tube could be identified, but the right ostia was not visible. A hysterosalpingography performed during surgery confirmed the image. Because of intravasation of contrast medium, proper imaging was limited, and the operation was ended. A second session was planned. At the outpatient department visit, the patient reported that she was menstruating again. The patient canceled the second procedure because of a regular menstrual cycle.

Findings

Postpartum curettage and/or digital exploration/evacuation are considered the standard surgical therapy when there is the suspicion of placental remnants or hemorrhage. It is unknown how often a secondary surgical procedure is performed and of the possible complications.

The reported cases show that secondary puerperal interventions can lead to serious complications. Performing a postpartum exploration/evacuation or curettage on suspicion of placental remnants can lead to adhesion formation—Asherman's syndrome. Therefore, caution is advised when performing intrauterine interventions in both patients with an earlier intrauterine intervention (cases 1 and 2) as in patients without (case 3). Although only a few studies are available in which the incidence of intrauterine adhesions after secondary puerperal intervention is assessed, they imply a serious clinical problem.

Curettage alone does not seem to predispose to adhesion formation, as in the nonpregnant uterus, intrauterine adhesions post-curettage are reported in 0.4–1.2% of patients [3]. Pregnancy, however, appears to be a contributing factor, as intrauterine adhesions have been reported in 2% after manual removal [10]. Also, curettage, exploration, or evacuation performed between 2 and 4 weeks after delivery leads to a substantial increase in adhesion formation varying between 29% and 37.5% [11–13]. The timing of surgical intervention also appears to be important as intervention after 24–48 h post-delivery appears to increase the risk of adhesion formation [12, 13]. Even more concerning and disturbing is that, besides the increase chance of adhesion formation, in 30–60%, the adhesions are of a severe stage [12, 14].

IUA formation is considered multifactorial, although the true pathophysiological process is still unknown. The specific characteristics of the puerperal uterus and time of intrauterine intervention are important predisposing factors in adhesion formation. The influence of other factors still remains obscure.

A possible explanation for the enhanced risk and severity of the reported adhesions is the fact that the endometrium of the gravid uterus is in a recovering state. The manipulation disturbs or influences the healing process in an irreparable way, implicating the ultimate result. Destruction of the basal layer of the endometrium, in the healing process probably is one of the key factors in the process leading to adhesion formation.

A second explanation could be the presence of an infection or inflammation. The prolonged presence of placenta tissue in the uterine cavity could enhance infection. Infection is a known situation with enhancement of adhesion formation [4]. In 56% of the patients after puerperium curettage, performed in the second to fourth week during puerperium, histological examination shows the presence of acute, subacute, or chronic inflammation without symptoms that would suggest endometritis [15]. Low estrogen state, including the puerperium, seems to significantly increase the risk of developing adhesions [12]. Lactation, also being a hypoestrogenic condition, could be an important additional factor in adhesion formation.

Instead of curettage, which is obviously performed blindly, evaluation of the uterine cavity can be conducted by hysteroscopy. Hysteroscopy is considered a reliable technique for identification of intrauterine pathology, including placental remnants [16]. Direct vision of the uterine cavity enables identification of placental remnants. In the absence of placental tissue, intervention and trauma to the endometrium can be prevented.

If placental remnants are present, hysteroscopic removal of placental remnants is a good alternative [16]. Hysteroscopy has the advantage of the placental remnants being evacuated selectively, minimizing trauma to surrounding endometrium and basal layer [17]. Hysteroscopic removal of placenta tissue can easily be performed without increase of complications. Both in the absence as in the presence of placental remnants, trauma to the endometrium is reduced compared to curettage. Reduction of trauma to the endometrium reduces the risk of adhesion formation. In view of the benefits, hysteroscopic evaluation should be the treatment of choice whenever a secondary intervention is performed on suspicion of placental remnants [18].

The prevention of intrauterine adhesions is important; adhesions are associated with menstrual and fertility disorders and complications during pregnancy and delivery. In order to minimize the amount of (unnecessary) surgical interventions in the puerperium, it is important to strictly maintain the indication for postpartum curettage and to consider medical evacuation. If a surgical intervention is necessary, preferable hysteroscopically, it should be performed in the gentlest manner, avoiding unnecessary trauma. Application of preventive matters for the prevention or reduction of adhesion can be considered, but only a minority of these products has been studied in women postpartum.

Conclusion

The gravid uterus is highly predisposed to adhesion formation. Besides the puerperal uterus, the time of postpartum curettage, evaluation, or exploration performance is crucial in the risk for adhesion formation.

When performing an intrauterine surgical intervention after more than 24–48 h, the chance of adhesion development significantly increases. An accurate indication is essential, and when performed, it should be in the gentlest manner, avoiding unnecessary trauma. Hysteroscopic treatment should be the preferred treatment; selective removal of placental remnants is possible with reduced trauma to the uterine cavity compared to curettage. Hysteroscopy minimizes the amount of unnecessary surgical intervention and trauma to the uterine cavity. Further research is necessary to analyze IUA formation and preventive measures.

Declaration of interest The authors report no conflicts of interest. The authors alone are responsible for the content and writing of the paper.

References

1. Fritsch H (1894) Ein Fall von volligen Schwund der Gebaumutterhohle nach Auskratzung. Zentralbl Gynaekol 18:1337–1342
2. Asherman JG (1948) Amenorrhoea traumatica (atretica). J Obstet Gynaecol Br Emp 55(1):23–30
3. Schenker JG, Margalioth EJ (1982) Intrauterine adhesions: an updated appraisal. Fertil Steril 37(5):593–610
4. Schenker JG (1996) Etiology of and therapeutic approach to synechia uteri. Eur J Obstet Gynecol Reprod Biol 65(1):109–13
5. Capella-Allouc S, Morsad F, Rongières-Bertrand C, Taylor S, Fernandez H (1999) Hysteroscopic treatment of severe Asherman's syndrome and subsequent fertility. Hum Reprod 14 (5):1230–3
6. Valle RF, Sciarra JJ (1988) Intrauterine adhesions: hysteroscopic diagnosis, classification, treatment, and reproductive outcome. Am J Obstet Gynecol 158(6):1459–70
7. March CM (1995) Intrauterine adhesions. Obstet Gynecol Clin North Am 22(3):491–505
8. Fernandez H, Al-Najjar F, Chauveaud-Lambling A, Frydman R, Gervaise A (2006) Fertility after treatment of Asherman's syndrome stage 3 and 4. J Minim Invasive Gynecol 13(5):398–402
9. Friedler S, Margalioth EJ, Kafka I, Yaffe H (1993) Incidence of post-abortion intra-uterine adhesions evaluated by hysteroscopy—a prospective study. Hum Reprod 8(3):442–4
10. Golan A, Raziel A, Pansky M, Bukovsky I (1996) Manual removal of the placenta—its role in intrauterine adhesion formation. Int J Fertil Menopausal Stud 41(5):450–1
11. Jensen PA, Stromme WB (1972) Amenorrhea secondary to puerperal curettage (Asherman's syndrome). Am J Obstet Gynecol 113(2):150–7
12. Westendorp IC, Ankum WM, Mol BW, Vonk J (1998) Prevalence of Asherman's syndrome after secondary removal of placental remnants or a repeat curettage for incomplete abortion. Hum Reprod 13(12):3347–50
13. Eriksen J, Kaestek C (1960) The incidence of uterine atresia after post-partum curettage. A follow-up examination of 141 patients. Dan Med Bull 7:50–1
14. Dawood A, Al-Talib A, Tulandi T (2010) Predisposing factors and treatment outcome of different stages of intrauterine adhesions. J Obstet Gynaecol Can 32(8):767–70
15. Smid I, Bedö T (1978) Curettage during puerperium and its late consequences. Zentralbl Gynäkol 100(14):916–20
16. Cohen SB, Kalter-Ferber A, Weisz BS, Zalel Y, Seidman DS, Mashiach S, Lidor AL, Zolti M, Goldenberg M (2001) Hysteroscopy may be the method of choice for management of residual trophoblastic tissue. J Am Assoc Gynecol Laparosc 8(2):199–202
17. Goldenberg M, Schiff E, Achiron R, Lipitz S, Mashiach S (1997) Managing residual trophoblastic tissue. Hysteroscopy for directing curettage. J Reprod Med 42(1):26–8
18. Ventolini G, Zhang M, Gruber J (2004) Hysteroscopy in the evaluation of patients with recurrent pregnancy loss: a cohort study in a primary care population. Surg Endosc 18(12):1782–4

19

Diagnostic hysteroscopy and saline infusion sonography in the diagnosis of intrauterine abnormalities

Heleen van Dongen · Anne Timmermans ·
Cathrien E. Jacobi · Trudy Elskamp ·
Cor D. de Kroon · Frank Willem Jansen

Abstract This study was conducted to assess whether women would prefer to undergo saline infusion sonography (SIS) or office hysteroscopy for the investigation of the uterine cavity. In a randomised controlled trial, 100 patients underwent SIS or office hysteroscopy for assessing patients' pain scores. After the investigation, 92 of them were asked to fill out an anonymous questionnaire addressing their preference regarding the method of evaluation and treatment of the uterine cavity. A control group, consisting of 50 women who never underwent SIS or office hysteroscopy, was also asked to complete an identical questionnaire. The questionnaire was completed by 113 women (83.7%). Twenty-four (21.2%) women would opt for SIS, whereas 52 (46.0%) would opt for office hysteroscopy, and 37 (32.7%) had no preference. If therapy would be necessary, 48.7% of the women would opt for an outpatient treatment, whereas 33.0% of the women would prefer treatment under general anaesthesia. Despite the fact that SIS is less painful, the majority of the women prefer office hysteroscopy.

H. van Dongen (✉) · T. Elskamp · C. D. de Kroon · F. W. Jansen
Department of Gynaecology, Leiden University Medical Center,
Albinusdreef 2,
2300 RC Leiden, The Netherlands
e-mail: H.van_Dongen@lumc.nl

A. Timmermans
Department of Gynaecology, University Medical Center Utrecht,
Utrecht, The Netherlands

C. E. Jacobi
Department of Medical Decision Making,
Leiden University Medical Center,
Leiden, The Netherlands

Additionally, therapy in an outpatient setting is preferred to a day case setting.

Keywords Preference · Intrauterine abnormalities · Hysteroscopy · Saline infusion sonography · Diagnosis · Outpatient

Background

Hysteroscopy is widely accepted to be the accurate standard for investigation of the uterine cavity [1, 2]. A meta-analysis showed that the diagnostic accuracy of saline infusion sonography (SIS) equals the accuracy of diagnostic hysteroscopy [3]. With the introduction of SIS, several authors showed that SIS provided less discomfort for patients compared to office hysteroscopy [4, 5]. However, since the development of smaller diameter hysteroscopic systems and the introduction of a 'vaginoscopic' approach to hysteroscopy (without speculum and tenaculum), patient compliance has improved considerably [6]. A great advantage of hysteroscopy over SIS is the possibility to perform a directed biopsy or a small surgical intervention in the same session. Moreover, gynaecological treatments in an outpatient setting have shown to be highly acceptable and popular with patients [7, 8].

Nevertheless, we recently showed in a randomised comparison of outpatient vaginoscopic hysteroscopy and SIS that the latter still is significantly less discomforting [9]. To follow up on this, we undertook a survey to determine which form of investigation (SIS or office hysteroscopy) women prefer and for what reasons.

Methods

This study was conducted at the Department of Gynaecology of Leiden University Medical Center (Leiden, The Netherlands) from January 2006 to July 2007. One hundred and forty-two women were approached to complete a questionnaire. Ninety two of these women were included in a randomised controlled trial comparing the pain scores of SIS and office hysteroscopy performed according to the vaginoscopic approach [9]. These women were randomly allocated to SIS or office hysteroscopy (solely for diagnostic purposes) and underwent one of these procedures. They were therefore not influenced by their doctor's choice or their own preferences. They received the questionnaire following the allocated investigation.

Another 50 women attending the general gynaecology outpatient clinic, for reasons other than the investigation of the uterine cavity, were randomly asked by their doctor to complete the questionnaire as well. All the women attending the outpatient clinic were eligible to participate in this control group irrespective of age, parity, general health or menopausal status. If they had previously undergone SIS or office hysteroscopy, they were excluded from analysis. Ethical approval for this study was obtained from the Leiden University Medical Center Ethics Committee.

Questionnaire

A questionnaire was designed and consisted of a general part and a problem-specific part. The general part addressed demographic data, including employment and number of children, and a brief medical history, including questions relating to the patient's past experience with outpatient procedures (e.g. colposcopy or mini-curettage). It also addressed the patients' preferred role in the decision-making process, including to what extent they would like to be informed about advantages and disadvantages.

The problem-specific part focused on the preference of SIS or hysteroscopy. The primary outcome measures of this questionnaire were preference for SIS or hysteroscopy in a diagnostic setting and preference for therapy in an outpatient or day case setting. Secondary outcome measures were factors influencing preference.

For this purpose, a full description with advantages and disadvantages of both investigations was provided (Appendix A). In an attempt to minimise bias, the descriptions were based on patient information of the Dutch Society of Obstetrics and Gynaecology. The order of the descriptions was randomly allocated. With reference to these descriptions, women were asked to state which of the two investigations they would choose if they needed an investigation of the uterine cavity (again) and what was most important in their decision and preferences, scored on

a Likert scale. Since controls had no experience with any of the investigations, these questions were rewritten for better understanding. Following this, women were specifically asked to what extent they would accept pain in exchange for certain advantages of the investigations and what the required benefit should be in terms of successful therapy. In addition, they were asked what level of pain they would expect to experience during both investigations, scored on a visual analogue scale (VAS) of 10 cm. Finally, they were asked in what setting (i.e. outpatient without anaesthesia or day case with general or regional anaesthesia) they would prefer treatment if during the investigation an abnormality would be found. To maximise the response rate, a reminder was sent by mail to the non-responders after 6 weeks.

The received information was entered in statistical software (SPSS, version 14; SPSS Inc., Chicago, IL). Patient characteristics of the study groups were analysed with one-way ANOVA in case of normally distributed, continuous variables and Pearson's chi-square test in case of dichotomous data. Confidence intervals for difference in means were calculated. Pearson's chi-square was also used to analyse differences of preference among the study groups. A paired-samples t test was used to compare expected VAS scores for both investigations. All tests were two-sided, and p values<0.05 were considered statistically significant.

Findings

Of the 142 women approached, 113 (79.6%) women completed the questionnaire: 79 in the trial and 34 in the control group. Of the trial patients, 38 (33.6%) underwent SIS and 41 (36.3%) underwent office hysteroscopy (Fig. 1).

Table 1 presents data on the personal characteristics of the participating women, stratified by study group. Twenty-four (21.2%) women would opt for SIS, whereas 52 (46.0%) would opt for office hysteroscopy, and 37 (32.7%) had no preference. Because preferences were strongly related to previous investigation, we present them by group as well (Fig. 2). The percentage of women preferring SIS or hysteroscopy differs significantly when women are stratified by the allocated investigation (hysteroscopy or SIS; Pearson's Chi-square, $p=0.003$). There were no differences found by social characteristics when stratified according to preference. Women preferring SIS expected to experience significantly less pain during SIS than during hysteroscopy (VAS scores 3.0 and 4.9, respectively; $p=0.006$), whereas women preferring hysteroscopy expected to experience similar pain levels during both investigations (VAS scores 3.1 and 3.5 for SIS and hysteroscopy, respectively; $p=0.120$). There were no significant differences of pain scores measured during the investigation the patients were allocated to (data from van Dongen et al. [9]) with regard to their postexamination

Fig. 1 Flowchart depicting received procedures and participation in preference study of women participating in randomised trial comparing pain scores

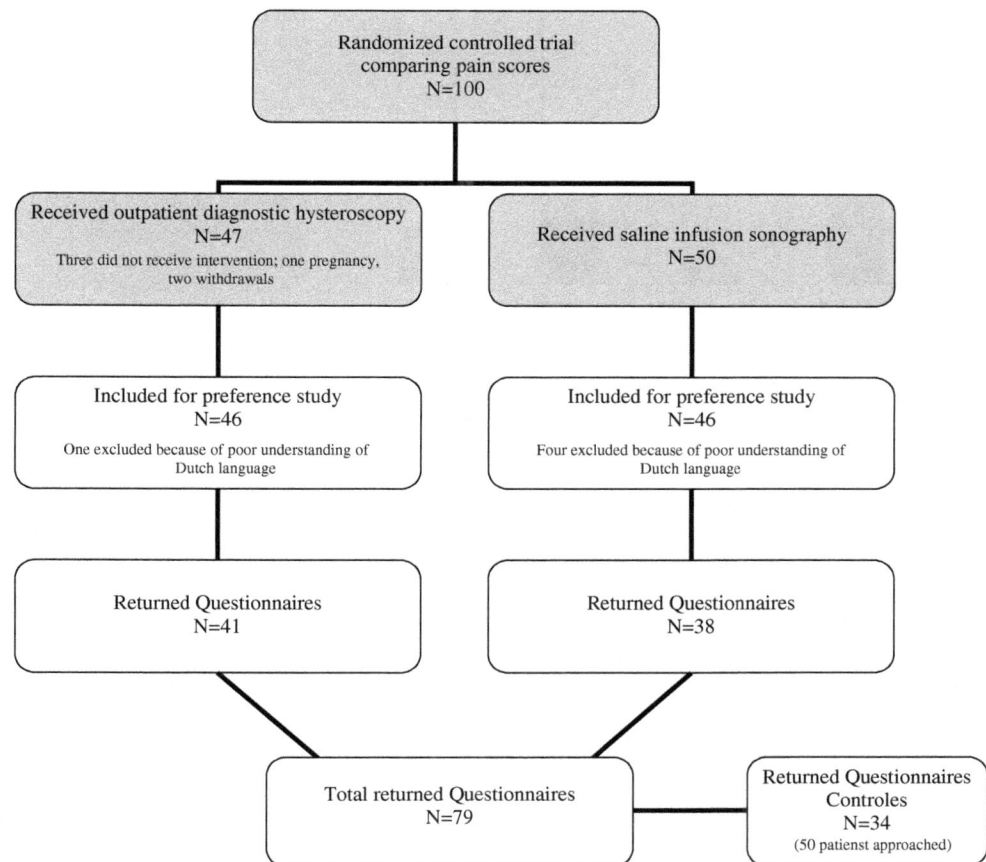

preferences (Table 2). The pain levels measured during both examinations differed significantly in favour of SIS [9].

Different aspects of preferences with regard to the investigation of the uterine cavity and possible necessitating therapy were scored on a Likert scale (0=unimportant, 5=very important) and are detailed in Table 3. Except for having or not having anaesthesia during therapy, every aspect was considered important. When stratifying the Likert scores by preference (SIS or office hysteroscopy), the following differences were found. Women with a preference for office hysteroscopy found it of utmost importance that diagnosis and therapy are offered in one visit ($p=0.004$), whereas women preferring SIS felt time to consider treatment options more important than women preferring office hysteroscopy ($p=0.014$). With regard to what extent women would accept pain in exchange for

Table 1 Patient characteristics stratified by study group

Outcome	SIS ($n=38$)	Office hysteroscopy ($n=41$)	Controls ($n=34$)	p value
Age in years (95%-CI)	45.0 (41.8–48.2)	44.7 (42.3–47.1)	42.2 (37.5–47.0)	0.484[a]
Employment	28 (73.7%)	32 (80.0%)	28 (82.4%)	0.901[b]
Married/living together	30 (78.9%)	34 (82.9%)	28 (82.4%)	0.795[b]
Children	30 (78.9%)	29 (70.7%)	20 (58.8%)	0.176[b]
Accessibility of hospital	35 (92.1%)	40 (97.6%)	32 (94.1%)	0.215[b]
Premenopausal	31 (81.6%)	34 (82.9%)	25 (73.5%)	0.564[b]
Postmenopausal	7 (18.4%)	7 (17.1%)	9 (26.5%)	0.564[b]
Previous surgery	31 (81.6%)	32 (78.0%)	26 (76.5%)	0.808[b]
Previous intervention in outpatient setting	23 (60.5%)	29 (70.7%)	21 (61.8%)	0.477[b]

SIS saline infusion sonography

[a] One-way ANOVA

[b] Pearson's Chi-square

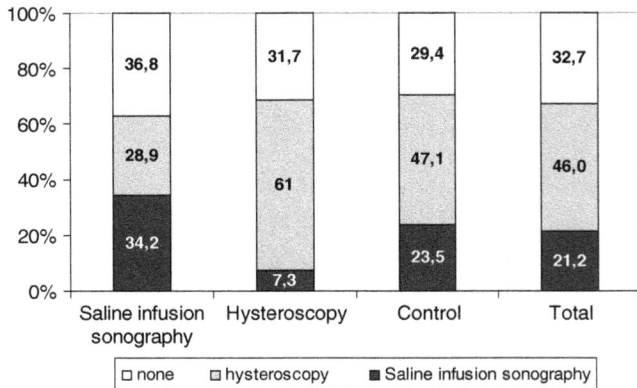

Fig. 2 Preferences in percentages of diagnostic investigation after carefully weighing advantages and disadvantages, stratified by study group. *SIS* saline infusion sonography

certain advantages of the investigation, sixty-eight (45.1%) women would accept more pain if the diagnostic investigation and therapy would be offered in one visit. This accounts for 22.7% of the women preferring SIS and 59.6% of the women preferring office hysteroscopy (*p*=0.02). The interviewed women who preferred hysteroscopy would accept hysteroscopy as diagnostic of first choice with a smaller chance of successful therapy than women specifically preferring SIS (Fig. 3).

If during the investigation of the uterine cavity an abnormality would be found, 55 (48.7%) women would opt for an outpatient treatment, and 38 (33.6%) women would opt for treatment under general anaesthesia. Twenty (15.9%) women had no preference.

Conclusion

In this preference study, we found that, given a choice, the majority of women would prefer to undergo office hysteroscopy for further investigation of the uterine cavity. This conclusion may be even stronger with the knowledge that the women participating in this study experienced more pain during office hysteroscopy compared to SIS [9]. In other words, pain scores had no effect on their preferences

Table 2 Mean pain scores (VAS in centimeters) stratified by preference

Allocated to	Mean pain scores by preference (95%-CI)			*p* value
	SIS	Office hysteroscopy	None	
SIS	2.2 (0.6–3.8)	2.6 (1.2–4.0)	3.5 (1.9–5.1)	0.431
Office hysteroscopy	6.0 (4.0–8.0)	3.1 (2.3–3.9)	3.9 (3.1–4.7)	0.057
Total	2.9 (1.3–4.5)	3.0 (2.2–3.8)	3.7 (2.9–4.5)	0.467

Table 3 Reason behind patient preferences for diagnostic investigation of the uterine cavity and subsequent therapy on a Likert scale

	Likert score median (25th–75th percentile)
Regarding diagnostic investigation	
Least discomfort as possible	4 (3–5)
Diagnosis and treatment in one session	4 (4–5)
Time to consider treatment options	4 (3–4)
Small risk failure investigation	4 (4–5)
Regarding therapy	
Short waiting time therapy	5 (4–5)
Small surgery risk	5 (4–5)
Anaesthesia during therapy	3 (3–4)
No anaesthesia during therapy	3 (3–4)
High chance therapy successful	5 (5–5)

1 very unimportant, *2* unimportant, *3* neutral, *4* important, *5* very important

afterwards. In women preferring SIS for uterine cavity assessment, the most important factor for their preference seems to be pain, while in women preferring hysteroscopy, other factors (e.g. immediate therapy) seemed to be of more importance in their preference.

A limitation of this study remains that we had to design a questionnaire specifically for this purpose because there were no validated questionnaires available. In order to minimise bias due to experience, we included women randomly allocated to SIS and office hysteroscopy who presumably had no strong preference beforehand and women with no history of uterine cavity investigation, which makes our design unique.

Another possible source of bias results from what is called cognitive justification—a phenomenon that makes people

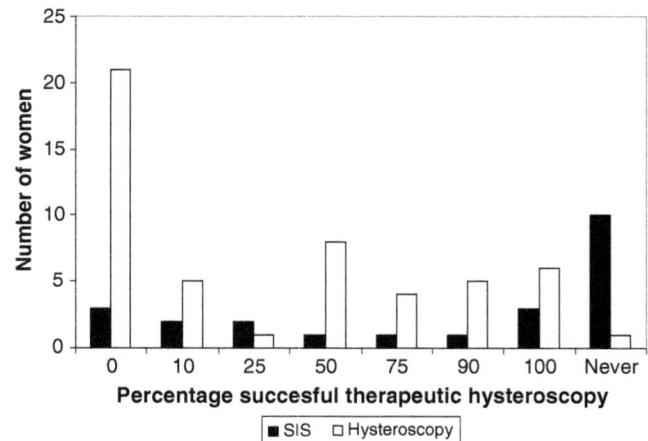

Fig. 3 Acceptance of hysteroscopy by the percentage of required successful hysteroscopic therapy among women preferring SIS and hysteroscopy. *SIS* saline infusion sonography

change their perceptions to make their situation seem better. Women were included in this study after undergoing SIS or office hysteroscopy, which might explain why the preference for the treatment they underwent was strongest. However, this accounts for both SIS and office hysteroscopy. Moreover, it is interesting that women of the control group preferred office hysteroscopy over SIS.

The most important reason for this preference was completeness of diagnosis and therapy in one visit. Additionally, our study showed that, apart from the diagnostic investigation, most women would prefer to undergo therapy in an outpatient setting rather than a day case setting. This is in concordance with previously published literature [7, 8, 10]. As proposed by Marsh et al. [8], we included in our questionnaire information about the risks and side effects of general anaesthesia in order to investigate whether the need for regional or general anaesthesia with day case hysteroscopy would influence their preference for an outpatient or day case approach. Surprisingly, this was not regarded of any importance in their preference.

Furthermore, most women prefer being informed about all advantages and disadvantages of diagnostic and therapeutic possibilities in general and prefer to participate in this decision. Considering this and the fact that a considerable part of the respondents preferred SIS and treatment under general anaesthesia, women should be informed of their options completely and not automatically be offered office hysteroscopy as the 'preferred' choice of investigation. Especially since the prevalence of intrauterine abnormalities after selection by transvaginal ultrasound examination is only 50% [11], and we do not know yet what the success rates are for treatment by office hysteroscopy.

In conclusion, we found that, given the choice, the majority of women would prefer office hysteroscopy over SIS. Additionally, if there was an indication for intrauterine surgery, an outpatient setting is preferred to a day case setting. Nevertheless, one third of the surveyed women would rather be treated under general anaesthesia. So, although our results support the establishment of outpatient one-stop clinics, the inpatient alternative should be offered as well.

Conflict of interest The authors report no conflict of interest. The authors alone are responsible for the content and writing of the paper.

Appendix A

Table 4 The descriptions of saline infusion sonography and office hysteroscopy

Saline infusion sonography	Office hysteroscopy
In general	In general
This procedure is used to determine the presence or absence of abnormalities in the uterine cavity.	This procedure is used to determine the presence or absence of abnormalities in the uterine cavity. Occasionally during this procedure, treatment will immediately follow a diagnosis.
Description of procedure	Description of procedure
The patient is seated in an examination chair with the legs resting on two knee supports. The doctor or investigator places a speculum in the vagina. A thin catheter (cross-sectional plane, 2 mm) is inserted through the neck of the womb into the womb, through which sterile normal saline solution is injected. When filled, a vaginal ultrasound is performed.	The patient is seated on an examination chair with the legs resting on two knee supports. The doctor inserts a thin telescope (cross-sectional plane, 4 mm) through the vagina and neck of the womb, into the womb (without using a speculum). Through the telescope, sterile saline solution is injected into the womb. Once the tip of the hysteroscope is in the womb, the inner wall is seen on a TV screen and can be evaluated.
Duration of procedure	Duration of procedure
15 min. Directly after the procedure, the patient may go home.	15 min. If subsequent therapy is required, an additional 15–30 min. Directly after the procedure, the patient may go home.
Anaesthesia	Anaesthesia
None	None
Therapy	Therapy
If an abnormality is found (50% of cases), a new appointment to treat it	If an abnormality is found (50% of cases) in a part of the cases, the

Table 4 (continued)

Saline infusion sonography	Office hysteroscopy
will be made. Depending on the type of abnormality, treatment will take place in the outpatient clinic by hysteroscopy (as described on the right). If this is not possible, treatment under general anaesthesia in the operating room may be required.	doctor will be able to remove it with a special instrument introduced through the telescope, e.g. removal of polyps or by taking biopsies for further analysis. If this is not possible, treatment under general anaesthesia in the operating room may be required.
Risk	Risk
Complications of SIS, 0.2% (1 out of 500; e.g. infection)	Complications of hysteroscopy, 0.4% (1 out of 250; e.g. infection, bleeding)
Failure of procedure	Failure of procedure
In 16% (16 out of 100) of the cases, the procedure will fail or will not provide enough information on the suspected pathology. In such cases, a new appointment will be made to perform a hysteroscopy in the outpatient clinic.	In 12% (12 out of 100) of the cases, the procedure will fail or will not provide enough information on the suspected pathology. In such cases, the hysteroscopy will be repeated under general anaesthesia in the operating room.

References

1. Clark TJ, Voit D, Gupta JK, Hyde C, Song F, Khan KS (2002) Accuracy of hysteroscopy in the diagnosis of endometrial cancer and hyperplasia: a systematic quantitative review. JAMA 288:1610–1621
2. van Dongen H, de Kroon CD, Jacobi CE, Trimbos JB, Jansen FW (2007) Diagnostic hysteroscopy in abnormal uterine bleeding: a systematic review and meta-analysis. BJOG 114:664–675
3. de Kroon CD, de Bock GH, Dieben SW, Jansen FW (2003) Saline contrast hysterosonography in abnormal uterine bleeding: a systematic review and meta-analysis. BJOG 110:938–947
4. Rogerson L, Bates J, Weston M, Duffy S (2002) A comparison of outpatient hysteroscopy with saline infusion hysterosonography. BJOG 109:800–804
5. Widrich T, Bradley LD, Mitchinson AR, Collins RL (1996) Comparison of saline infusion sonography with office hysteroscopy for the evaluation of the endometrium. Am J Obstet Gynecol 174:1327–1334
6. Bettocchi S, Selvaggi L (1997) A vaginoscopic approach to reduce the pain of office hysteroscopy. J Am Assoc Gynecol Laparosc 4:255–258
7. Kremer C, Duffy S, Moroney M (2000) Patient satisfaction with outpatient hysteroscopy versus day case hysteroscopy: randomised controlled trial. BMJ 320:279–282
8. Marsh F, Taylor L, Kremer C, Black J, Duffy S (2002) Delivering an effective outpatient service in gynaecology: an assessment of patient preference. Gynaecol Endosc 11:337–343
9. van Dongen H, de Kroon CD, van den Tillaart S, Louwe L, Trimbos-Kemper T, Jansen FW (2008) A randomized comparison of office vaginoscopic hysteroscopy with saline infusion sonography: a patient compliance study. BJOG 115:1232–1237
10. Ferry J, Rankin L (1994) Low cost, patient acceptable, local analgesia approach to gynaecological outpatient surgery. A review of 817 consecutive procedures. Aust N Z J Obstet Gynaecol 34:453–456
11. Towbin NA, Gviazda IM, March CM (1996) Office hysteroscopy versus transvaginal ultrasonography in the evaluation of patients with excessive uterine bleeding. Am J Obstet Gynecol 174:1678–1682

20

Indications of diagnostic hysteroscopy

**Angelos Daniilidis · A. Pantelis · K. Dinas ·
T. Tantanasis · P. D. Loufopoulos · S. Angioni · F. Carcea**

Abstract Plenty of authors propose outpatient hysteroscopy as the gold standard diagnostic method for the evaluation of endometrial pathology. This statement has been strengthened in the recent years due to the wide use of smaller diameter hysteroscopic devices, which have made the dilation of the cervix and the use of anesthesia unnecessary. The main purpose of this paper is to summarize the indications of diagnostic hysteroscopy. In this review, we used the most recent publications in MEDLINE and Cochrane Library in order to specify the indications of diagnostic hysteroscopy and the experience that have been obtained till today in the management of certain pathological uterine conditions. The key words we used were diagnostic hysteroscopy, abnormal uterine bleeding, infertility, endometrial cancer. Hysteroscopy provides an accurate method of evaluation and direct visualization of the endometrial cavity and moreover directed biopsy and sampling of suspected lesions. Last years with the continuous development in the hysteroscopy devices, plenty of women benefit surgical hysteroscopy techniques for uterine abnormalities. Hysteroscopy is useful for the diagnosis in patients with abnormal uterine bleeding, with endometrial cancer and in infertile women. Hysteroscopy has the unique advantage of combining a thorough procedure with great diagnostic accuracy. The only disadvantage is that hysteroscopy requires specific teaching and training and has a long learning curve.

Keywords Diagnostic hysteroscopy · Abnormal uterine bleeding · Infertility · Endometrial cancer

A. Daniilidis · A. Pantelis · K. Dinas · T. Tantanasis ·
P. D. Loufopoulos · F. Carcea
2nd Department of Obstetrics and Gynecology,
Aristotle University of Thessaloniki,
Evosmos, Greece

S. Angioni
Department of Obstetrics and Gynecology,
University Hospital Don Calabria,
Cagliari, Italy

A. Daniilidis (✉)
Department of Obstetrics and Gynecology,
Aristotle University of Thessaloniki,
9 Smirnis, 56224,
Evosmos, Thessaloniki, Greece
e-mail: angedan@hotmail.com

Introduction

Diagnostic hysteroscopy is an accurate and less invasive method for the evaluation of common gynecological disorders such as premenopausal or postmenopausal abnormal uterine bleeding (AUB), endometrial hyperplasia, endometrial cancer, and infertility. Although hysteroscopy as an invasive method is available for the past two decades, the management and the investigation of the uterine pathology till recently, involved dilatation and curettage (D&C) of endometrial cavity under general anesthesia for the majority of gynecologists. A variety of innovations in hysteroscopic instrumentation and techniques, provide accurate evaluation and direct visualization of the endometrial cavity and moreover directed biopsy and sampling of suspected lesions with great safety. The introduction of smaller diameter hysteroscopes has allowed diagnostic hysteroscopy to become an outpatient procedure. Other methods, less invasive, for evaluating the female reproductive tract with a prevalent use are the transvaginal ultrasonography (TVS) with saline infusion sonography or without saline infusion into the endometrial cavity, hysterosalpingography (HSG), and the blind endometrial sampling with pipelle. The main advantage of hysteroscopy is that it combines a more reliable method with greater diagnostic accuracy because of direct visualization. The only disadvantage of hysteroscopy is that it acquires specific teaching and training and has a longer learning curve.

The main purpose of this paper is to summarize the indications of diagnostic hysteroscopy according to the current literature and papers published in MEDLINE and Cochrane library.

Hysteroscopy in patients with abnormal uterine bleeding

AUB is probably the most common abnormal condition in gynecological practice especially for women over the age of 45 years old. It also affects almost 25% of reproductive aged women. Plenty of diagnostic techniques (such as TVS, TVS with saline solution infusion, D&C, and endometrial biopsy) have been widely used in order to evaluate women with AUB. In recent years, hysteroscopy has been widely used as an outpatient office procedure in combination with direct biopsy after visualization of the endometrial cavity. Plenty of authors till today have managed to demonstrate the great potential of hysteroscopy as the gold standard method for the investigation of women with such pathology. Barati et al. have announced that in a sum of 147 women with AUB and normal TVS, 32 of them (21.8%) were hysteroscopically abnormal, and cervical canal polyp has been described as the commonest lesion that has been misdiagnosed by TVS [1]. Endometrial or cervical polyps can be treated better by hysteroscopy since D&C has proved to be less effective [2]. A few years earlier, Refaie et al. evaluated 112 pre- and postmenopausal women with AUB in order to assess if an outpatient hysteroscopy affects the decision making of treatment. The authors concluded that half of the women had abnormal uterine cavities with most common findings the submucous myomas and endometrial polyps and that hysteroscopical investigation of AUB could lead to the most appropriate treatment, without unnecessary major surgical intervention [3]. Bettocchi et al. have proved the efficacy of office hysteroscopy treatment in benign intrauterine pathologies in menopausal women. He has enrolled in his study a sum of 925 menopausal women with AUB in a period of 5 years and divided them into two investigation groups according to the endometrial thickness (group 1 <4 mm, group 2 >4 mm). The conclusion was that the diagnostic value of hysteroscopy yielded 99–100% specificity and sensitivity respectively for both groups [4]. In an attempt of some authors to summarize the results of diagnostic hysteroscopy, a systematic review has been published by H Van Dongen et al. In this study, 17 articles in a meta-analysis have been enrolled and it has been proposed that diagnostic hysteroscopy for women with AUB

is both accurate and feasible in the detection of intrauterine anomalies with a success rate estimated approximately at 96.9% (SD 5.2%, range 83–100%) [5].

Summarizing, we can assume that the most frequent hysteroscopic findings in patients with AUB are the submucous myomas, polyps, and endometrial hyperplasia, either benign or malignant, in about 60–70% of the cases. Moreover, diagnostic hysteroscopy as a method is even more valuable and with greater success rates, in the identification of AUB in perimenopausal and postmenopausal women with no specific risk of cancer progression.

Hysteroscopy in patients with endometrial cancer

The most common type of pelvic malignancy still remains the endometrial cancer. This type of malignancy causes abnormal genital bleeding usually as a first symptom in most of the cases, thus, the early investigation of such symptom is of great importance for woman's survival and progress. Unfortunately, some of women with endometrial adenocarcinoma remain asymptomatic. Endometrial hyperplasia is deemed as a precursor of endometrial cancer. The most important sign of endometrial cancer or endometrial hyperplasia is the endometrial thickness in an ultrasound exam. Unfortunately, ultrasound exam has very low specificity in the differentiation of the type of endometrial hyperplasia as soon as directed biopsy of the suspected uterus still remains a prerequisite for an appropriate control. An endometrial thickness greater than 4 mm requires further evaluation in postmenopausal women with AUB [6–8]. Hysteroscopy not only can clearly and accurately display the appearance of endometrial cancer but also demonstrates any possible involvement of the lower uterine segment and cervix. Cordeiro and her colleagues summarized hysteroscopic findings in 245 postmenopausal women with increased endometrial thickness in TVS and compared the diagnostic outcomes regarding the presence or absence of AUB [9]. In this study, the investigators suggested that sensitivity, specificity, positive predictive, and negative predictive value of hysteroscopy for endometrial carcinoma was 94.1%, 98.95%, 88.9%, and 99.5%, respectively. Also, the concordance between hysteroscopic findings and histological diagnosis was 89.9%. The specificity and negative predictive value of hysteroscopy for diagnosing cancer were similar to other authors [10].

In all this continuing debate about the value and the accuracy of hysteroscopy in the diagnosis of serious endometrial disease (cancer and hyperplasia), plenty of answers have been given by a systematic quantitative review that has been announced by JT Clark and co partners. In this review, 65 papers have been isolated and the results were the following: The overall sensitivity and specificity of hysteroscopy for endometrial cancer was 86.4% and 99.2%, respectively. The variation in sensitivity was much greater than the variation in specificity of diagnostic hysteroscopy in endometrial disease (cancer and hyperplasia), and finally concluded that as a method, diagnostic hysteroscopy is safe with low incidence of serious complications, with high accuracy in diagnosing endometrial cancer rather than excluding it, and with high accuracy in diagnosing endometrial disease (cancer and hyperplasia) mainly in postmenopausal women rather than in premenopausal [11].

Another great debate enrolls the hypothesis of dissemination of cancer cells after diagnostic hysteroscopy in women with endometrial cancer. Some investigators have proposed that distention of the endometrial cavity with saline solution or CO_2 during the hysteroscopic procedure can, under certain circumstances, disseminate endometrial cancer cells to the abdominal cavity and change both the prognosis and the course of treatment. There are several conflicted arguments and concerns about this hypothesis. On the one hand, it is well-known that all examination methods (bimanual examination, D&C, and even hysterectomy) may lead to migration of endometrial cancer cells through the fallopian tubes to systemic circulation and peritoneal cavity without increasing the incidence of metastasis. Tanizawa et al. in 1,040 women with endometrial cancer examined by hysteroscopy, found no significant differences in the presence of intraperitoneal tumor cells compared to patients evaluated by a different method [12]. Taddei et al. demonstrated that hysteroscopy evaluation of the extent of endometrial carcinoma could lead to an individualized therapeutic program and have a beneficial effect on survival rates [13]. Nagele et al. in a prospective randomized self-controlled study showed that there was no significant difference in the spreading of endometrial cells after hysteroscopy either by the use of natural solution or by the use of CO_2 for uterine distention. Only transtubal dissemination has occurred in about 25% of the patients [14]. Finally, de Sousa Damiao et al., after they have diagnosed endometrial cancer in 72 women, concluded that the hysteroscopic evaluation of endometrial cancer, if it is performed under low pressure of CO_2, does not cause spread of malignant endometrial cells into the peritoneal cavity [15]. On the other hand, Takac et al., after a retrospective study on 146 patients with endometrial cancer, emphasized that hysteroscopy significantly increases the risk of positive peritoneal cytology in women with endometrial cancer in comparison with D&C [16]. Revel et al. only a few years earlier have mentioned an increased risk of peritoneal contamination by malignant cells after hysteroscopy but with no evidence for these women to face worse prognosis comparing to patients who have undergone other diagnostic procedures [17]. Polyzos and his colleagues very recently analyzed nine clinical trials with 1,015 women with histologically proven endometrial carcinoma who either underwent or not preoperative hysteroscopy evaluation. Hysteroscopy resulted in a significantly higher rate of malignant peritoneal cytology compared to no hysteroscopy, especially if the distention medium was isotonic sodium chloride and if the inflated media pressure reached or exceeded 100 mmHg [18].

To summarize, it seems that there is a slightly higher percentage of positive peritoneal cytology in women with endometrial cancer who have been evaluated preoperatively with hysteroscopy under high pressure (>100 mmHg) probably due to a transtubal reflux of endometrial cells into the peritoneal cavity. These cells although appear a functional viability, in clinical practice, they seem to disappear in a short time and do not affect the patient's overall outcome. In cases that endometrial cancer is suspected, decrease of intrauterine pressure (less than 80 mmHg) possibly provides security for these patients in order to be evaluated preoperatively with diagnostic hysteroscopy with no negative influence to their prognosis [19] (Table 1).

Hysteroscopy in infertile patients

According to the WHO guidelines, HSG is recommended to all infertile women in order to be evaluated properly for the uterine malformations that are responsible for infertility problems [20]. The goal of uterine cavity evaluation is to detect uterine malformations such as polyps, myomas, or uterine septums that can negatively influence the embryo implantation [21]. There is an ongoing debate regarding the value of routine hysteroscopy before an in vitro fertilisation (IVF) attempt. Hysteroscopic examination seems to be superior in the evaluation of these patients than HSG [21]. Barati et al. have enrolled in a study women with unexplained infertility and women with infertility because of uterine factor. He investigated them either by TVS and HSG, or by TVS, HSG, and hysteroscopy. There was a 38.8% positive finding in office hysteroscopy despite of normal TVS and HSG. He concluded that office hysteroscopy should be a part of routine work in the evaluation of infertile women [22]. Kumar and his colleagues compared the diagnostic efficacy of HSG and hysteroscopy in assessment of uterine factor in infertile women in a 2-year study in which 60 patients were subjected to HSG and hysteroscopy as well. They have showed specificity of HSG as 90% and false negative value as 40%. They have mentioned the significant role of HSG as a screening procedure but it must be supplemented by hysteroscopy although it is an observer-dependent technique [23]. Koskas et al. evaluated hysteroscopically 556 women with difficulty to conceive after 1 year of unprotected intercourse and

Table 1 Summary of studies regarding endometrial cancer investigations and hysteroscopy

Hysteroscopy in endometrial cancer	Year of study	Number of women	Type of publication	Summary of publication—Findings.
Tanizawa O et al.	1991	1,040	Observational	No significant differences in the presence of intraperitoneal tumor cells.
Taddei GL et al.	1994	235	Observational	Hysteroscopic evaluation of endometrial cavity and cervical canal in women with endometrial adenocarcinoma has beneficial effects on woman's survival rates.
Fay TN et al.	1999	83	Multicenter randomized double-blind control trial.	Hysteroscopic assessment of endometrial cavity efficient in the detection of pathological intrauterine lesions but only moderately successful determining physiological endometrial changes.
Nagele F et al.	1999	30	Prospective randomized self-controlled study	No significant difference in the spreading of endometrial malignant cells either by CO_2 or N/S as a distention media for hysteroscopy.
Clark TJ et al.	2002	26,346	Systemic quantitative review	The diagnostic accuracy of hysteroscopy is high for endometrial cancer and moderate for endometrial disease.
Revel A et al.	2004		Systemic review	An increased risk of peritoneal contamination of malignant cells after hysteroscopy but with no evidence for the patients to face worsen prognosis.
Takac I et al.	2007	146	Retrospective randomized trial	Diagnostic hysteroscopy significantly increases the risk of positive peritoneal cytology but not the risk of adnexal, abdominal or retroperitoneal lymph node metastases in women with endometrial cancer.
De Sousa Damiao et al.	2009	76	Prospective longitudinal study	If hysteroscopy is performed under a low pressure of CO_2, no spread of endometrial cells occur into the peritoneal cavity.
Polyzos NP et al.	2010	1,015	Systematic review and meta-analysis	Hysteroscopy resulted in a significantly higher rate of malignant peritoneal cytology especially if the distention medium was N/S and the inflated media pressure exceeded 100 mmHg.

Table 2 Summary of studies regarding infertility investigations and hysteroscopy

Hysteroscopy in infertility	Year of study	Number of women	Type of publication	Summary of publication—Findings
Valle RF	1980	142	Observational	Hysteroscopy before IVF more superior than HSG
Barati M et al.	2009	107	Observational	There was a 38.8% positive finding in office hysteroscopy despite of normal TVS and HSG in infertile women.
Kumar et al.	2003	60	Observational retrospective	Mentioned the significant role of HSG as a screening procedure but it must be supplemented by hysteroscopy although it is an observer-dependent technique.
Koskas et al.	2010	556	Clinical study	Evaluated hysteroscopically 556 women incapable to conceive and found that first line office hysteroscopy for infertility shows abnormal findings ranged from 30% to more than 60%
Bosteels et al.	2010	1,410	Systemic review	Removal of endometrial polyps doubles the pregnancy rate compared with diagnostic hysteroscopy and polyp biopsy in women who undergo IUI. Diagnostic hysteroscopy in the cycle preceding subsequent IVF attempt almost doubles the pregnancy rates
El-Toukhy et al.	2008	1,691	Meta analysis	Remarkable evidence of benefit from hysteroscopy in increasing the chance of pregnancy in a subsequent IVF cycle.

found that first-line office hysteroscopy for infertility showed abnormal findings which ranged from 30% at women 30 years old to more than 60% at women more than 42 years old. Thus, they have proposed an additional argument that office hysteroscopy must be part of first-line exams in infertile women regardless of age [24]. Very recently, Bosteels et al. revealed a systemic review about the effectiveness of hysteroscopy in subfertile women without other gynecological symptoms. The investigators detected that removal of endometrial polyps doubles the pregnancy rate compared with diagnostic hysteroscopy and polyp biopsy in women who undergo IUI. They also mentioned the lack of randomized controlled trials on hysteroscopic treatment of intrauterine adhesions and also that diagnostic hysteroscopy in the cycle preceding subsequent IVF attempt almost doubles the pregnancy rates in women with at least two failed IVF attempts in comparison with women starting IVF immediately [25]. In order to reveal the impact of hysteroscopy in patients with two or more failed IVF cycles, El-Toukhy et al. have announced a systemic review and meta-analysis in 2008 in which 1,691 women divided into two groups participated; one of hysteroscopy and one control group. According to the authors, there was a remarkable evidence of benefit from hysteroscopy in increasing the chance of pregnancy in a subsequent IVF cycle [26].

According to the experience of all these authors, there were lesions detected by hysteroscopy in about 30% of subfertile women reported as normal by HSG and about 50% of subfertile women reported as normal in transvaginal ultrasound. It is clear that diagnostic hysteroscopy not only defines intrauterine lesions such as polyps, submucous myomas, and adhesions, with great accuracy, but also it makes them amenable to surgery by operative hysteroscopy instead of many traditional surgical approaches (Table 2). Nevertheless, for women with recurrent IVF failure, there is some evidence of benefit from hysteroscopy and increasing the success of embryo transfer in subsequent IVF cycle.

Conflict of interest The authors report no conflicts of interest. The authors alone are responsible for the content and writing of the paper.

References

1. Barati M, Masihi S, Moramezi F, Salemi S (2008) Office hysteroscopy in patients with abnormal uterine bleeding and normal transvaginal ultrasonography. Int J Fertil Steril 4:175–178
2. Cravello L, Stolla V, Bretelle F, Roger V, Blanv B (2000) Hysteroscopic resection of endometrial polyps: a study of 195 cases. Eur J Obstet Gynecol Reprod Biol 93:131–134
3. Refaie A, Anderson T, Cheah S (2005) Out-patient hysteroscopy: findings and decision making for treatment of abnormal uterine bleeding in pre- and post-menopausal women. Mid East Fertil Soc Journ
4. Bettocchi S, Nappi L, Ceci O, Santoro A, Fattizzi N, Nardelli C et al (2004) The role of office hysteroscopy in menopause. J Am Assoc Gynecol Laparosc 11:103–106
5. van Dongen H, de Kroon CD, Jakobi CE, Trimbos JB, Jansen FW (2007) Diagnostic hysteroscopy in abnormal uterine bleeding: a systematic review and meta-analysis. BJOG 114:664–675
6. Bree RL, Bowerman RA, Bohm-Velez M, Benson CB, Doubilet PM, DeDreu S et al (2000) US evaluation of the uterus in patients with postmenopausal bleeding: a positive effect on diagnostic decision making. Radiology 216:260–264
7. Dijkhuizen F, Mol BWJ, Brolman HAM, Heintz APM (2000) The accuracy of endometrial sampling in the diagnosis of patients with endometrial carcinoma and hyperplasia. Cancer 89:1765–1772
8. Smith-Bindman R, Kerlikowske K, Feldstein VA, Subak L, Scheidler J, Segal M et al (1998) Endovaginal ultrasound to exclude endometrial cancer and other endometrial abnormalities. J Am Med Assoc 280:1510–1517
9. Cordeiro A, Condeco R, Leitao C, Sousa F, Coutinho S, do Carmo S et al (2010) Office hysteroscopy after ultrasonographic diagnosis of thickened endometrium in postmenopausal patients. Obstet Gynecol Surv 2:95–96
10. Fay TN, Khanem N, Hosking D (1999) Out-patient hysteroscopy in asymptomatic postmenopausal women. Climacteric 2:263–267
11. Clark TJ, Voit D, Gupta JK, Hyde C, Song F, Khan KS (2002) Accuracy of hysteroscopy in the diagnosis of endometrial cancer and hyperplasia: a systematic quantitative review. JAMA 288:1610–1621
12. Tanizawa O, Miyake A, Suqimoto O (1991) Re-evaluation of hysteroscopy in the diagnosis of uterine endometrial cancer. Nippon Sanka Fujinka Gakkai Zasshi Jun 43:622–626
13. Taddei GL, Moncini D, Scarselli G, Tantini C, Bargelli G (1994) Can hysteroscopic evaluation of endometrial carcinoma influence therapeutic treatment? Ann N Y Acad Sci 734:482–487
14. Nagele F, Wieser F, Deery A, Hart R, Magos A (1999) Endometrial cell dissemination at diagnostic hysteroscopy: a prospective randomized cross-over comparison of normal saline and carbon dioxide uterine distention. Hum Reprod 14:2739–2742
15. de Sousa Damiao R, Lopes RG, Dos Santos ES, Lippi UG, da Fonseca EB (2009) Evaluation of the risk of spreading endometrial cell by hysteroscopy: a prospective longitudinal study. Obstet Gynecol Int 397079
16. Takac I, Zegura B (2007) Office hysteroscopy and the risk of microscopic extrauterine spread in endometrial cancer. Gynecol Oncol 107:94–98
17. Revel A, Tsafrir A, Anteby SO, Shushan A (2004) Does hysterectomy produce spread of endometrial cancer cells? Obstet Gynecol Surv 59:280–284
18. Polyzos NP, Mauri D, Tsioras S, Messini CI, Valachis A, Messinis IE (2010) Intraperitoneal dissemination of endometrial cancer cells after hysteroscopy: a systematic review and meta-analysis. Int J Gynecol Cancer 20:261–267
19. Koutlaki N, Dimitraki M, Zervoudis S, Skafida P, Nikas I, Mandratzi J et al (2010) Hysteroscopy and endometrial cancer. Gynecol Surg 7:335–341
20. Rowe PC, Hargreave T, Mellows H. WHO Manual for the standardized investigation and diagnosis of the infertile couple (1993) The Press Syndicate of the University of Cambridge, Cambridge, UK
21. Valle RF (1980) Hysteroscopy in the evaluation of female infertility. Am J Obstet Gynecol 137:425–431
22. Barati M, Zargar M, Masihi S, Borzoo L, Cheraghian B (2009) Office hysteroscopy in infertility. Int J Fertil Steril 3:17–20
23. Kumar S, Awasthi RT, Gokhale N (2003) Assessment of uterine factor in infertile women: hysterosalpingography vs. hysteroscopy. MJAFI 60:39–41

24. Koskas M, Mergui JL, Yazbeck C, Uzan S, Nizard J (2010) Office hysteroscopy for infertility: a series of 557 consecutive cases. Obstet Gynecol Int 168096:1–4

25. Bosteels J, Weyers S, Puttemans P, Panayiotidis C, Van Herendael B, Gomel V et al (2010) The effectiveness of hysteroscopy in improving pregnancy rates in subfertile women without other gynaecological symptoms: a systematic review. Hum Reprod Update 16:1–11

26. El-Toukhy T, Sunkara SK, Coomarasamy A, Grace J, Khalaf Y (2008) Outpatient hysteroscopy and subsequent IVF cycle outcome: a systematic review and meta-analysis. Reprod Biomed Online 16:712–719

21

Reliability of out-patient hysteroscopy in one-stop clinic for abnormal uterine bleeding

Atef M. Darwish · Ezzat H. Sayed ·
Safwat A. Mohammad · Ibraheem I. Mohammad ·
Hoida I. Hassan

Abstract This study aims to estimate the effect of adding office hysteroscopy to the preoperative diagnostic work-up in abnormal uterine bleeding on the diagnostic accuracy. It is a prospective comparative diagnostic trial at a tertiary care referral facility and a university hospital. There were a total of 295 patients, more than 35 years old, with abnormal uterine bleeding. The patients had vaginal sonography, office hysteroscopy, and office endometrial biopsy on one-stop bases. The diagnostic accuracy of each method in diagnosing focal lesion and endometrial hyperplasia was measured as the main outcome of this paper. Combined hysteroscopy and biopsy were taken as the gold standard for diagnosing focal lesion while endometrial biopsy alone was the gold standard for diagnosing endometrial hyperplasia. Office hysteroscopy was superior to other methods for diagnosing focal lesion with about half of the focal lesions failing to be diagnosed with the other two methods. Office hysteroscopy was superior to vaginal sonography in diagnosing endometrial hyperplasia. Office hysteroscopy is an indispensable tool for diagnosing abnormal uterine bleeding and without its use, half of the focal lesions could be missed. Office setting and the one-stop approach greatly facilitate the use of the combination of office hysteroscopy with vaginal sonography and office endometrial sample.

A. M. Darwish (✉) · E. H. Sayed · S. A. Mohammad ·
I. I. Mohammad
Department of Obstetrics and Gynecology,
Woman's Health University Hospital,
71111 Assiut, P.O. Box: (1) Assiut, Egypt
e-mail: atef_darwish@yahoo.com

H. I. Hassan
Department of Pathology, Faculty of Medicine, Assiut University,
Assiut, Egypt

Keywords Office hysteroscopy · Uterine bleeding ·
Ultrasonography · Biopsy

Introduction

Abnormal uterine bleeding (AUB) is any vaginal bleeding unrelated to normal menstruation and represents a major gynecological problem in about 20% of all gynecological referrals [1]. Anatomic and histologic causes predominate after the age of 35 years which made the American College of Obstetrics and Gynecology recommend endometrial biopsy as a part of investigating any woman with AUB above 35 years and sometimes earlier if there is a risk factor [2]. In addition to a careful clinical examination, the traditional approach for diagnosis of AUB comprises both transabdominal ultrasonography (TAS) and transvaginal ultrasonography (TVS), and endometrial sampling. Ultrasonography, especially TVS, is generally accepted as an initial investigation of these patients as it is well tolerated, least invasive, easy to do, and gives idea about the uterine anatomy (the wall and the lining) and the adnexa with little cost. These diagnostic tools share some common disadvantages in the form of failure to diagnose minute causes that are not commonly seen, to localize the exact site of the lesion causing bleeding, to define its relationship to tubal ostea specially in infertile women and lastly to guide biopsy aid. For cavitary disorders, hysteroscopy is the gold standard for diagnosis of AUB which is widely performed as office hysteroscopy (OH) procedure with the possibility of see and treat in the setting. OH is a well-tolerated procedure and equally accepted as hysteroscopy under general anesthesia [3]. There is no consensus however that OH should be included in the initial evaluation of patients with AUB or be restricted to those with abnormalities at TVS. This study

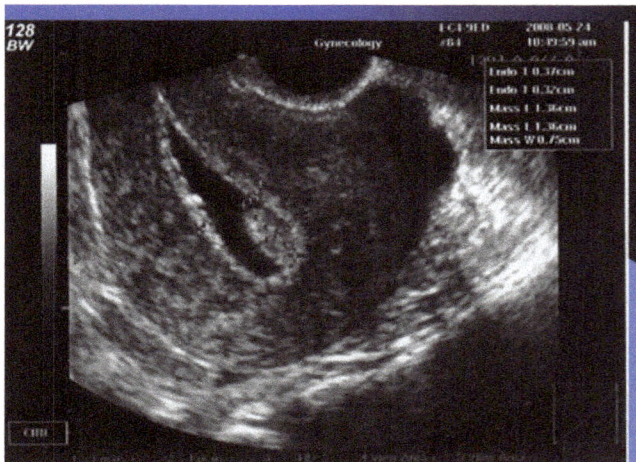

Fig. 1 Transvaginal sonohysterographic appereance of an endometrial polyp

aims to estimate the effect of adding OH to the preoperative diagnostic work-up in AUB on the diagnostic accuracy.

Materials and methods

After obtaining the acceptance of the ethics committee of the Assiut Faculty of Medicine, this study was conducted in the outpatient hysteroscopy unit of Woman's Health University Hospital from August 2006 to May 2011. It included women with AUB of 35 years or older. Exclusion criteria included suspected pregnancy, active pelvic infection, severe comorbidity, e.g., severe cardiac, neurologic, or chest disease, recent initiation of contraception in the previous 3 months, or cervical neoplasm. The patients were examined at the day of presentation on one-stop bases irrespective of the day of the cycle. All patients had clear description of the study and were asked to participate. An informed consent was taken from those who agreed.

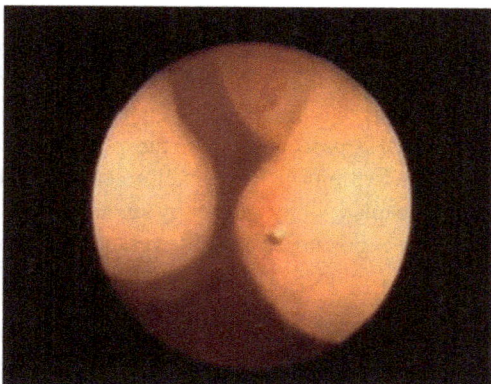

Fig. 3 Strawberry appearance of the congested endometrium

The included patients were subjected to complete history taking and meticulous physical examination. Both TAS and TVS were thereafter performed using a Medison 128 BW machine (MEDISON COR, South Korea). The uterus was examined in the saggital and coronal views for endometrial thickness, focal cavitary or intramural masse(s), evidence of adenomyosis uteri [4], or adnexal mass(s).

The endometrium was considered thick when it was 5 mm or more in postmenopausal patients and in premenopausal patients of 8 mm or more and 10 mm or more cutoff levels was tested. Because it was not possible in all cases to clearly discriminate between polyp and submucous myoma, focal lesion was used to describe either of them. Abnormal endometrium was used to describe endometrial line with which was either thick and/or shows signs of focal lesion. In case of suspicious diagnosis when TVS could not exactly differentiate intracavitary from intramural lesions, a quick office sonohysterography was performed according to our simplified technique [5] as shown in Fig. 1. TVS was performed by an ultrasonography team but sonohysterography was performed by the first author.

OH was done using posterior wall Sims' speculum to expose the cervix where the anterior lip is grasped with

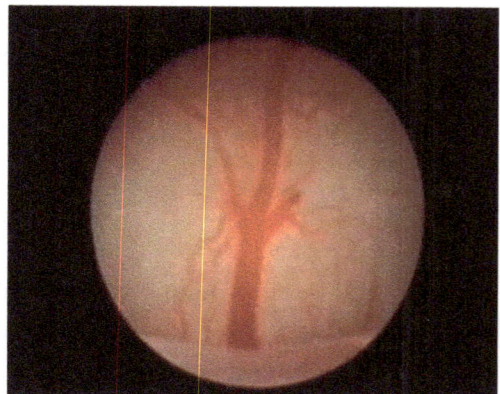

Fig. 2 Kissing endometrial polyp

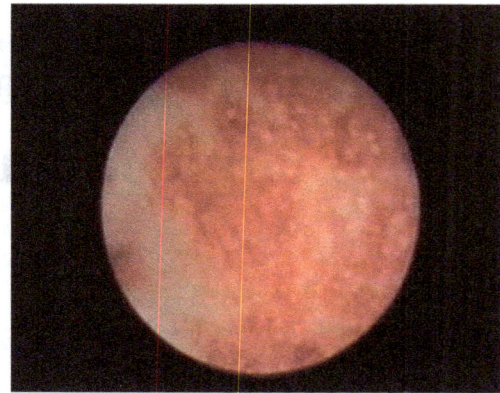

Fig. 4 Telangiectatic vessel of the endometrium

Fig. 5 Office sampling

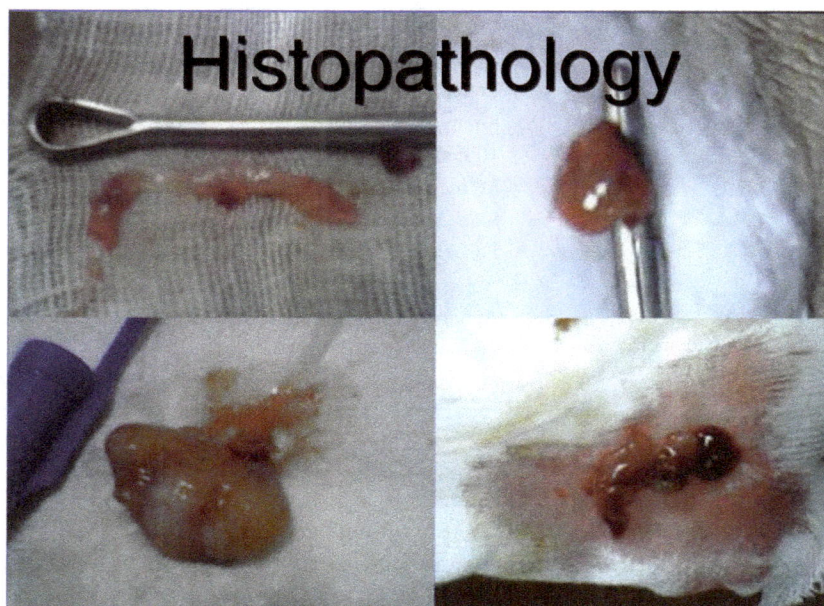

single-toothed tenaculum without any premedication or local anesthesia. We used 2.9° mm 30° rigid scope with 4 mm single flow sheath (Promis, Germany) and the uterus was distended with normal saline at 100 mmHg generated from a pneumatic cuff of sphygmomanometer. We used 250-W halogen light source for the video OH. The scope was introduced gently through the cervical canal without previous dilatation using the saline to expand the way in front of the scope. The cervical canal was examined for polypi, Nabothian cysts, or micropolypi suggestive of chronic cervicitis. The uterine cavity was examined systematically (panoramic view) starting by its anterior and posterior walls; the fundus, and the borders and examination was considered complete if the both tubal ostia were reached describing any gross pathology, e.g., polyp, myoma, growth, etc. (Fig. 2).

Focused OH was then performed to describe endometrial appearance (atrophic, normal thick, papillary, suspicious of atypical hyperplasia or cancer), vasculature (normal, congestion, petechiae, ecchymosis, or abnormal suspicious vascular pattern), and color (whitish, pink, reddish, or dark red; Figs. 3 and 4). The scope was finally gradually withdrawn with confirmation of previous findings. Then a 5-mm uterine curette or a 4-mm Novak curette with suction was introduced in multiprous uterus or nulliprous uterus, respectively, for endometrial biopsy (office sample, OS) from the anterior and/or the posterior walls of the uterus just below the fundus and directed towards any suspicious area previously defined on hysteroscopic examination (Fig. 5).

The statistical analysis was done using SPSS 16 program. Categorical date were described as percentages and

	Global	35–40	40 or more	Menopausal	Sig.
Mean age (years)	45.3 (7.9)	36.4 (1.5)	45.6 (4.2)	55.6 (8.3)	NA
Parity	6.3 (3.1)	4.7 (2.2)	6.6 (3)	7.6 (3.3)	0.000
Abortions	1.3 (1.5)	0.9 (1.2)	1.4 (1.6)	1.3 (1.5)	0.06
Nulliparity	3.1%	4.3%	2.9%	1.8%	0.72
Contraceptive use	21%[a]	30%	17%	NA	0.04[a]
Progestin treatment	37%	37%	39%	31%	0.5
Previous D&C	31%	27%	36%	20%	0.051
Hypertension	18.6%	4.3%	19.4%	35%	0.000
DM	10%	4.3%	8.2%	22%	0.003
BMI	30.6 (6.3)	28.4 (6)	30.7 (5.7)	33 (7.4)	0.000
Obesity(BMI>/=30)	51%	37%	53%	62%	0.000

Table 1 Characteristics of the study patients

[a]Comparisons were made between premenopausal groups only.

NA Not applicable

Table 2 Transvaginal sonographic findings.

	Global	35–40	40 or more	Menopausal	Sig.
Endometrial thickness (mm)	10.9±5.7	9.7±5.2	10.3 (4.8)	14.2 (7.6)	0.000
8 mm or more	67%	59%	64%	87.3%[b]	0.001
10 mm or more	51%	34%	46%	87.3%[b]	0.000
Myometrial thickness (cm)	1.9 (0.5)	1.8 (0.4)	2 (0.5)	1.7 (0.4)	0.000
Signs of adenomyosis	41%	27%	52%	24%	0.000
Focal lesion	21%	16%	21%	29%	0.187
Abnormal endometrium 8 mm[a]	74%	67%	73%	87.3%[b]	0.032
Abnormal endometrium 10 mm	60%	43%	59%	87.3%[b]	0.000
Fibroid	17%	10%	21%	13%	0.072
Ovarian mass	6.4%	8.6%	5.9%	5.5%	0.81

[a]Either thick endometrium or focal lesion

[b]At 5 mm cut off level

compared with chi square and exact Fischer tests. Continuous data were described as mean±SD or median (according to data distribution) and compared using t test, Man–Whitney test, and analysis of variance test with least significant difference post hock test when appropriate. Correlation was used when appropriate. The diagnostic performance is calculated using 2×2 tables using EB as the gold standard for diagnosing hyperplasia or cancer and the combined hysteroscopy and biopsy for diagnosing focal lesion.

Results

The characteristics of the study patients are shown in Table 1. Only five cases (1.7%) had failed OH with success rate of (295/300) 98.3% while 15 cases had failed OS with success rate of (295/310) 95%. The results of TVS, OH, and EB examinations are summarized in Tables 2, 3, and 4. Abnormal findings tended to increase with age with more prevalence of precancerous and cancerous lesions in the postmenopausal group.

Table 3 Office hysteroscopic findings

	Global	35–40	40 or more	Menopausal	Sig.
Appearance					
Atrophic	2%	1.4%	1.8%	3.6%	0.64
Normal	58.3%	66%	59%	43.6%	0.02
Thick	32.5%	30%	33%	36.4%	0.62
Plypoid	4.4%	2.9%	5.3%	3.6%	0.67
Suspecious	2.7%	0%	0.6%	13%	0.000
Vasculature					
Normal	24%	21%	25%	22%	0.76
Congestion	41%	47%	37%	47%	0.22
Petechiae and Ecchymosis	29%	30%	33.5%	16%	0.052
Abnormalvessles	5.4%	1.4%	4.1%	15%	0.003
Polyp	15%	5.7%	14%	29%	0.001
Submucous myomas	13%	5.7%	16%	12.7%	0.1
Either	25%	11.4%	26%	40%	0.001
Abnormal hysteroscopy	55%	39%	56%	71%	0.001
Blood clots	17.3%	24.3%	14%	18%	0.163
Adhesions	3.7%	2.9%	4.7%	1.8%	0.56
Access to tubal ostia					
Both	77.3%	87%	76.5%	67.3%	0.097
One	10.5%	7.1%	11.1%	12.75	0.097
Neither	12.2%	5.7%	12.4%	20%	0.097
Fluid volume (cc)	311 (115)	309 (133)	309 (107)	320 (116)	0.828

Table 4 Results of endometrial biopsy

	Global (%)	35–40 (%)	40 or more (%)	Menopausal (%)	Sig.
Insufficient	2.4	2.9	2.9	0	0.439
Proliferative	35.4	41.4	38.8	18.2	0.005
Secretory	13	21.4	12.4	5.5	0.029
Simple hyperplasia	34.2	24.3	35.3	43.6	0.045
Atypical hyperplasia	3.4	1.4	1.8	10.9	0.003
Cancer	1.4	0	0	7.3	0.000
Others					
Atrophy	4	2.9	3.5	5.4	0.732
Endometritis	2	1.4	1.8	3.6	0.169
TB endometritis	0.7	1.4	0.6	0	0.342
Polyp	2.4	1.4	1.2	5.5	0.03
Submucous myoma	2.4	1.4	2.9	3.6	0.274
Remnants of conception	1.4	2.9	1.2	0	0.372
Menstruating	0.3	0	0.6	0	0.23

Table 6 Patient and physician satisfaction with the different procedures

	TVS	OH	EB	Sig.
Duration (min)	3.47 (0.78)	3.6 (0.97)	2.14 (0.33)	0.000
Pain score	1.4 (0.5)	3.25 (0.8)	4.67 (1)	0.000
Patient acceptance				
Easy	85.1%	23.1%	2.7%	0.000
Fair	14.6%	61.7%	39.7%	0.000
With difficulty	0.3%	15.3%	48.5%	0.000
Not accepted	0%	0%	4.1%	0.000
Not at all	0%	0%	0.3%	0.000
The procedure				
Easy	95%	44.1%	14%	0.000
Uncomfortable	5%	37.3%	23.4%	0.000
Painful	0%	18.6%	62.7%	0.000
Vagal reaction	0%	1.7%	5.4%	0.01
Physician satisfaction	9.7 (0.5)	9.6 (0.9)	NA	0.8

The diagnostic performance of the different methods in for either focal lesion or hyperplasia and cancer is shown in Table 5. OH showed better accuracy and agreement with histologic diagnosis of hyperplasia or cancer with larger area under the curve (AUC). It was much better than VUS and EB in diagnosing focal lesions with much better accuracy and agreement and larger AUC. The patient response to every procedure together with physician satisfaction is summarized in Table 6.

Discussion

Thanks for the development in optics that allowed the use of small caliber instruments that could pass through the cervix without the need of dilatation. This allowed the use of hysteroscopy in the office in a one-stop setting where all the investigations needed could be done at the time of presentation with the possibility of see-and-treat policy [6]. The addition of office hysteroscopy to vaginal sonography in the initial evaluation of abnormal uterine bleeding was associated with decrease number of visits with shorter duration to diagnosis [7]. In a qualitative trial, most women preferred office hysteroscopy for varying reasons as they could cope without anesthesia, dislike of general anesthesia, do not like to wait, or do not like to be admitted to hospital [8].

This study was performed by the conventional OH; but nowadays, we perform all OH with the vaginoscopic approach which seems less painful and well tolerated by the patients. Nevertheless, in this study, we did not use any pre

Table 5 Diagnostic performance of different methods in diagnosing hyperplasia and focal lesions

	SN%	SP%	PPV%	NPV%	DA%	PLR	NLR	Kap.	AUC
Focal lesion									
Focal lesion at US	42	87	55	80	75	3.2	0.67	0.31	0.65
Abnormal US 8 mm	85	30	32	84	45	1.2	0.5	0.1	0.574
Abnormal US 10 mm	81	47	37	87	57	1.5	0.4	0.21	0.643
OH myoma or polyp	91	100	100	97	98	91	0.09	0.94	0.96
EB	17	100	100	69	78	17	0.83	0.24	0.59
Hyperplasia and cancer									
Thick end. 8 mm	82	42	48	78	58	1.4	0.43	0.22	0.612
Thick end 10 mm	74	63	56	79	67	2	0.41	0.36	0.674
OH thick or suspicious endometrium	76	83	75	84	80	4.5	0.29	0.6	0.77
Abnormal OH	85	65	61	87	73	2.4	0.23	0.47	0.73

or intraprocedure analgesia or anesthesia as most studies suggests that OH in experienced hands is a well-tolerated technique and requires the use of analgesics only in selected patients [9]. Office hysteroscopy was well tolerated by our patients with mean pain score of 3.25 ± 0.8 which is comparable to previous studies with a range of 3–4.8 with variable caliber of the hysteroscopes used [10–14]. The procedure also has high patient acceptance with 85% of patients had easy or faire acceptance and in the other 15% it was accepted with some difficulty. The corresponding figures were 88.7% and 83% with others [11, 13]. The addition of office hysteroscopy to the initial evaluation was associated with decrease number of visits. Our results are intermediate in comparison to previous trials regarding hysteroscopic diagnosis of endometrial hyperplasia with 80% diagnostic accuracy. Some trials had low-diagnostic accuracy of 59% [15], others had comparable accuracy of 73% [16], 79% [17], and 81% [18] while others had higher accuracy of 90% [19] or 96% [20]. This could be explained partially by difference in patient population as Loizzi et al. [21] had a sensitivity of 100% in a population of postmenopausal women with bleeding and thick endometrium. It was found that combining endometrial biopsy and finding of focal lesion in vaginal sonography missed about 50% of focal lesions in our trial. Vaginal sonography had 42% sensitivity in detecting focal lesions. Previous studies had very wide range of sensitivity ranging from 12% to 86% [22, 23], with many of them having very near figures to our study ranging from 39% to 50% [24, 25]. This was also the case for endometrial biopsy which detected only 17% of focal lesions and this also was comparable to previous trials with detection rate varying from 11% to 19% [19, 26].

Considering low-resource countries like Egypt with high parity and consequently very high load of obstetric cases (the average rate of deliveries in our hospital is 18,000 per year), it is crucial to decrease the inpatient case load with adopting policies like one-stop outpatient service. This also much decrease the costs associated with the inpatient service.

In conclusion, the addition of office hysteroscopy in initial evaluation of women with abnormal uterine bleeding appears very beneficial as it allows complete diagnosis in fewer visits within shorter duration with the possibility of see-and-treat action and subsequently saving of the inpatient hospital resources especially in low-resource high-load countries. Regarding endometrial pathology, if performed alone, OH is superior to TVS in all diagnostic indices except being less sensitive. If combined with TVS, OH improves all diagnostic indices. As regards intrauterine lesions, OH is superior to TVS, OS, and even histopathology in detection of IU lesions. Future research should focus on comparing the diagnostic accuracy of OH to 4-D ultrasonography or MRI.

References

1. Collins S, Arulkumeran S, Hayes K, et al. eds. (2008) Normal menstruation and its disorders. In: Oxford handbook of obstetrics and gynecology. Oxford, OUP, 483–500
2. ACOG (2002) Guidelines for wome's health care, 2nd edn. ACOG, Washington
3. Kremer C, Duffy S, Moroney M (2000) Patient satisfaction with outpatient hysteroscopy versus day case hysteroscopy: randomized controlled trial. BMJ 320:279–282
4. Darwish AM, Makhlouf AM, Youssof AA, Gadalla HA (1999) Hysteroscopic myometrial biopsy in unexplained abnormal uterine bleeding. Eur J Obstet Gynecol Reprod Biol 86(2):139–143
5. Darwish AM, Youssef AA (1999) Screening sonohysterography in infertility. Gynecol Obstet Invest 48(1):43–47
6. Siristatidis C, Chrelias C (2011) Feasibility of office hysteroscopy through the "see and treat technique" in private practice: a prospective observational study. Arch Gynecol Obstet 283 (4):819–823
7. Böttcher B, Brown VA (2002) Postmenopausal bleeding: management by transvaginal ultrasound scan or outpatient hysteroscopy? Gynaecol Endosc 11:245–249
8. Morgan M, Dodds W, Wolfe Ch, Raju S (2004) Women's views and experiences of outpatient hysteroscopy: implications for a patient-centered service. Nurs Heal Sci 6:315–320
9. Cicinelli E (2010) Hysteroscopy without anesthesia: review of recent literature. J Minim Invasive Gynecol 17(6):703–708
10. Diniz DB, Depes Dde B, Pereira AM, David SD, Lippi UG, Baracat FF, Lopes RG (2010) Pain evaluation in office hysteroscopy: comparison of two techniques. Rev Bras Ginecol Obstet 32 (1):26–32
11. McIlwaine K, Readman E, Cameron M, Maher P (2009) Outpatient hysteroscopy: factors influencing post-procedure acceptability in patients attending a tertiary referral centre. Aust N Z J Obstet Gynaecol 49(6):650–652
12. van Dongen H, de Kroon CD, van den Tillaart SA, Louwé LA, Trimbos-Kemper GC, Jansen FW (2008) A randomised comparison of vaginoscopic office hysteroscopy and saline infusion sonography: a patient compliance study. BJOG 115 (10):1232–1237
13. Van den Bosch T, Verguts J, Daemen A, Gevaert O, Domali E, Claerhout F, Vandenbroucke V, De Moor B, Deprest J, Timmerman D (2008) Pain experienced during transvaginal ultrasound, saline contrast sonohysterography, hysteroscopy and office sampling: a comparative study. Ultrasound Obstet Gynecol 31(3):346–351
14. Cordeiro A, Condeço R, Leitão C, Sousa F, Coutinho S, Docarmosilva M, Bernardo MJ, Mira R (2009) Office hysteroscopy after ultrasonographic diagnosis of thickened endometrium in postmenopausal patients. Gynecol Surg 6:317–322
15. Ekin M, Karayalçın R, Özcan S, Özcan U (2007) Transvaginal ultrasonography and office hysteroscopic findings and their hystopathologic correlation in asymptomatic and symptomatic postmenopausal women. Med J Bakirköy 3:2
16. Lasmar RB, Barrozo PR, de Oliveira MA, Coutinho ES, Dias R (2006) Validation of hysteroscopic view in cases of endometrial hyperplasia and cancer in patients with abnormal uterine bleeding. J Minim Invasive Gynecol 13(5):409–412
17. Wang CJ, Mu WC, Yuen LT, Yen CF, Soong YK, Lee CL (2007) Flexible outpatient hysterofibroscopy without anesthesia: a feasible and valid procedure. Chang Gung Med J 30 (3):256–262

18. Paschopoulos M, Lolis ED, Alamanos Y, Koliopoulos G, Paraskevaidis E (2001) Vaginoscopic hysteroscopy and transvaginal sonography in the evaluation of patients with abnormal uterine bleeding. J Am Assoc Gynecol Laparosc 8(4):506–510

19. Angioni S, Loddo A, Milano F, Piras B, Minerba L, Melis GB (2008) Detection of benign intracavitary lesions in postmenopausal women with abnormal uterine bleeding: a prospective comparative study on outpatient hysteroscopy and blind biopsy. J Minim Invasive Gynecol 15(1):87–91

20. Ceci O, Bettocchi S, Pellegrino A, Impedovo L, Di Venere R, Pansini N (2002) Comparison of hysteroscopic and hysterectomy findings for assessing the diagnostic accuracy of office hysteroscopy. Fertil Steril 78(3):628–631

21. Loizzi V, Bettocchi S, Vimercati A, Ceci O, Rossi C, Marello F, Greco P (2000) Hysteroscopic evaluation of menopausal women with endometrial thickness of 4 mm or more. J Am Assoc Gynecol Laparosc 7(2):191–195

22. Timmermans A, Gerritse MB, Opmeer BC, Jansen FW, Mol BW, Veersema S (2008) Diagnostic accuracy of endometrial thickness to exclude polyps in women with postmenopausal bleeding. J Clin Ultrasound 36(5):286–290

23. Georgantopoulou C, Simm A, Roberts M (2008) Transvaginal saline hysterosonography: a comparison with local anaesthetic hysteroscopy for the diagnosis of benign lesions associated with menorrhagia. Gynecol Surg 5:27–34

24. Pasqualotto EB, Margossian H, Price LL, Bradley LD (2000) Accuracy of preoperative diagnostic tools and outcome of hysteroscopic management of menstrual dysfunction. J Am Assoc Gynecol Laparosc 7(2):201–209

25. Mukhopadhayay S, Bhattacharyya SK, Ganguly RP, Patra KK, Bhattacharya N, Barman SC (2007) Comparative evaluation of perimenopausal abnormal uterine bleeding by transvaginal sonography, hysteroscopy and endometrial biopsy. J Indian Med Assoc 105(11):624, 626, 628

26. Verrotti C, Benassi G, Caforio E, Nardelli GB (2008) Targeted and tailored diagnostic strategies in women with perimenopausal bleeding: advantages of the sonohysterographic approach. Acta Biomed 79(2):133–136

22

Ectopic pregnancy: when is expectant management safe?

**Sharon P. Rodrigues · Kirsten J. de Burlet ·
Ellen Hiemstra · Andries R. H. Twijnstra ·
Erik W. van Zwet · Trudy C. M. Trimbos-Kemper ·
Frank W. Jansen**

Abstract This study was conducted to evaluate expectant management in asymptomatic patients with an initial serum beta-hCG titer of <2,500 IU/l and to determine the independent ability of initial serum beta-hCG titers and trend of serum beta-hCG to predict successful expectant management. A cohort of patients (N=418) with suspected ectopic pregnancy (EP) between January 1991 and July 2008 is described. Three groups were defined: group I (n=182), immediate surgical intervention (<24 h); group IIa (n=130), unsuccessful expectant management (surgical intervention during follow-up), and group IIb (n=99), successful expectant management (spontaneous regression of trophoblast). Hospital protocol was not complied in 35 cases (Table 1). Beta-hCG levels >3,000 IU/l occur in our expectant management group; however, none of these cases were successful. Unnecessary surgery was prevented in 14% (n=7) of asymptomatic patients with initial beta-hCG of >2,000 IU/l. The success rate of expectant management was 49%, without a rise in complication rate or number of acute cases. In conclusion, the initial serum beta-hCG cutoff level of 2,000 IU/l is not a rigid upper limit for accepting expectant management in suspected EP and best practice is case specific. In asymptomatic patients, the serum beta-hCG cutoff level of at least 2,500 IU/l can be used for expectant management. This cutoff could be higher, but interpretation is limited due to censure in follow-up inherent to the predefined clinical protocol. There is no gain in including patients for expectant management with initial serum beta-hCG level >3,000 IU/l.

Keywords Suspected ectopic pregnancy · Expectant management · Management · Beta-hCG · Cutoff

S. P. Rodrigues · K. J. de Burlet · E. Hiemstra ·
A. R. H. Twijnstra · T. C. M. Trimbos-Kemper · F. W. Jansen (✉)
Department of Gynecology,
K6-76, Leiden University Medical Center,
PO Box 9600, 2300 RC Leiden, the Netherlands
e-mail: F.W.Jansen@lumc.nl

E. W. van Zwet
Department of Medical Statistics,
Leiden University Medical Center,
Leiden, The Netherlands

Introduction

Despite the availability of accurate diagnostic algorithms for the detection of ectopic pregnancy (EP), choosing the best treatment when EP is suspected can still pose a dilemma in daily practice. This dilemma arises in particular when patients without any clinical symptoms are diagnosed with EP. The latter tends to happen more often due to the availability of sensitive serum beta human chorionic gonadotrophin (beta-hCG) tests and high-resolution endovaginal ultrasonography that allows us to detect EP in early pregnancy even before clinical symptoms have the chance to set in [1, 2]. Consequently, early intervention has become a possibility and could potentially prevent serious complications. However, a considerable number of the EPs can also resolve spontaneously and treatment is not always necessary [3–5]. Inherently, early detection and quick intervention could result in overtreatment.

A recent cost analysis showed that diagnosing EP in a single visit could potentially save around £ 1 million per year in Scotland [6]. Because of this, the authors suggest that diagnosis of EP should be improved and that a single serum biomarker or other imaging modalities should be developed. However, this could also lead to a higher rate of overtreatment. Besides, the unnecessary exposure to risks in overtreatment and the expenses of this treatment could undo the gained savings. Therefore, modifications should ideally focus on predicting the need for future treatment earlier in the diagnostic pathway.

Various treatments for EP have been studied, i.e., surgical intervention (laparoscopy/laparotomy), medical treatment, and expectant management. Expectant management has only been advised in a selective group of patients, i.e., asymptomatic patients with relatively low (<2,000 IU/l) and diminishing serum beta-hCG levels [4, 5, 7, 8]. However, for over 10 years, asymptomatic patients with suspected EP and an initial serum beta-hCG titer below 2,500 IU/l were treated with expectant management. This study was designed to evaluate this policy and to determine the independent ability of initial serum beta-hCG titers and trend of serum beta-hCG titers in the prediction of successful expectant management.

Methods

This study describes a cohort of patients with suspected EP between January 1991 and July 2008 at the Leiden University Medical Center, Leiden, The Netherlands. Suspected EP was defined as patients with a serum beta-hCG above 1,500 IU/l and no ultrasonographic signs of intrauterine pregnancy or patients with abdominal pain and/or blood loss combined with a positive urine pregnancy test (i.e., beta-hCG >50 IU) without signs of intrauterine pregnancy. Clinical symptoms, ultrasonography results, and serum beta-hCG values of these patients were registered. Patients with a heterotopic pregnancy or medical treatment of EP were excluded. After inclusion, patients were categorized according to their management type: either in the group of immediate treatment (within 24 h) by surgical intervention (group I) or in the group of expectant management when follow-up of beta-hCG and clinical signs took place (group II; Fig. 1). Some patients in group II required surgery during follow-up (group IIa; unsuccessful expectant management), while others had a spontaneous regression of throphobast (group IIb; successful expectant management).

Data analysis was performed with SPSS 16.0. Patient characteristics were compared with Chi-square/Cramer's V, except for age, which was analyzed with one-way ANOVA. Beta-hCG values were compared for every group combination with the Mann–Whitney test. For the comparison of complications between the intervention groups, patients in group I who presented with pain were excluded because of a presumed association between acute presentation (symptoms of acute pain and/or peritoneal irritability objectified by the treating physician) and higher complication rates. Furthermore, their acute presentation was not preventable, in contrast to patients in group IIa. For patients in group IIa, the choice to initially refrain from surgery includes a risk of future acute presentation and thus potentially an increased risk of complications.

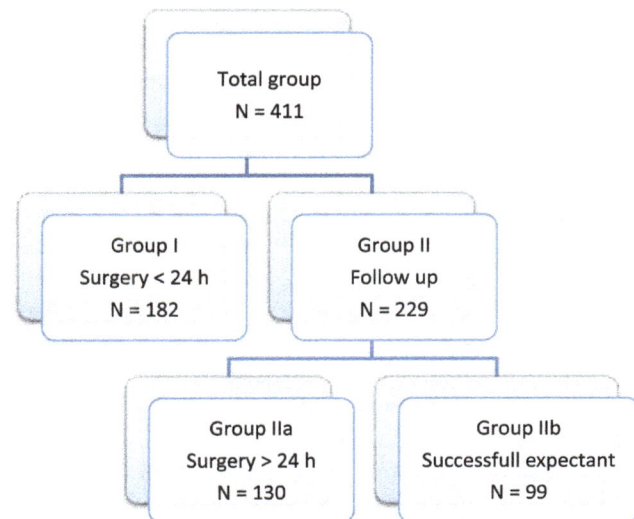

Fig. 1 Categorization of patients in groups according to their management type. *Group I* immediate treatment (within 24 h) by surgical intervention; *Group IIa* unsuccessful expectant management (surgery >24 h); *Group IIb* successful expectant management

Therefore, patients with pain in group IIa were not excluded for comparison of complications (Chi-square/Cramer's V).

To compare the course of serum beta-hCG levels among the groups, the ratio of each consecutive beta-hCG concentration to the initial concentration was calculated. The ratios in group IIb (successful expectant management) were compared to the ratios in the group IIa (unsuccessful expectant management) at predetermined time points. Therefore, the ratio at the time of surgery (group IIa) was compared to the highest ratio during follow-up (group IIb) (independent samples *t* test).

The optimal beta-hCG cutoff was determined for asymptomatic patients using a receiver operating characteristics (ROC) curve. Patients with hemodynamic instability or presenting with acute pain at initial presentation were excluded from this analysis because surgical intervention was obliged irrespective of the serum beta-hCG values. Success rate of expectant management was determined as the percentage of successes (IIb) of the total expectant management group (II). Finally, a logistic regression model was fitted for the probability of receiving surgery at some time during the diagnostic pathway based on initial serum beta-hCG level and an increase or decrease in beta-hCG between the initial measurement and the second measurement.

Results

In the present study, 416 patients with suspected EP were identified. Five patients with a heterotopic pregnancy were excluded. None of the patients had medical treatment. Altogether, 411 patients were included (Fig. 1), of whom 182 patients needed surgical intervention within 24 h (group I) because of hemodynamic instability and/or acute pain ($N=$ 149) or a serum beta-hCG level exceeding 2,500 IU/l ($N=33$). Initially, 229 patients were asymptomaic and therefore eligible for expectant management (group II). Surgical intervention during follow-up was required in 130 patients because of no signs of spontaneous resolution, excessive pain, or hemodynamic instability (group IIa). In 99 patients, the EP regressed spontaneously (group IIb). During laparoscopy, no EP could be identified in one case (group I) which during follow-up culminated in an intrauterine gravidity. In all other surgical cases, EP was confirmed with pathology findings. In group IIb, a spontaneous abortion could not be excluded in 16 cases; however, EP remained the final diagnosis.

The distribution of the initial serum beta-hCG levels of asymptomatic patients in the three management groups shows that hospital protocol was not complied in 35 cases (Table 1). One patient with an initial serum beta-hCG level of 1,809 IU/l had a laparoscopy within 24 h because ultrasonography showed a vital EP. And 34 patients with initial serum beta-hCG levels above 2,500 IU/l were managed expectantly of whom 2 (5.5%) were managed expectantly with success (serum beta-hCG levels, 2,735 and 2,799 IU/L). Table 2 displays general characteristics of the three groups. Patient characteristics were similar, whereas initial serum beta-hCG titers differed significantly. Both intervention groups (from group I only patients without symptoms) had a comparable number of laparotomies and conversion rates. Neither time nor length of surgery differed significantly. Furthermore, the incidence of acute presentation and complication rates were similar in both groups, except for conversion due to heavy blood loss which occurred once in group I and not in group IIa (Table 3).

The ROC curve did not indicate an optimal trade-off between sensitivity and specificity for successful expectant management. The best trade-off reached was at a serum beta-hCG cutoff level of 1,275.5 IU/L with a sensitivity of 65.3% and specificity of 87.1%. None of the successful expectant management cases had an initial beta-hCG level above 3,000 IU/l, while there were cases with an initial beta-hCG level above 3,000 in the unsuccessful group (IIa).

Table 1 Distribution of initial serum beta-hCG levels

Initial beta-hCG titer	Group I Immediate intervention	Group IIa Unsuccessful expectant management	Group IIb Successful expectant management	Total
<2,000	1	88	92	181
2,000–2,500	0	10	5	15
>2,500	32	32	2	66
Total	33	130	99	262

Initial serum beta-hCG distribution of patients without severe pain or hemodynamic instability in the three management groups

The calculated mean ratio, based on the highest beta-hCG value during follow-up in group IIb, was 1.11 (99% confidence interval (CI), 0.99–1.22). The mean ratio, based on the beta-hCG value which indicated surgery in group IIa, was 2.53 (99% CI, 1.56–3.50), which is significantly higher ($p=<.001$).

Success rate of expectant management was 49%. In 14% ($n=7$) of the cases with an initial serum beta-hCG above 2,000 IU/l, expectant management was successful (Table 1). However, there were also nine cases in this group who presented with severe symptoms during follow-up and therefore needed surgery. Of these nine cases, seven had an initial serum beta-hCG level above 2,500 IU/l (six above 3,750 IU/l and one of 2,671 IU/l). The other two had initial beta-hCG levels of 2,360 and 2,364 IU/l, respectively. If an initial beta-hCG cutoff level of 2,000 IU/l had been used for expectant management, success rate would have been 50%.

Figure 2 illustrates the estimated probabilities of eventual surgery at a given beta-hCG level as a result of the logistic regression model. The second visit is taken into account by defining a dummy variable which indicates a rising (red line) or declining (blue line) beta-hCG. The figure shows for example that if an 80% chance of surgery is used as cutoff, theoretically, patients with an initial serum beta-hCG level of 2,400 IU/l or higher should have surgery and patients with an initial serum beta-hCG level below 2,400 IU/l are eligible for follow-up. Using a cutoff of 90% certainty at the second visit, according to this model, surgery is advised in patients with an initial serum beta-hCG level of 2,000 IU/l or higher which is rising, while a declining beta-hCG level under these restrictions could be interpreted as acceptable.

Discussion

An initial serum beta-hCG cutoff level of 2,500 IU/l for expectant management can be used for asymptomatic patients with suspected ectopic pregnancy. This is also suggested by a small prospective study by Lurie et al. [9] in which patients with rising serum beta-hCG levels were successfully managed expectantly and a serum beta-hCG cutoff level of 2,500 IU/l was used. However, the current protocol of the Dutch Society of Obstetrics and Gynecology states that expectant management is justified in asymptomatic patients with a serum beta-hCG value until 2,000 IU/l. By raising beta-hCG cutoff from 2,000 to 2,500 IU/l in our clinic, unnecessary surgery was prevented in 14% of the patients eligible for expectant management, while complication rates and the number of patients with acute presentation are comparable in both intervention groups.

Previous studies have used receiver operating characteristics (ROC) curves to determine an optimal serum beta-hCG cutoff level for diagnosis of EP (2,000 IU/l in asymptomatic

Table 2 Group characteristics

	Group I Immediate intervention	Group IIa Unsuccessful expectant management	Group IIb Successful expectant management	P
N	182	130	99	
Age (years) [a]	31.9±4.8	31.4±4.4	31.7±5.5	NS
Parity [b]	0 (0–5)	0 (0–4)	1 (0–4)	NS
Previous abortions [b]	0 (0–7)	0 (0–2)	0 (0–3)	NS
Previous miscarriages [b]	0 (0–6)	0 (0–10)	0 (0–10)	NS
History tubal pathology [c]	33 (18%)	34 (26%)	19 (19%)	NS
History infertility [c]	44 (24%)	42 (32%)	19 (19%)	NS
Amenorrhea at first visit (weeks) [a]	6.30±1.6	6.26±1.9	6.18±2.1	NS
Number of days till second visit [a]	N/A	2.6±1.6	2.8±2.2	NS
Initial beta-hCG level (IU/l) [d]	3834 (89–100414)	1403 (58–20858)	530 (34–2799 IU/l)	<.001
Observational period (days) [d]	N/A	6.3 (2–21)	28.8 (3–95)	

General characteristics of the three management groups

NS not significant, *N/A* not applicable

[a] Mean ± SD

[b] Median (range)

[c] Number of cases (percentage of intervention group)

[d] Mean (range)

patients) [1]. These studies do not consider spontaneous resolution of EP. We also aimed to determine an optimal serum beta-hCG cutoff level for expectant management in asymptomatic patients suspected of EP with a ROC curve. The result shows that a serum beta-hCG cutoff level of 1,275.5 IU/L gives the optimal trade-off between sensitivity and specificity. However, the results of this (and other similar) ROC curve(s) should be interpreted with caution because of the design of the study. When serum beta-hCG levels rise above 2,500 IU/l,

patients become eligible for laparoscopy and follow-up of serum beta-hCG concentration is censured. Although the probability that these cases would become acute is presumed to be very high, the true outcome remains unknown. To determine the true optimal cutoff, ideally patients should be managed expectantly until symptoms of acute pain and/or peritoneal irritability arise. However, exposing patients to such potential risks would be unethical, and thus, such a study is unlikely to ever be done.

Table 3 Characteristics and complications of the intervention groups

	Group I (*N*=33) Immediate intervention	Group IIa (*N*=130) Unsuccessful expectant management	P	Test
Laparotomies[a]	4	11	NS	Cramer's V
Time surgery took place	Time of surgery during the day		NS	Cramer's V
Length of surgery (hh:mm)[b]	01:02±00:03	01:04±00:02	NS	Mann–Whitney
Tubal rupture [a]	0	1	NS	Cramer's V
Persistent trophoblast [a] (No decline of beta-hCG levels)	0	9	NS	Cramer's V
Conversions [a]	2	9	NS	Cramer's V
Heavy blood loss (>1 l) [a]	1	2	NS	Cramer's V
Conversions due to heavy blood loss [a]	1	0	<.05	Cramer's V

Comparison of the characteristics and complications of the two intervention groups. As explained in the "Methods" section, only asymptomatic patients of group I are analyzed (because of a presumed association between acute presentation and higher complication rates), whereas in group IIa, all patients are analyzed (because an increased risk is a direct consequence of expectant management)

[a] *N*

[b] Mean ± SD

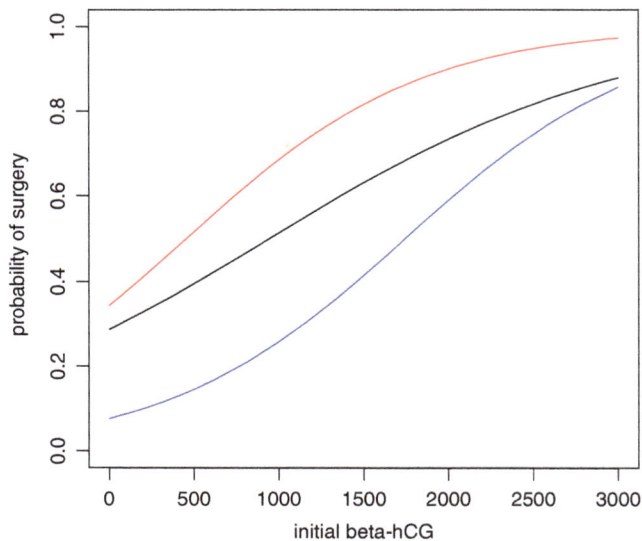

Fig. 2 Estimated probability of surgery. The *black line* represents the first visit. The *red line* indicates patients with a rising beta-hCG at the second visit, and the *blue line* indicates patients with a declining beta-hCG

The success rate of expectant management in this study was 49%. Previous studies have shown great variety in success rates (46.7–92%) [4, 5, 8, 10]. This variety is most likely explained by differences in inclusion criteria and protocols used. Selection criteria for expectant management in previous studies were much stricter. Most studies only include patients with low and stable or decreasing serum beta-hCG levels. In our study, patients with increasing serum beta-hCG concentration were allowed to remain expectant and the cutoff level of initial serum beta-hCG was 2,500 IU/l, which is higher than generally used in previous studies. Logically, a higher cutoff level of beta-hCG will lead to a lower sensitivity explaining a higher number of patients with an unsuccessful expectant policy. However, this protocol also leads to a higher specificity resulting in lower numbers of unnecessary surgery. Altogether in this study, seven patients (14%) were spared unnecessary surgery without observing an overall increase in complications or acute presentation. In our opinion, this justifies the lower success rate.

Korhonen et al. have shown a rise in serum beta-hCG in 49% of the patients requiring surgical intervention [8]. This supports our observation in serum beta-hCG trend, i.e., increase in beta-hCG ratio in the unsuccessful expectant group and decrease in the successful expectant management group. In the unsuccessful expectant management group, the mean beta-hCG ratio at intervention was 2.5 (99% CI, 1.56–3.50), whereas at the highest point, the mean beta-hCG ratio was 1.1 (99% CI, 0.99–1.22) in the successful expectant management group. This finding suggests that if expectant management is chosen for, a rise of initial beta-hCG concentration by one and a half should be interpreted as an indication for surgical intervention. Of course, the before mentioned censure in follow-up

when serum beta-hCG levels rise above 2,500 IU/l also influences this result. However, we reasoned that prolonged follow-up of these patients would probably lead to an even higher serum beta-hCG level. By respecting lower levels, we are likely to stay on the safe side of the limit, but we should keep in mind that these limits are not rigid. Table 2 illustrates that the upper limit of our protocol was not obliged rigidly. Serum beta-hCG levels even above 3,000 IU/l occur in our expectant management group. However, none of these cases were successful. Furthermore, 67% (N=6) of the cases with an initial serum beta-hCG level above 2,000 IU/l, who also developed acute symptoms during follow-up, had an initial serum beta-hCG above 3,000 IU/l. This implies that there is absolutely no gain in including patients for expectant management when initial serum beta-hCG levels are above 3,000 IU/l.

Since EP is expensive to diagnose and exclude, mainly due to the many assessment visits needed [6], determining the appropriate treatment early in the diagnostic pathway could potentially save a lot of costs. The logistic regression model could be indicative in early decision making. However, because the model is drawn up solely from the presented cohort, conclusions about absolute cutoff levels cannot be made. Interpretation of the calculated probabilities should be left in the hands of the gynecologist with knowledge of the specific case. Overall, the model shows that an increase in serum beta-hCG level at the second visit strongly raises the probability of having surgery during follow-up. Although a decrease of serum beta-hCG level at the second measurement evidently lowers the chance of culminating into an acute surgical case, these patients should still be observed with caution, especially in those with a high initial serum beta-hCG level (i.e., >2,500 IU/l) who, despite a decreasing serum beta-hCG level during follow-up, still have a high chance of culminating into an acute situation. This is also illustrated by the published cases of patients with rupture of EP while serum beta-hCG level is disappearing [11, 12]. A recent study showed that a serum beta-hCG level of >1,500 IU/l is associated with a higher rate of tubal rupture than a beta-hCG level of <1,500 IU/l [13]. Therefore, frequent follow-up and clear patient instructions are necessary for safe expectant management.

Although today medical treatment with methotrexate is gaining popularity, as it can be a good alternative for surgery, this was not in the scope of the current study. Multiple-dose systemic treatment with methotrexate has been shown to be as effective as surgical treatment, whereas single-dose treatment is less effective. However, health-related quality of life was more severely impaired after systemic methotrexate. Furthermore, systemic multiple-dose treatment is only cost-effective in patients with a serum beta-hCG level of <3,000 IU/l, or a single-dose treatment in patients with a serum beta-hCG level of <1,500 IU/l [7, 14, 15]. Because of these reasons, in some clinics, such as the study clinic, methotrexate as treatment of EP has not been implemented as standard treatment.

Conclusion

The often advised initial serum beta-hCG cutoff level of 2,000 IU/l should not be handled as a rigid upper limit for accepting expectant management in asymptomatic patients with suspected ectopic pregnancy. However, there seems to be no gain in including patients for expectant management with initial serum beta-hCG levels above 3,000 IU/l. Because of the heterogeneity in patient profiles, the best treatment option is case specific. Besides the clinical symptoms and initial serum beta-hCG level, the second serum beta-hCG measurement (i.e., rising or declining) and trend in serum beta-hCG concentration are also very indicative for the management choice.

Declaration of interest The authors report no conflicts of interest. The authors alone are responsible for the content and writing of the paper.

References

1. Mol BW, Hajenius PJ, Engelsbel S, Ankum WM, Van der Veen F, Hemrika DJ, Bossuyt PM (1998) Serum human chorionic gonadotropin measurement in the diagnosis of ectopic pregnancy when transvaginal sonography is inconclusive. Fertil Steril 70:972–981
2. Mol BW, van der Veen F, Bossuyt PM (1999) Implementation of probabilistic decision rules improves the predictive values of algorithms in the diagnostic management of ectopic pregnancy. Hum Reprod 14:2855–2862
3. Balasch J, Barri PN (1994) Treatment of ectopic pregnancy: the new gynaecological dilemma. Hum Reprod 9:547–558
4. Shalev E, Peleg D, Tsabari A, Romano S, Bustan M (1995) Spontaneous resolution of ectopic tubal pregnancy: natural history. Fertil Steril 63:15–19
5. Ylostalo P, Cacciatore B, Sjoberg J, Kaariainen M, Tenhunen A, Stenman UH (1992) Expectant management of ectopic pregnancy. Obstet Gynecol 80:345–348
6. Wedderburn CJ, Warner P, Graham B, Duncan WC, Critchley HO, Horne AW (2010) Economic evaluation of diagnosing and excluding ectopic pregnancy. Hum Reprod 25:328–333
7. Hajenius PJ, Mol F, Mol BW, Bossuyt PM, Ankum WM, van der Veen F (2007) Interventions for tubal ectopic pregnancy. Cochrane Database Syst Rev 1:CD000324
8. Korhonen J, Stenman UH, Ylostalo P (1994) Serum human chorionic gonadotropin dynamics during spontaneous resolution of ectopic pregnancy. Fertil Steril 61:632–636
9. Lurie S, Katz Z, Goldshmit R, Gotlibe Z, Insler V (1994) Expectant management of suspected ectopic pregnancies even with rising beta-subunit human chorionic gonadotropin levels. A clinical prospective study. Arch Gynecol Obstet 255:125–129
10. Elson J, Tailor A, Banerjee S, Salim R, Hillaby K, Jurkovic D (2004) Expectant management of tubal ectopic pregnancy: prediction of successful outcome using decision tree analysis. Ultrasound Obstet Gynecol 23:552–556
11. Hochner-Celnikier D, Ron M, Goshen R, Zacut D, Amir G, Yagel S (1992) Rupture of ectopic pregnancy following disappearance of serum beta subunit of hCG. Obstet Gynecol 79:826–827
12. Tulandi T, Hemmings R, Khalifa F (1991) Rupture of ectopic pregnancy in women with low and declining serum beta-human chorionic gonadotropin concentrations. Fertil Steril 56:786–787
13. Downey LV, Zun LS (2011) Indicators of potential for rupture for ectopics seen in the emergency department. J Emerg Trauma Shock 4:374–377
14. Mol F, Mol BW, Ankum WM, Van der Veen F, Hajenius PJ (2008) Current evidence on surgery, systemic methotrexate and expectant management in the treatment of tubal ectopic pregnancy: a systematic review and meta-analysis. Hum Reprod Update 14:309–319
15. van Mello NM, Mol F, Mol BW, Hajenius PJ (2009) Conservative management of tubal ectopic pregnancy. Best Pract Res Clin Obstet Gynaecol 23:509–518

23

The FAST-EU trial: 12-month clinical outcomes of women after intrauterine sonography-guided transcervical radiofrequency ablation of uterine fibroids

Hans Brölmann[1] · Marlies Bongers[2] · José Gerardo Garza-Leal[3] · Janesh Gupta[4] · Sebastiaan Veersema[5] · Rik Quartero[6] · David Toub[7,8]

Abstract The FAST-EU Trial was designed to establish the effectiveness and confirm the safety of transcervical intrauterine sonography-guided radiofrequency ablation with the VizAblate™ System in the treatment of symptomatic uterine fibroids. This was a multicenter, prospective, single-arm trial involving academic and community hospitals in the United Kingdom, the Netherlands, and Mexico. Women with qualifying uterine fibroids and heavy menstrual bleeding underwent intrauterine sonography-guided transcervical radiofrequency ablation (RFA) with the VizAblate System; anesthesia was individualized. Patients were required to have up to five fibroids from 1 to 5 cm in diameter. The primary trial endpoint was the percentage change in perfused fibroid volume, as assessed by contrast-enhanced MRI at 3 months by an independent core laboratory. Secondary endpoints, evaluated at 6 and 12 months, included safety, percentage reductions in the Menstrual Pictogram (MP) score, and the Symptom Severity Score (SSS) subscale of the Uterine Fibroid Symptom-Quality of Life (UFS-QOL) questionnaire, along with the rate of surgical reintervention for abnormal uterine bleeding and the mean number of days to return to normal activity. Additional assessments included the Health-Related Quality of Life (HRQOL) subscale of the UFS-QOL, nonsurgical reintervention for abnormal uterine bleeding, anesthesia regimen, patient satisfaction, and pain during the recovery period. An additional MRI study was performed at 12 months on a subgroup of patients. Fifty patients (89 fibroids) underwent transcervical radiofrequency ablation with the VizAblate System. At 3 and 12 months, perfused fibroid volumes were reduced from baseline by an average of 68.1 ± 28.6 and 67.4 ± 31.9 %, respectively, while total fibroid volumes were reduced from baseline by an average of 54.7 ± 37.4 and 66.6 ± 32.1 %, respectively (all $P<.001$ compared with baseline; Wilcoxon signed-rank test). At 12 months, mean MP score and SSS decreased by 53.8 ± 50.5 and 55.1 ± 41.0 %, respectively; the mean HRQOL score increased by 277 ± 483 %. There were four surgical reinterventions (8 %) within 12 months. This is the first report of the 12-month follow-up for patients in the FAST-EU Trial. In concert with previously reported 3- and 6-month endpoint data, the 12-month results of the FAST-EU Trial suggest that in addition to substantially reducing the perfused and total volume of targeted uterine fibroids, the VizAblate System is safe and effective through 12 months in providing relief of abnormal uterine bleeding associated with submucous, intramural, and transmural fibroids.

Keywords Fibroids · Radiofrequency ablation · VizAblate · Intrauterine sonography · Ultrasound

✉ David Toub
   dtoub@mac.com

[1] Vrije Universiteit Medisch Centrum, Amsterdam, Netherlands

[2] Máxima Medisch Centrum, Veldhoven, Netherlands

[3] Universidad Autónoma de Nuevo León, Monterrey, Nuevo Leon, Mexico

[4] Birmingham Women's Hospital, Birmingham, UK

[5] Sint Antonius Ziekenhuis, Nieuwegein, Netherlands

[6] Medisch Spectrum Twente, Enschede, Netherlands

[7] Gynesonics, Inc., Redwood City, CA 94063, USA

[8] Albert Einstein Medical Center, 5501 Old York Road, Philadelphia, PA 19141, USA

Introduction

Uterine fibroids are highly prevalent and the primary indication for over 200,000 hysterectomies performed annually in the USA [1, 2]. While various fibroid treatments exist, they have limitations, such as being invasive, requiring general anesthesia, or being not optimally suited for treatment of both intramural and submucous myomata.

Radiofrequency ablation (RFA) involves the placement of one or more needle electrodes into a solid tumor in order to deliver thermal energy, resulting in thermal fixation and coagulative necrosis within the treated tissue [3, 4]. Recent studies have been performed using RFA in conjunction with simultaneous, real-time sonography to guide volumetric ablations, resulting in volume reduction and symptom improvement [3, 5, 6].

The VizAblate System (Gynesonics; Redwood City, CA) combines radiofrequency ablation with intrauterine sonography and is CE-marked and commercially available in the European Union. VizAblate permits real-time imaging and transcervical treatment of uterine fibroids, including those that are not amenable to hysteroscopic resection such as type 3, type 4, and types 2–5 (transmural) fibroids as well as large type 1 and type 2 myomata [7]. The Fibroid Ablation Study-EU (FAST-EU) was designed to examine the safety and effectiveness of transcervical radiofrequency ablation of uterine fibroids under intrauterine sonography guidance with the VizAblate System. The trial endpoints, reached at 3 and at 6 months, have previously been reported [8]. This paper presents the 12-month efficacy and safety results of women treated under the FAST-EU Trial.

Patients and methods

This was a prospective, single-arm, multicenter trial. The primary endpoint was the percentage change in target fibroid perfused volume as assessed by contrast-enhanced MRI by an independent core laboratory at baseline and at 3 months. Additional endpoints, reached at 6 months, included safety, percentage reductions in the Menstrual Pictogram (MP) score and the Symptom Severity Score (SSS) subscale of the Uterine Fibroid Symptom-Quality of Life (UFS-QOL) questionnaire, the rate of surgical reintervention for abnormal uterine bleeding, and the mean number of days to return to normal activity. The Health-Related Quality of Life (HRQOL) subscale of the UFS-QOL questionnaires, along with anesthesia regimen, patient satisfaction, and recovery pain, was also assessed.

Patients were enrolled across seven sites in three nations: Mexico (one site), the United Kingdom (two sites), and the Netherlands (four sites). The trial included women with one to five uterine fibroids of FIGO types 1, 2, 3, 4, and 2–5 (transmural) measuring between 1 and 5 cm in maximum diameter. Fibroids that did not contain an edge within the inner half of the myometrium were not counted in this total and were not targeted for ablation, as they were believed to be less likely to materially contribute to abnormal uterine bleeding

(AUB). At least one fibroid was required to indent the endometrial cavity.

Patients were 28 years of age or older and not pregnant, with regular, predictable menstrual cycles and heavy menstrual bleeding for at least 3 months. A Menstrual Pictogram score ≥120 was also required for inclusion along with a baseline UFS-QOL SSS ≥20. The Menstrual Pictogram was first described by Wyatt and colleagues and is a variant of the Pictorial Blood Loss Assessment Chart (PBAC) that patients complete to provide a visual assessment of menstrual blood loss during a single cycle [9, 10]. Unlike the original PBAC described by Higham and colleagues, the Menstrual Pictogram includes a greater range of icons representing different saturations of sanitary products, clots, and losses in a toilet and also distinguishes different absorbency levels of sanitary napkins and tampons [11].

Exclusions included a desire for future fertility, the presence of one or more type 0 fibroids, cervical dysplasia, endometrial hyperplasia, active pelvic infection, clinically significant adenomyosis (>10 % of the junctional zone measuring more than 10 mm in thickness as measured by MRI), and the presence of one or more treatable fibroids that were significantly calcified (defined as <75 % fibroid enhancement by volume on contrast-enhanced MRI). Screening included transvaginal sonography, as well as hysteroscopy or hysterosonography, contrast-enhanced MRI, endometrial biopsy, and a pregnancy test.

All records were de-identified and only the range of each patient's age was documented, as per clinical trial requirements in the Netherlands. Women were followed at 7–14 days, 30 days, 3 months, 6 months, and 12 months post-treatment. All MRI studies were forwarded to an independent core laboratory (MedQIA, Los Angeles, CA, USA) for quality control and interpretation to reduce variability in the measurements; the core laboratory also developed standardized imaging protocols for use at the individual trial sites, credentialed the sites, and trained MRI technologists at each trial site. Fibroid measurements consisted of the total voxel volume and perfused voxel volume via contrast-enhanced MRI at the specified time points.

Procedure

The VizAblate System, as well as its use, has previously been described in detail and includes a reusable intrauterine ultrasound (IUUS) probe and a single-use, articulating radiofrequency ablation handpiece that are combined into an integrated treatment device that is inserted transcervically (Fig. 1) [8]. A custom graphical interface provides the gynecologist with a real-time, image-guided treatment system that indicates the borders of the thermal ablation (Ablation Zone) as well as the border beyond which tissues are safe from ablation (Thermal Safety Border). Because the deployment path is

Fig. 1 The VizAblate treatment device

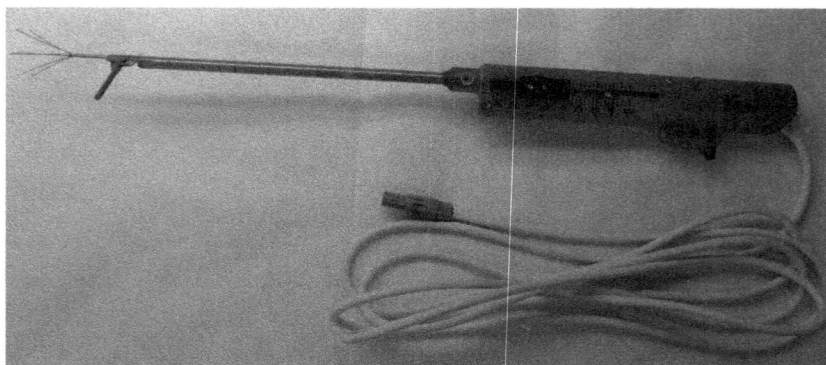

predictable relative to the ultrasound image, one can plan the ablation location and size before introducing any electrode elements into a fibroid. Additionally, the guidance software provides graphics that allow the gynecologist to maintain a safe margin from the ablation to the serosal margin and extra-uterine viscera. Mechanical stops provide definitive tactile limits, ensuring that the needle electrodes are deployed to the proper distance to achieve the ablation size as selected by the gynecologist. The radiofrequency generator modulates power (up to 150 W) to maintain a constant temperature of 105 °C at the needle electrode tips, and the ablation time is preset based on the ablation size. Depending on the width of the ablation, the distance from the Ablation Zone to the Thermal Safety Border will vary from 6.0 to 9.5 mm.

In this trial, the method of anesthesia was chosen by each investigator based on individual patient characteristics in consultation with an anesthesiologist. Treated fibroids received one or more ellipsoidal ablations under real-time intrauterine sonographic guidance, ranging from 1 to 4 cm in width and 2 to 5 cm in length. The number of ablations, along with their sizes, was at the discretion of the investigator and was chosen in order to maximize the ablation volume of the fibroid while maintaining the Thermal Safety Border within the uterine serosal margin.

Statistical analysis

The primary endpoint was the percentage change in target fibroid perfused volume at 3 months. The null hypothesis for the primary trial endpoint at 3 months was H_0: probability of success <50 % versus the alternative H_a: probability of success ≥50 %. A sample of 40 patients was sufficient to detect this difference of 22 % in probability of success with a power of 82 % using a one-group chi-square test with a 0.05 two-sided significance level. Allowing for an expected drop-out rate of 20 % at the 12-month follow-up visit, the minimum recommended sample size for the initial trial protocol was 48. The primary trial endpoint success criterion was achievement of >30 % reduction in mean target fibroid perfused volume in at least 50 % of patients at 3 months.

The data in this report consist of the Full Analysis dataset. This includes all patients enrolled who provided a baseline fibroid volume assessment and received treatment with the VizAblate System. Patients who received a surgical reintervention were considered treatment failures, and their subsequent data was imputed using the last observation carried forward (LOCF) method. Missing data was not imputed for patients who conceived or who neglected to complete a questionnaire.

All statistical analyses were performed with SAS 9.3 (SAS, Cary, NC). Values were considered significant at the level of $\alpha=0.05$. The Wilcoxon signed-rank test was used to test if a change was significantly different from 0.

Ethics

The protocol was approved by the Ethics Committees of the respective institutions as well as by the Federal Commission for Protection against Health Risks (COFEPRIS) in Mexico. All enrolled patients provided written informed consent for treatment with the VizAblate System prior to enrollment. The trial overview was published on ClinicalTrials.gov (identifier: NCT01226290) and conducted in accordance with Standard ISO 14155 (Clinical investigation of medical devices for human subjects – Good clinical practice) of the International Organization for Standardization (ISO), the Helsinki Declaration of 1975, as revised in 2008, and the ethical standards of applicable national regulations and institutional research policies and procedures governing human experimentation.

Results

Patients

Fifty patients were treated in the FAST-EU trial at seven sites. Baseline characteristics for all treated patients are provided in Table 1. Anesthesia was provided as noted in Table 2.

Table 1 Baseline subject characteristics

Subjects treated	50
Most frequent age range	41–45 years of age[a]
Mean Menstrual Pictogram (MP) score	423±253 (range 119–1582)
Mean UFS-QOL SSS	61.7±16.9 (range 28.1–100.0)
Mean UFS-QOL HRQOL score	34.3±19.0 (range 0.0–73.3)
Total number of target fibroids identified on MRI	118
Mean number of target fibroids per patient	2.4±1.7 (range 1–7)[b]
Mean diameter of target fibroids	2.9±1.4 cm (range 1.0–6.9 cm)
Mean perfused fibroid volume	18.3±20.6 cm^3 (range 0.3–77.0 cm^3)
Mean total (perfused+nonperfused) fibroid volume	18.8±21.4 cm^3 (range 0.3–77.0 cm^3)

UFS-QOL Uterine Fibroid Symptom-Quality of Life Questionnaire, *SSS* Symptom Severity Score subscale, *HRQOL* Health-Related Quality of Life subscale

[a] Subject ages were specified as a range by each site to protect subject privacy

[b] Two small additional fibroids, beyond the upper limit of 5 target fibroids/patient, were identified on review of one MRI series after treatment

One patient (three fibroids) was excluded from analysis of the primary endpoint. This patient was deemed by the core MRI laboratory to have had unusable imaging for making precise baseline fibroid measurements, although eligibility based on fibroid diameter ≤5 cm and location was not in question. This patient was treated as she met the eligibility requirements and her treatment could contribute to patient-reported and safety data for the trial. Consequently, while 92 fibroids were ablated, accurate baseline volume measurements could only be performed for 89. One patient reported a pregnancy at the time of her 6-month follow-up visit and was thus excluded from the 6- and 12-month analyses. While all patients provided baseline MP data, one patient each at 3, 6, and 12 months declined to submit a Menstrual Pictogram. One patient did not turn in her baseline HRQOL portion of the UFS-QOL; her HRQOL data was not included in the analysis. A flow diagram depicting sample sizes for MRI and patient-reported outcomes at baseline and 3-, 6-, and 12 months is provided in Fig. 2.

The protocol required a baseline and 3-month MR study for the primary endpoint analysis (reduction in perfused fibroid volume). Approximately 14 months after the first patient was treated, the protocol was amended to add an MR evaluation at 12 months in order to provide longer-term information about the effects of transcervical RFA. Twenty-eight patients (58.3 %) provided their informed consent to undergo another MR examination with contrast enhancement at 12 months post-ablation and underwent such imaging.

Effects on fibroid volume

Characteristics of fibroids that were ablated are shown in Table 3, and results of fibroid ablation on total and perfused volume at 3 and 12 months are provided in Table 4. Fibroids are classified in Table 3 as per the FIGO classification system [12]. Radiofrequency ablation with the VizAblate System was associated with statistically significant reductions (68.1 and 54.7 %, respectively) in both total and perfused fibroid volumes at 3 and 12 months. Seventy-nine of 89 treated fibroids (88.8 %) in all 49 patients with measurable MRI data met the primary trial endpoint success criterion at 3 months (achievement of >30 % reduction in mean target fibroid perfused volume at 3 months in at least 50 % of patients). By 12 months post-ablation (*n*=28 patients; 43 fibroids), treated fibroids experienced a mean reduction in total fibroid volume of 66.6± 32.1 % (*P*<.001). Thirty-seven fibroids (86.0 %) in 100 % of the 28 patients imaged at 12 months demonstrated >30 % reduction in perfused fibroid volume at 12 months.

Patient-reported outcomes

Patient-reported secondary endpoint data through 12 months are provided in Table 5. The mean MP score declined through 12 months, with mean and median reductions of 53.8 and 72.3 % at 12 months, respectively (all *P*<.001). By 3 months post-ablation, 44 of 49 patients (89.8 %) experienced a reduction in menstrual blood loss as reflected by their Menstrual

Table 2 Anesthesia provided to FAST-EU subjects

Anesthesia option	No. of subjects
General anesthesia alone	15 (30.0 %)
Conscious sedation alone	15 (30.0 %)
Spinal anesthesia alone	8 (16.0 %)
Conscious sedation+epidural anesthesia	8 (16.0 %)
Epidural anesthesia alone	2 (4.0 %)
Paracervical blockade alone	1 (2.0 %)
General anesthesia+epidural anesthesia	1 (2.0 %)

Fig. 2 Patient flow diagram

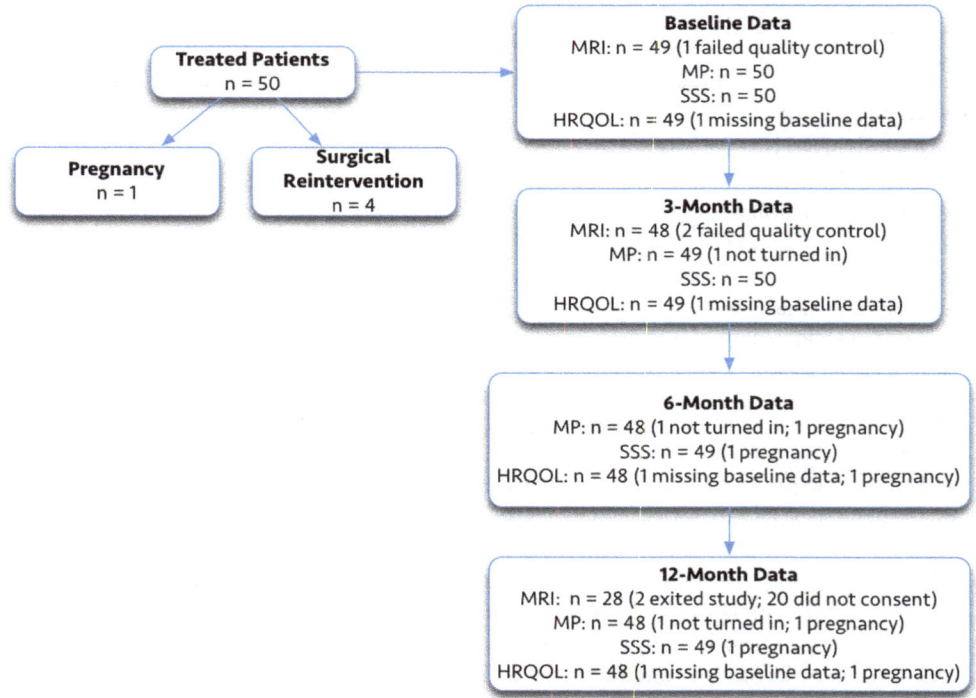

Pictogram scores. Of these 49 patients at 3 months, 28 (57.1 %) had >50 % reduction in MP scores; this proportion increased to 35 of 48 patients (72.9 %) at 6 months and was realized by 31 of 48 patients (64.6 %) at 12 months. The proportion of patients achieving >50 % bleeding reduction at 6 months was not significantly different from the proportion at 12 months ($P=.095$).

Lukes and colleagues reported that a 22 % or greater reduction in menstrual blood loss was meaningful to the majority of women [13]. In the FAST-EU Trial, 37 of 49 (75.5 %) patients had achieved such clinically meaningful reductions in menstrual bleeding by 3 months. This increased to 41 of 48 patients (85.4 %) at 6 months and 38 of 48 patients (79.2 %) at month 12, which was not significantly different from 6 months ($P=.175$).

As shown in Table 5, the reductions in the transformed SSS subscale of the UFS-QOL questionnaire at 3, 6, and 12 months were statistically significant, as were the increases in the transformed HRQOL subscale. Patients experienced a 55.1 % reduction in SSS at 12 months, corresponding to a mean reduction in transformed SSS of 35.3 points from baseline. At all post-ablation time points studied, the majority of patients experienced at least a clinically significant 10-point reduction in SSS (82 % of patients at 3 months, 86 % at 6 months, 78 % at 12 months).

Adverse events

There were 34 adverse events deemed possibly, probably, or definitely related to the VizAblate System or overall

Table 3   Characteristics of ablated fibroids

Total number of ablated target fibroids[a]	92
Mean number of ablated target fibroids per subject	1.8±1.1 (range 1–5)
Total number of type 0 ablated fibroids	0
Total number of type 1 ablated fibroids	14
Total number of type 2 ablated fibroids	42
Total number of type 3 ablated fibroids	3
Total number of type 4 ablated fibroids	25
Total number of type 2–5 (transmural) ablated fibroids	8
Mean diameter of ablated fibroids	3.2±1.4 cm (range 1.1–6.9 cm)

[a] Includes three fibroids that were ablated in a subject whose MRI data was not evaluable with regard to precise fibroid measurements

Table 4 Reduction in mean perfused and total fibroid volumes through 12 months

	Baseline	3 months	% Reduction from baseline	P value[a]	12 months[b]	% Reduction from baseline	P value[a]
No. of ablated fibroids	89	89			43		
No. of subjects	49	49			28		
Perfused fibroid volume (cm^3)	18.3±20.6 9.5 (0.3–77.0)	5.8±9.6 1.6 (0.0–45.7)	68.1±28.6 % 76.9 % (−33.3 to 100 %)	<.001	6.6±11.3 1.0 (0.0–56.1)	67.4±31.9 % 73.3 % (−32.7 to 100 %)	<.001
Total fibroid volume (cm^3)	18.8±21.4 9.5 (0.3–77.0)	8.0±12.0 1.9 (0.0–56.3)	54.7±37.4 % 62.5 % (−85.7 to 100 %)	<.001	6.8±11.4 1.2 (0.0–56.1)	66.6±32.1 % 73.3 % (-32.7–100 %)	<.001

Data are mean±standard deviation; median (range)

[a] Wilcoxon signed-rank test, null hypothesis of no change

[b] A 12-month MRI study was added through a protocol amendment after several patients had been treated, and 28 patients provided informed consent to undergo this additional imaging study

procedure over a 12-month period. These included seven women with dysmenorrhea, six with abnormal uterine bleeding above baseline, four with pelvic pain and/or cramping, two urinary tract infections (both within 30 days of treatment), and one fibroid expulsion that had no significant consequences. There were two readmissions within 30 days of the procedure. One patient was admitted overnight on post-procedure day #9 to receive parenteral antibiotics for lower abdominal pain believed secondary to cystitis (one of the two instances of urinary tract infection previously noted) and was discharged on the following day. Another patient developed bradycardia down to 38 bpm shortly after the procedure and was kept overnight in the hospital for successful treatment with atropine and observation.

Surgical reintervention

Four patients (8 %) underwent surgical reintervention, all after 6 months post-ablation. One patient underwent hysteroscopy and nonresectoscopic endometrial ablation (ThermaChoice®; Ethicon, Somerville, NJ) at 10 months. At the time of her endometrial ablation, hysteroscopy confirmed the presence of a normal endometrial cavity; no residual fibroid tissue was noted. Two patients, both treated by the same investigator, underwent hysteroscopic myomectomy at 6.5 and 7 months post-ablation, respectively, due to AUB felt secondary to fibroid sloughing. In both cases, the ablated fibroids had a 70–85 % reduction in perfused volume at 3 months. A fourth patient underwent total abdominal hysterectomy at 11 months secondary to abnormal uterine bleeding above baseline. The patient was noted post-operatively to have had an abnormal bleeding duration at baseline that had not been reported in her menstrual history, constituting a protocol violation. The patient may have had a component of anovulation contributing to her abnormal uterine bleeding.

Pregnancy

There was a single pregnancy reported within the first 6 months after ablation with the VizAblate System. The patient presented with 12 weeks of amenorrhea at her 6-month trial visit, had a positive pregnancy test at that time, and delivered a live-born male infant at term via elective repeat Cesarean section [14].

Return to normal activity, patient satisfaction, and pain during recovery

Forty-eight patients provided results of a 10-point visual analogue scale (VAS) regarding their pain during the recovery period (up to 14 days post-treatment). On average, they reported a mean VAS score of 3.0±1.7 (median 3.0, range 0–9). Forty-seven patients completed a recovery diary relating to how long it took them to return to their normal activities of daily life. On average, return to normal activity took 4.4± 3.1 days (median 4.0 days, range 1–14 days). There was an overall satisfaction rate of 87.8 % (43/49 patients) at 12 months; 69.4 % were "very satisfied," 10.2 % were "satisfied," and 8.2 % were "somewhat satisfied," with their treatment. At 12 months, 49 patients provided a mean scoring of 8.8±2.4 out of 10 in terms of how likely they would be to recommend the treatment to a friend or relative.

Discussion

It is of particular importance to determine how well patients fared beyond the previously reported 3- and 6-month endpoints from the FAST-EU Trial. The results outlined in this report confirm and extend the results of the 3- and 6-month endpoints and demonstrate that intrauterine sonography-

Table 5 Improvement in patient-reported outcomes through 12 months

	Baseline	3 months	Change from baseline	% Change from baseline	P value[a]	6 months	Change from baseline	% Change from baseline	P value[a]	12 months	Change from baseline	% Change from baseline	P value*
MP	50 423±253 361 (119–1582)	49 202±202 170 (0–1011)	49 221±290 191 (–700, 1265)	49 45.2±57.9% 56.9% (–225–100%)	<.001	48 181±209 107 (0–1011)	48 244±302 191 (–700, 1307)	48 51.9±59.8% 68.6% (–225–100%)	<.001	48 173±200 85 (0–786)	48 243±296 217 (–343, 1543)	48 53.8±50.5% 72.3% (–103–100%)	<.001
SSS	50 61.7±16.9 60.9% (28.1–100%)	50 31.7±20.1 31.3% (0.0–93.8%)	50 30.0±22.2 31.3 (–18.8, 84.4)	50 46.7%±32.8% 52.5% (–33.3–100%)	<.001	49 25.1±19.3 18.8 (0.0–78.1)	49 36.7±22.6 37.5 (–6.3, 75.0)	49 57.6±31.4% 66.7% (–22.2–100%)	<.001	49 26.6±24.0 21.9 (0.0–78.1)	49 35.3±26.9 37.5 (–18.8, 93.8)	49 55.1±41.0% 62.5% (–66.7–100%)	<.001
HRQOL	49 34.3±19.0 30.2 (0.0–73.3)	49 76.4±22.2 83.6 (5.2–100)	49 42.1±25.6 40.5 (–7.8, 95.7)	49 336±846% 123% (–11.1–5550%)	<.001	48 79.5±22.7 85.3 (0.9–100)	48 44.5±26.7 45.3 (–5.2, 96.6)	48 266±475% 118% (–28.6–2800%)	<.001	48 80.7±24.7 91.4 (0.9–100)	48 45.7±30.5 45.7 (–33.6, 96.6)	48 277±483% 127% (–54.2–2800%)	<.001

Data are number of subjects; mean±standard deviation; median (range)

MP Menstrual Pictogram, SSS Symptom Severity Score, HRQOL Health-Related Quality of Life

[a] Wilcoxon Signed-Rank Test, null hypothesis of no change

guided transcervical radiofrequency ablation of fibroids provides significant reductions in fibroid volume and bleeding symptoms through 12 months.

Transcervical radiofrequency ablation avoids many of the potential complications associated with a laparoscopic or open procedure for the treatment of fibroids. There are no incisions, eliminating the potential for wound infection, seroma, and hematoma. The peritoneal cavity is not entered nor is the serosa penetrated or coagulated, so that intraperitoneal adhesiogenesis is unlikely. There is no overt risk of ureteral injury, unlike hysterectomy. In contrast to operative hysteroscopy, only a small quantity of hypotonic fluid is used for acoustic coupling, no large venous sinuses are exposed, and intrauterine pressure is not raised to levels above mean arterial pressure, avoiding the risk of significant fluid intravasation. The integral intrauterine sonography probe permits real-time visualization of the myometrium and serosa, providing a perspective of the myometrium and intramyometrial pathology that are not achievable with a hysteroscope and enabling treatment of intramural and transmural fibroids as well as larger submucous myomata.

The trial success criterion was >30 % reduction in mean target fibroid perfused volume at 3 months in at least 50 % of patients. This success criterion stems from the MR-guided focused ultrasound data of Stewart and colleagues, which found that sustained relief of fibroid symptoms up to 24 months is associated with nonperfused volume ratios >20 % after hyperthermic ablation [15]. Initially, it was not known if total fibroid volume would be significantly reduced at that early time point, which was the rationale for using reduction in perfused fibroid volume (measured via contrast-enhanced MRI) as the primary endpoint as opposed to reduction in total fibroid volume. In the FAST-EU Trial, contrast-enhanced MRI demonstrated significant mean reductions at 3 months in both the volume of perfused fibroid tissue as well as in total fibroid volume at 3 months (68.1 and 54.7 %, respectively). At 12 months, patients demonstrated significant reductions (67.4 and 66.6 %, respectively) in mean perfused and total fibroid volumes. It has been previously demonstrated that hyperthermic ablation of >20 % of a fibroid may provide sustained relief from fibroid symptoms [15].

There were statistically significant reductions in menstrual blood loss, as evidenced by 45.2, 51.9, and 53.8 % reductions in the menstrual pictogram at 3, 6, and 12 months, respectfully, as well as significant improvements in both subscales of the UFS-QOL questionnaire. The majority of patients (57.1–72.9 %, depending on time point) realized more than a 50 % reduction in their menstrual pictogram scores, with 75.5 % of patients achieving a clinically meaningful reduction in menstrual bleeding as early as 3 months after treatment. Similarly, 78–86 % patients realized at least a 10-point reduction in SSS (depending on time point), with a mean reduction from baseline of 35.3 points at 12 months; a 10-point reduction in SSS represents a moderate effect size and was required by the US Food and Drug Administration for the approval of MRgFUS [16].

Patients typically experienced mild or no pain through the first post-ablation visit. Return to normal activity was just over 4 days and patient satisfaction was high (87.8 %). Two patients (4 %) were hospitalized overnight, one for abdominal pain secondary to apparent cystitis and the other for observation after bradycardia that responded to atropine. Neither event was deemed to have been related to the VizAblate System upon review by an independent medical advisory board.

This trial has several noteworthy attributes. Care was taken to exclude women with abnormal uterine bleeding secondary to anovulation through strict adherence to the inclusion criterion regarding the menstrual history. Additionally, at least one fibroid was required to have indented the endometrial cavity, making it more likely that a patient's bleeding symptoms are largely or exclusively secondary to fibroids rather than another etiology. A core MRI facility was used to reduce variability and bias in MRI imaging quality, interpretation, and measurements relative to the primary trial endpoint. In addition, the use of multiple clinical sites included academic medical centers as well as community hospitals to provide a more realistic assessment of the use of the VizAblate System in different treatment locations.

As a nonrandomized single-arm trial that does not directly compare against another fibroid treatment, this trial cannot be used to compare treatment with VizAblate to standard fibroid therapy. Only a subset of patients (28/48 eligible; 58.3 %) underwent MRI at 12 months. Finally, follow-up was limited to 12 months; longer surveillance and greater numbers of patients will be required to establish definitive efficacy and safety data. Toward that end, a larger clinical trial is underway.

Conclusions

These results from the FAST-EU Trial demonstrate that the initial endpoint results reported at 3 and 6 months were sustained in the treated population through 12 months. Patients realized significant reductions in perfused and total fibroid volume, menstrual bleeding, overall symptoms, and improvements in quality of life. The data demonstrate the potential of intrauterine sonography-guided, transcervical radiofrequency ablation with the VizAblate System as a promising uterus-preserving technology for the treatment of submucous, intramural, and transmural fibroids without incisions or the need for general anesthesia.

Acknowledgments The authors would like to acknowledge Mark Holdbrook, PhD, for expert guidance with statistical analysis.

Conflict of interest This is a Gynesonics-initiated trial, which is fully sponsored by Gynesonics. Drs. Brölmann, Bongers, Veersema, Quartero, and Gupta have no personal conflicts of interest to disclose; their respective institutions received reimbursement from Gynesonics for expenses incurred in the performance of this trial. Dr. Garza is a consultant for Gynesonics. Dr. Toub is Medical Director of Gynesonics.

Informed consent Informed consent was obtained from all patients included in the trial.

Contributions of the Authors Doctors Bongers, Brölmann, Gupta, Veersema, Quartero, and Garza-Leal were responsible for the conception and design of the study, data collection, patient recruitment, and preparation of the manuscript and were the responsible surgeons. Dr. Toub was responsible for the conception and design of the study, data collection, data analysis and interpretation, statistical analysis, and preparation of the manuscript.

References

1. Baird DD, Dunson DB, Hill MC et al (2003) High cumulative incidence of uterine leiomyoma in black and white women: ultrasound evidence. Am J Obstet Gynecol 188(1):100–7
2. Dembek CJ, Pelletier EM, Isaacson KB et al (2007) Payer costs in patients undergoing uterine artery embolization, hysterectomy, or myomectomy for treatment of uterine fibroids. J Vasc Interv Radiol 18(10):1207–13
3. Ghezzi F, Cromi A, Bergamini V et al (2007) Midterm outcome of radiofrequency thermal ablation for symptomatic uterine myomas. Surg Endosc 21(11):2081–5
4. Luo X, Shen Y, Song WX et al (2007) Pathologic evaluation of uterine leiomyoma treated with radiofrequency ablation. Int J Gynaecol Obstet 99(1):9–13
5. Cho HH, Kim JH, Kim MR (2008) Transvaginal radiofrequency thermal ablation: a day-care approach to symptomatic uterine myomas. Aust N Z J Obstet Gynaecol 48(3):296–301
6. Iversen H, Lenz S (2008) Percutaneous ultrasound guided radiofrequency thermal ablation for uterine fibroids : A new gynecological approach. Ultrasound Obstet Gynecol 32(3):325
7. Garza-Leal JG, Toub D, León IH et al (2011) Transcervical, intrauterine ultrasound-guided radiofrequency ablation of uterine fibroids with the VizAblate System: safety, tolerability, and ablation results in a closed abdomen setting. Gynecol Surg 8(3):327–334
8. Bongers M, Brolmann H, Gupta J et al (2015) Transcervical, intrauterine ultrasound-guided radiofrequency ablation of uterine fibroids with the VizAblate(R) System: three- and six-month endpoint results from the FAST-EU study. Gynecol Surg 12(1):61–70
9. Wyatt KM, Dimmock PW, Walker TJ et al (2001) Determination of total menstrual blood loss. Fertil Steril 76(1):125–31
10. Higham JM, O'Brien PM, Shaw RW (1990) Assessment of menstrual blood loss using a pictorial chart. Br J Obstet Gynaecol 97(8):734–9

11. Warrilow G, Kirkham C, Ismail KMK et al (2004) Quantification of menstrual blood loss. Obstetrician & Gynaecologist 6(2):88–92

12. Munro MG, Critchley HO, Broder MS et al (2011) FIGO classification system (PALM-COEIN) for causes of abnormal uterine bleeding in nongravid women of reproductive age. Int J Gynaecol Obstetrics 113(1):3–13

13. Lukes AS, Muse K, Richter HE et al (2010) Estimating a meaningful reduction in menstrual blood loss for women with heavy menstrual bleeding. Curr Med Res Opin 26(11):2673–8

14. Garza-Leal JG, León IH, Toub D (2014) Pregnancy after transcervical radiofrequency ablation guided by intrauterine sonography: case report. Gynecol Surg 11(2):145–149

15. Stewart EA, Gostout B, Rabinovici J et al (2007) Sustained relief of leiomyoma symptoms by using focused ultrasound surgery. Obstet Gynecol 110(2 Pt 1):279–87

16. Stewart EA, Rabinovici J, Tempany CM et al (2006) Clinical outcomes of focused ultrasound surgery for the treatment of uterine fibroids. Fertil Steril 85(1):22–9

24

Proposal of a modified transcervical endometrial resection (TCER) technique for menorrhagia treatment: Feasibility, efficacy, and patients' acceptability

Pietro Litta · Luigi Nappi · Pasquale Florio ·
Luca Mencaglia · Mario Franchini · Stefano Angioni

Abstract The aim of this study is to evaluate the feasibility, efficacy, safeness, and patients' acceptability of a modified transcervical endometrial resection (TCER) technique for the treatment of menorrhagia. Eighty-four premenopausal women with menorrhagia after careful investigation and 2 months therapy with GnRHa underwent a modified TCER. It was performed with a standard dual channel, 26 French irrigating resectoscope (Karl Storz, GmbH, Germany) after cervix dilatation to 10 mm and sorbitol mannitol solution used as distension medium. The modified technique was based on the resection of the endometrium and of the first myometrial layers only on the anterior and posterior walls, without treating fundus and cornual areas as usually performed. Endometrial resection was performed to a depth of 4 to 5 mm. Clinical and hysteroscopic follow-up was performed for 60 months. Early and late complications, changing in bleeding patterns, and patients' satisfaction were recorded. Sixty-four out of 73 patients that completed the 60 months improved. Eumenorrhea was achieved in 68.5 %, hypomenorrhea in 5.5 %, and amenorrhea in 13.7 %. Most of the patients (86.3 %) showed satisfaction at the follow-up interview. Control hysteroscopy showed that post modified TCER uterine cavity maintained the possibility of macroscopic and histopathology investigation during follow-up. Modified TCER is a technique easy to perform and effective in the long-term resolution of menorrhagia. In particular, it avoids the formation of synechiae and the shrinkage of the uterine cavity that may be the cause of various long-term complications, such as the delay in the diagnosis of endometrial carcinoma onset.

Keywords Menorrhagia · AUB · Endometrial resection · Minimally invasive surgery · Hysteroscopy

P. Litta
Department of Gynecological Science and Human Reproduction,
University of Padua, Padua, Italy

L. Nappi
Department of Medical and Surgical Sciences, Institute of Obstetrics
and Gynaecology, University of Foggia, Foggia, Italy

P. Florio
U.O.C. Obstetrics & Gynecology, "San Giuseppe" Hospital, Empoli,
Italy

L. Mencaglia
Section of Gynecology, Centro Oncologico Fiorentino, Sesto
Fiorentino, Italy

M. Franchini
Palagi Freestanding Unit, Florence, Italy

S. Angioni (✉)
Department of Surgical Sciences, Section of Obstetrics &
Gynecology, University of Cagliari, Azienda Ospedaliero
Universitaria, Blocco Q, SS554, Monserrato, Cagliari, Italy
e-mail: sangioni@yahoo.it

Introduction

Hysteroscopic transcervical endometrial resection (TCER) is a minimally invasive surgical technique developed in recent years with the purpose of removing the entire thickness of the endometrium lining of the uterus [1]. Indeed, to suppress menstruation successfully, it is essential to remove the full thickness of this lining together with the superficial myometrium, including the deep endometrial basal glands which are believed to be the primary foci for endometrial regrowth [1, 2]. However, TCER is not always completely successful and, in some cases, additional surgical treatment is required, thus limiting the benefits related to the reduced trauma and post-operative complications to the woman. The risk of failure and the expense of multiple treatments opened a debate whether endometrial ablation should replace or not hysterectomy [3], or if it might be an effective therapy for women with hyperplasia, with abnormal uterine bleeding, with high risk for medical therapy or hysterectomy [4]. The emerging clinical opinion is that TCER is an effective and safe alternative to hysterectomy that should be offered to women with menorrhagia for the relief of their heavy menstrual bleeding, together with the caution that there should be the possibility of further surgery, either repeat endometrial ablation or hysterectomy [5].

Matter of discussion related to TCER is also the putative occurrence of other problems related to the endometrial injury, as in the case of immediate (vascular or metabolic type complications (fluid overload) and perforation), or delayed complications (as in the case of the development of partial intrauterine dense adhesions and/or total obliteration of the cavity) [5–12]. Therefore, the ideal method of TCER associating high efficacy to nice tolerability and low incidence of complications is still far from being achieved. In the present study, we evaluated short- and long-term outcomes associated with a new TCER technique to treat menorrhagia that differ from the standard one in the fact that uterine fundus and cornual areas are not removed in the modified technique.

Materials and methods

Subjects

For this prospective cohort study, we consecutively enrolled from October 2, 2000 to September 24, 2005 all women suffering of menorrhagia who referred to our tertiary centers of women health care. The diagnosis of menorrhagia was performed by means of a pictorial blood loss assessment chart, adjusted to our needs in patients describing a history of heavy menstrual blood loss over several consecutive cycles [13]. A scoring system ranging from 1 to 10 was used, with 1 = slightly soiled tampon, 5 = moderately soiled, and 10 = heavily soiled. Sanitary napkins were assigned ascending scores from 1 to 20. A total score more than 100 for each pictorial chart was meant as a confirmed diagnosis of menorrhagia [14]. We considered for the study only patients who had performed a full clinical evaluation including colposcopy and Papanicolaou test, transvaginal ultrasonography, and hysteroscopy with endometrial biopsy [15]. Exclusion criteria were the following: not confirmed diagnosis of menorrhagia, uterine size >12 cm, presence of large organic intrauterine lesions (endometrial polyp >3 cm, submucous myomas G0>2 cm or submucous myomas G1 and G2); desire of future pregnancy, cervical and endometrial pre- and malignant conditions or adnexal pathologies; and debilitating medical condition. Any medical hormonal treatment was suspended at least 1 month before enrollment. All procedures followed were in accordance with the ethical standards of the responsible committee on human experimentation (institutional and national) and with the Helsinki Declaration of 1975, as revised in 2000. Informed consent was obtained from all patients for being included in the study.

Surgical procedure: modified TCER

All the women underwent therapy with GnRH analogs (Leuprolide Acetate 3.75 mg) for 2 months (every 28 days) before surgery, as in standard practice [6]. All procedures were performed under general anesthesia, with induction by propofol 2 mg kg^{-1} and spontaneous ventilation with a mixture of 60 % nitrous oxide and 40 % oxygen isofluothane, or spinal anesthesia in selected patient [16]. Hysteroscopic MTCER was performed with a standard dual channel, 26 French irrigating resectoscope (Karl Storz, GmbH, Germany) after that cervix was dilated to 10 mm. The uterine cavity was distended with sorbitol mannitol solution used as distension medium, and a suction-irrigating unit (Endomat, Karl Storz, GmbH, Germany) was used to provide positive pressure (120 mmHg) and continuous outflow suction control (0.5 bar). Fluid balance was carefully monitored throughout the procedure that was interrupted if fluid deficit was over 1,000 cm^3. Surgical time was recorded starting at resectoscope introduction inside the uterus and ending at its last removal.

Compared to the technique described by Wortman and Dagget [2], our modified TCER began on either anterior or posterior uterine wall and was based on the resection of the anterior cardinal strip of tissue followed by resection of the posterior and the two lateral cardinal strips without treating fundus and cornual areas (Fig. 1). The conventional TCER approach consists in the treatment of fundal and cornual areas by the equatorial loop and/or the use of the rollerball electrode. Endometrial resection was performed to a depth of 4 to 5 mm, and endomyometrial strips were removed from the cavity and sent for histological assessment. The procedure was scheduled for a 1-day surgery.

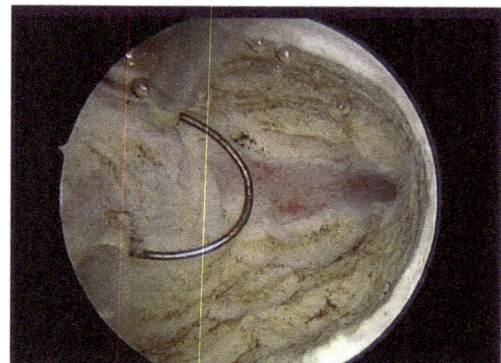

Fig. 1 Resection of the anterior cardinal strip of tissue followed by resection of the posterior and the two lateral cardinal strips without treating fundus and cornual areas

Office hysteroscopy

Control hysteroscopy was scheduled at 3, 12, 24, and 60 months after the surgery. It was performed by using vaginoscopic approach, with a continuous-flow hysteroscope using Telescope 2.9 mm (HOPKINS II Forward-Oblique Telescope 30°; Karl Storz, Tuttlingen, Germany) [17, 18]. The uterine cavity was distended with temperate saline solution and irrigated using an electronic irrigation pump (Hysteromat, Karl Storz®, Karl Storz, Tuttlingen, Germany). Examination was performed in an office setting, without anesthesia or cervical dilatation.

Main outcomes of the study

Outcome measures referred to changes in bleeding patterns, safeness, and patients' acceptability. In details, after modified TCER, women underwent office hysteroscopy for uterine cavity evaluation (with endometrial biopsy) 3, 12, 24, and 60 months after TCER, and simultaneously, patients were asked about the amelioration or persistence of bleeding, duration of amenorrhea, improvement of dysmenorrhea, and if they need any hormonal or surgical treatment for heavy bleeding after modified TCER.

Modified TCER was considered successful when it was associated with amenorrhea, hypomenorrhea, and eumenorrhea. A women was defined as amenorrheic when reporting persistent ceasing of menstruation after surgery. Eumenorrhea referred to regular menstrual cycle with average length of 28 days (range, 21–35 days), lasting on average for 4 days (range, 1–8 days) and of normal quantity (flowing less than 80 mL per cycle). Hypomenorrhea referred to menstruations regular in frequency but poor in quantity and/or lasting less than 2 days [1]. Resection was considered non-effective when the patient reported persistence or relapse of menorrhagia.

Interviews were done at the time of every follow-up hysteroscopy, and data were related to patients' subjective experiences related/consequent to modified TCER and their health status concerning endometrial status.

Statistical analysis

All data were analyzed with Prism software (GraphPad Software Inc., San Diego, CA, USA) and expressed as mean $\pm$SD. The Kolmogorov-Smirnov test was used to evaluate whether values had a Gaussian distribution, in order to choose between parametric and non-parametric statistical tests. Therefore, the unpaired t test was used to compute statistical significance, and χ-square and Fisher exact test to analyze differences between proportions. Statistical significance was assumed for values of $P<0.05$.

Results

Some patients were not included in the study. Exclusion criteria were the following: not confirmed diagnosis of menorrhagia (26 women), uterine size >12 cm (10 patients), presence of large organic intrauterine lesions (endometrial polyp >3 cm, submucous myomas G0>2 cm, and submucous myomas G1 and G2) (15 patients); desire of future pregnancy (eight patients), cervical, and endometrial pre- and malignant conditions or adnexal pathologies (10 patients).

Eighty-four patients out of 153 (age 45.37$\pm$4.02) entered the study. The clinical study protocol consisted of modified TCER, followed by the assessment of endometrial cavity by office diagnostic hysteroscopy 3, 12, 24, and 60 months after the surgery. Table 1 shows clinical and demographic details of the population evaluated in the study. Endometrial resection was successfully performed in all patients enrolled. No one of the patients had early or late complications. In 24 out of 84 patients, endometrial resection was associated with the simultaneous removal of small polyps ($n=15$) or myomas ($n=9$) (data not shown). In any case, the time required for endometrial resection with associated polypectomy (13.31$\pm$6.09 min) or myomectomy (14.7$\pm$8.2 min) did not differ when compared to the endometrial resection alone (11.91$\pm$4.15 min; $P>0.05$), as well as the time spent for cervical dilatation and the infusion volume needed for uterine distension (data not shown). In 11 cases (13 %), adenomyosis was evidenced by histopathologic examination.

Follow-up outcomes: clinical findings

Eleven women dropped out (13.1 %) and did not complete the first year of follow-up, while 73 (86.9 %) patients completed the follow-up for at least 60 months (Table 2) and 61 (83.6 %) of these reached a 84-month follow-up. During the observational time interval, bleeding patterns were observed in eumenorrhea in 50 out of 73 women (68.5 %), hypomenorrhea in four patients (5.5 %), and amenorrhea in 10 subjects (13.7 %) (Table 2). None of them reported spotting, neither dysmenorrhea onset or worsening, nor medium-/

Table 1 Anthropometric and surgical data related to the population prospectively evaluated

Age (years)	45.37$\pm$4.02
Gravida	2.3$\pm$1.2
Parity	2.4$\pm$1.2
BMI (kg/m^2)	28.7$\pm$3.3
Mean operating time (min)	12.4$\pm$1.8
Cervical dilatation (min)	1.4$\pm$0.4
Infusion volume (mL)	2,500$\pm$550
Fluid deficit (mL)	250$\pm$110

Data are reported as mean$\pm$SD

Table 2 Data related to the clinical findings retrieved at follow-up after modified TCER in women prospectively evaluated

Patients underwent MTCER (n; %)	84 (100 %)
Follow-up completed after 3 months (n; %)	84 (100)
Follow-up completed after 60 months (n; %)	73 (86.9)
Bleeding patterns after TCER	
Eumenorrhea (n; %)	50/73 (68.5)
Hypomenorrhea (n; %)	4/73 (5.5)
Amenorrhea (n; %)	10/73 (13.7)
Menorrhagia (n; %)	7/73 (9.6)
Recurrence of AUB/DUB (n; %)	2/73 (2.7)

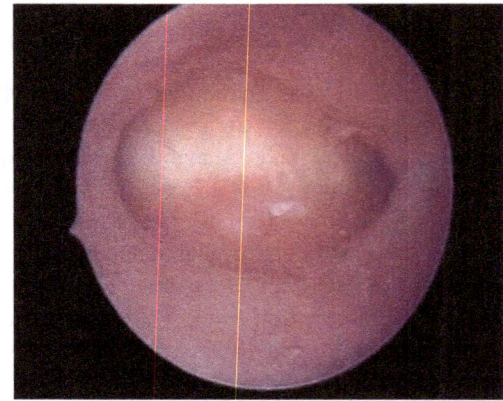

Fig. 2 Hysteroscopic appearance of endometrial cavity at 3-month follow-up after MTCER. None of the patients were found to have intrauterine adhesions

long-term complications such as pregnancy or complications putatively related to the development of intra-cavitary adhesions, such as hematometra and/or cornual hematometra, as observed at diagnostic office hysteroscopy.

Seven (9.6 %) patients continued to have menorrhagia, and among them, two of the 11 cases were with adenomyosis (18.2 %). Three patients underwent laparoscopic hysterectomy (n=3) after an average interval of 6 months (range, 1–11 months), two patients underwent hormonal treatment by means of levonorgestrel-based intrauterine device, and the remaining two women underwent 4-month GnRH analog administration (n=2) (data not shown). In these patients, a second modified TCER was not performed because patients refused such a type of treatment.

In addition, AUB recurred in two women (2.7 %) after 12 and 60 months after endometrial resection (Table 2). They underwent a new modified TCER or laparoscopic hysterectomy (for the women in whom recurrence occurred 60 months after modified TCER) (data not shown).

Follow-up outcome: data from interview

At the end of 3-month follow-up, 63 women (86.3 %) stated they were satisfied by the surgery so much that they would recommend it to women with menorrhagia, whereas the remaining 10 patients (13.7 %) would not, for reasons mainly related to the fear of general anesthesia (n=8; 80.0 %) or office hysteroscopy in the follow-up (n=2; 20 %). None of the patients had symptoms or conditions invalidating and/or limiting their quality of life (data not shown).

Follow-up outcome: hysteroscopic findings

Considering findings recorded at hysteroscopic follow-up, none of the patients was found to have intra-uterine adhesions or cavity contracture after 3 months. It was possible to evaluate the entire cavity, including the cornual area and the tubal ostia in all patients (Fig. 2). The same findings were obtained

at all time points in the follow-up, even if the uterine cavity at the hysteroscopic evaluation performed after 12, 24, and 60 months from endometrial resection was markedly reduced to a narrow tube as a result of fibrosis and contracture (Fig. 3). In any case, the entire uterine cavity, including the cornual areas, was found to be open and the tubal ostia were visualized at all time points of follow-up. In addition, histological evaluation of endometrial biopsy annually performed failed to found cancerous or pre-cancerous endometrial lesions (data not shown).

Discussion

The present study first refers on the clinical efficiency and patients' perception of a new endometrial resection technique, by using which menorrhagia was resolved in the majority of patients, without surgical complications, no intrauterine adhesions formation in the follow-up, no fluid overload syndrome, short operative time, and a high degree of patients' satisfaction.

The reasons that led us to devise such a new technique are related to the fact that the *conventional* hysteroscopic TCER is

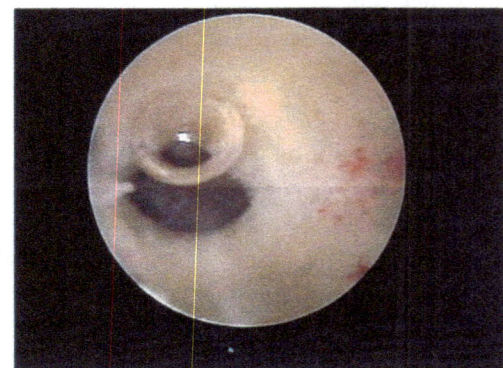

Fig. 3 A narrowing of the cavity is evidenced at 60 months but it does not hinder to evaluate the entire cavity, including the cornual area

sometime associated to clinical problems, like surgical (perforation of the uterus), vascular complications or fluid overload syndrome [5–12]. Moreover, like resectoscopic myomectomy, TCER is a surgical procedure suggested only to experienced surgeons [19]. Consequently, our aim was to simplify and to accelerate the procedure maintaining the success rate and possibly decreasing the complications in order to make it accessible even to less experienced gynecologists. In addition, we intended to decrease the occurrence of intrauterine adhesions, contractures, and/or hematometra [12, 20–22]. These last side effects are due to the fact that after the endometrium is destroyed or resected, the myometrium is exposed and intrauterine walls, collapsing on each other, have a natural tendency to grow together. The final result is the intrauterine contracture and marked reduction of the endometrial cavity to a narrow tubular structure as a result of fibrosis that often obstructs the cornual area. This mechanism is responsible for the occurrence of synechiae in 40 % of women submitted to total TCER [2] that may limit the access to the uterine cavity, hematometra, that usually localizes in the fundus of the uterus, or obstruction of the cornual area in 13 % of cases [11, 22, 23]. The persistence in these obstructed areas of islands of endometrial tissue may cause retrograde menstruation or symptomatic cornual hematometra, with an incidence of even 18 %, causing painful distention of the uterus [24]. The potential of all these complications may limit the clinical efficacy of hysteroscopic TCER and can require hysterectomy. In our technique, the resection of the endometrium and of the first myometrial layers was limited only on the anterior and posterior and lateral walls, without treating fundal and cornual areas by using the rollerball, as usually performed [1, 2] The initial hypothesis was that preserving endometrial mucosa of the fundal and cornual areas could decrease the risk of synechiae or focal hematometra facilitating the long-term uterine inspection [15, 25]. The possibility that this approach could result in menorrhagia or bleeding persistence due to the endometrial mucosa not removed was not shown by our study. Moreover, in our case series, we failed to detect intrauterine adhesions at all evaluated time points after 12, 24, and 60 months and it was possible to carry out an endometrial biopsy sampling for histological evaluation despite the presence of some cavity contracture in the long-term follow-up. As possible explanation, one may propose that the integrity of corneal and fundal areas might sustain intrauterine walls.

On this regard, the work of McCausland and McCausland was pioneering, since recommending ablation of only one wall of the uterine cavity and avoiding the cornual areas reduced the incidence of adhesions formation after TCER [26]. Moreover, other authors have already proposed the resection of the entire upper uterine fundus, but sparing the isthmus and the immediate supraisthmic region to prevent hematometra caused by stenosis at the level of the cervical isthmus [27].

Findings obtained in the long-term follow-up of the present study showed the absence of intrauterine adhesions and/or hematometra: no patient reported, both in the hysteroscopic and clinical verification, the appearance or worsening of dysmenorrhea, and none of them had long-term complications ascribable to the development of intrauterine synechiae such as cornual hematometra. These findings lead us to suggest that the modified TCER we are proposing is able to avoid the formation of synechiae or shrinkage of the uterine cavity.

The second clinical matter that merits discussion refers to the absence in our study of intra- and peri-operative complications (uterine perforation, hemorrhage, excess fluid absorption, and thermic damages to peri-uterine structures). Cornual myometrium is indeed notoriously thin and thus with low resistance, therefore representing the critical area for any procedure performed at uterine fundus. Deciding not to treat such zone, we simplified the procedure making uterine perforations or thermic damages to peri-uterine structures improbable or at least less frequent compared to the conventional technique. Nevertheless, in modified TCER, the exposure of a smaller surface of the myometrium and the short operating time needed may together contribute to reduce absorption of hypotonic, electrolyte-free non-conductive distention solution, consequently not allowing the development of the overload syndrome [28].

It could be criticized that the residual endometrial tissue not removed in uterine fundus and cornual areas may be the site of putative pre- or markedly malignant lesions. We took care of this criticism, and so, we submitted our patients to an endometrial surveillance by endometrial biopsy under hysteroscopic guidance. Our follow-up hysteroscopies consented to visualize and collect samples from fundus and corneal areas in every patient. On the contrary, in the conventional TCER technique, the habitual collapse of the uterine walls and the formation of synechiae may hinder endometrial biopsy. Whether such a problem does not seem to affect low-risk population (i.e., patients with pre-ablation biopsy negative for hyperplasia and negative medical history for common risk factors for uterine neoplasia) [29], modified TCER may represent a valid therapeutic option for those patients considered at increased risk of developing hyperplasia and endometrial carcinoma. The unquestionable advantage of TCER, as opposed to new-generation destructive ablation methods, is to provide additional tissue for histological examination of the endometrium so that it is possible to detect any presence of micro foci of neoplasia or a high risk for it in the resected material previously not diagnosed in pre-surgical biopsy [30]. On the other hand, patients with increased risk of hyperplasia or endometrial neoplasia frequently are also at higher risk for major surgery, such is hysterectomy. Indeed, cardiovascular diseases, severe obesity, chronic nephropathies, coagulopathies, and hepatopathies are often co-existent with a history of meno- or metrorrhagia and also imply a high surgical and anesthesiological risks. The modified TCER we propose can be even more suitable for those "complex" patients, since it would have the advantage to be performed more quickly, with less intra- and peri-operative complications that the endometrial resection used so far.

In conclusion, despite the limitation due to the small sample size, our data on complications and the low (11.3 %) prevalence of bleeding persistence after operative hysteroscopy would suggest that modified TCER is a technique easy to perform, effective in the resolution of long-term menorrhagia and useful in patients with high surgical and anesthesiological risks. In addition, this new approach allows avoiding the formation of synechiae and the shrinkage of the uterine cavity that may be the cause for various long-term complications, such as the delay in the diagnosis of endometrial carcinoma onset.

Informed consent All procedures followed were in accordance with the ethical standards of the responsible committee on human experimentation (institutional and national) and with the Helsinki Declaration of 1975, as revised in 2000. Informed consent was obtained from all patients for being included in the study.

Conflict of interest Pietro Litta, Luigi Nappi, Pasquale Florio, Luca Mencaglia, Mario Franchini, and Stefano Angioni declare that they have no conflict of interest.

References

1. Magos AL, Baumann R, Lockwood GM, Turnbull AC (1991) Experience with the first 250 endometrial resection for menorrhagia. Lancet 337:1074–1078
2. Wortman M, Daggett A (1994) Hysteroscopic endomyometrial resection: a new technique for the treatment of menorrhagia. Obstet Gynecol 83:295–299
3. Farquhar CM, Steiner CA (2002) Hysterectomy rates in the United States 1990–1997. Obstet Gynecol 99:229–234
4. Vilos GA, Harding PG, Ettler HC (2002) Resectoscopic surgery in women with abnormal uterine bleeding and nonatypical endometrial hyperplasia. J Am Assoc Gynecol Laparosc 9:131–137
5. Lethaby A, Penninx J, Hickey M, Garry R, Marjoribanks J (2013) Endometrial resection and ablation techniques for heavy menstrual bleeding. Cochrane Database Syst Rev 8, CD001501
6. Litta P, Merlin F, Pozzan C, Nardelli GB, Capobianco G, Dessole S, Ambrosini A (2006) Transcervical endometrial resection in women with menorrhagia: long-term follow-up. Eur J Obstet Gynecol Reprod Biol 125:99–102
7. MacLean-Fraser E, Penava D, Vilos GA (2002) Perioperative complication rates of primary and repeat hysteroscopic endometrial ablations. J Am Assoc Gynecol Laparosc 9:175–177
8. Papadopoulos NP, Magos A (2007) First-generation endometrial ablation: roller-ball vs loop vs laser. Best Pract Res Clin Obstet Gynaecol 21(6):915–929
9. Paschopoulos M, Polyzos NP, Lavasidis LG, Vrekoussis T, Dalkalitsis N, Paraskevaidis E (2006) Safety issues of hysteroscopic surgery. Ann N Y Acad Sci 1092:229–234
10. Perino A, Castelli A, Cucinella G, Biondo A, Pane A, Venezia R (2004) A randomized comparison of endometrial laser intrauterine thermotherapy and hysteroscopic endometrial resection. Fertil Steril 82(3):731–734
11. Boujida VH, Philipsen T, Pelle J, Joergensen JC (2002) Five-year follow-up of endometrial ablation: endometrial coagulation versus endometrial resection. Obstet Gynecol 99(6):988–992
12. Propst AM, Liberman RF, Harlow BL, Ginsburg ES (2000) Complications of hysteroscopic surgery: predicting patients at risk. Obstet Gynecol 96(4):517–520
13. Higham JM, O'Brian PMS, Shaw RW (1990) Assessment of menstrual blood loss using a pictorial chart. Br J Obstet Gynaecol 97: 734–739
14. De Angelis C, Carnevale A, Santoro G, Nofroni I, Spinelli M, Guida M, Mencaglia L, Di Spiezio Sardo A (2013) Hysteroscopic findings in women with menorrhagia. J Minim Invasive Gynecol 20(2):209–214
15. Angioni S, Loddo A, Milano F, Piras B, Minerba L, Melis GB (2008) Detection of benign intracavitary lesions in postmenopausal women with AUB. A prospective study on outpatients hysteroscopy and blind biopsies. J Minim Invasive Gynecol 15(1):87–91
16. Florio P, Puzzutiello R, Filippeschi M, D'Onofrio P, Mereu L, Morelli R, Marianello D, Litta P, Mencaglia L, Petraglia F (2012) Low-dose spinal anesthesia with hyperbaric bupivacaine with intrathecal fentanyl for operative hysteroscopy: a case series study. J Minim Invasive Gynecol 19(1):107–112
17. Di Spiezio Sardo A, Bettocchi S, Spinelli M, Guida M, Nappi L, Angioni S, Sosa Fernandez LM, Nappi C (2010) Review of new office-based hysteroscopic procedures 2003–2009. J Minim Invasive Gynecol 17:436–448
18. Daniilidis A, Pantelis A, Dinas K, Tantanasis T, Loufopoulos PD, Angioni S, Carcea F (2012) Indications of diagnostic hysteroscopy, a brief review of the literature. Gynecol Surg 9(1):23–28
19. Litta P, Conte L, De Marchi F, Saccardi C, Angioni S (2014) Pregnancy outcome after hysteroscopic myomectomy. Gynecol Endocrinol 30(2):149–152
20. Overton C, Hargreaves J, Maresh M (1997) A national survey of the complications of endometrial destruction for menstrual disorders: the MISTLETOE study. Minimally Invasive Surgical Techniques–Laser, EndoThermal or Endoresection. Br J Obstet Gynaecol 104(12): 1351–1359
21. Hart R, Magos A (1997) Endometrial ablation. Curr Opin Obstet Gynecol 9(4):226–232
22. Wortman M, Daggett A (2001) Reoperative hysteroscopic surgery in the management of patients who fail endometrial ablation and resection. J Am Assoc Gynecol Laparosc 8(2): 272–277
23. Tapper AM, Heinonen PK (1995) Hysteroscopic endomyometrial resection for the treatment of menorrhagia–follow-up of 86 cases. Eur J Obstet Gynecol Reprod Biol 62(1):75–79
24. McCausland AM, McCausland VM (2002) Frequency of symptomatic cornual hematometra and postablation tubal sterilization syndrome after total rollerball endometrial ablation: a 10-year follow-up. Am J Obstet Gynecol 186:1274–1280
25. Litta P, Merlin F, Saccardi C, Pozzan C, Sacco G, Fracas M, Capobianco G, Dessole S (2005) Role of hysteroscopy with endometrial biopsy to rule out endometrial cancer in postmenopausal women with abnormal uterine bleeding. Maturitas 50(2): 117–123
26. McCausland AM, McCausland VM (1999) Partial rollerball endometrial ablation: a modification of total ablation to treat menorrhagia without causing complications from intrauterine adhesions. Am J Obstet Gynecol 180:1512–1521
27. Perino A, Cittadini E, Colacurci N, De Placido G, Hamou J (1990) Endometrial ablation: principles and technique. Acta Eur Fertil 21(6): 313–317

28. Witz CA, Silverberg KM, Burns WN, Schenken RS, Olive DL (1993) Complications associated with the absorption of hysteroscopic fluid media. Fertil Steril 60(5):745–756

29. Neuwirth RS, Loffer FD, Trenhaile T, Levin B (2004) The incidence of endometrial cancer after endometrial ablation in a low-risk population. J Am Assoc Gynecol Laparosc 11(4): 492–494

30. Ahonkallio SJ, Liakka AK, Martikainen HK, Santala MJ (2009) Feasibility of endometrial assessment after thermal ablation. Eur J Obstet Gynecol Reprod Biol 147(1):69–71

25

Transcervical, intrauterine ultrasound-guided radiofrequency ablation of uterine fibroids with the VizAblate System: safety, tolerability, and ablation results in a closed abdomen setting

Jose Gerardo Garza-Leal · David Toub · Iván Hernández León ·
Lorena Castillo Saenz · Darrin Uecker · Michael Munrow · Diane King ·
Jordan Bajor · James Coad

Abstract This was a single-site cohort study to evaluate the safety of a new transcervical device (VizAblate™) combining real-time intrauterine sonography with radiofrequency (RF) ablation for the treatment of fibroids. Nineteen women with uterine fibroids received treatment with the VizAblate System in a closed abdomen setting prior to hysterectomy. Twelve of these subjects underwent an immediate abdominal hysterectomy after radiofrequency ablation (acute group), while the remaining seven underwent hysterectomy on post-ablation days 16 and 17 (subacute group). Uteri were sectioned and stained with the viability stain triphenyltetrazolium chloride (TTC) to quantify fibroid ablation dimensions and assess the serosa for thermal injury. Subjects in the subacute group were treated with the VizAblate System under conscious sedation; they provided pain and tolerability data for the interval from ablation through hysterectomy, and indicated overall procedural satisfaction. Twenty-two ablations ranging from 1.8 to 36.2 cm^3 were created among 19 subjects within 20 fibroids and one region of adenomyosis. There were no complications or thermal serosal injury. For subjects in the subacute group receiving one ablation, the mean total procedure time was 25.8 ± 6.0 min (range 18–32 min). All subjects in the subacute group were discharged within 2 h of the VizAblate procedure. For fibroids≤5 cm, $67.2\%\pm27.0\%$ of the fibroid volume was ablated (range 15–100%; median 75%). Transcervical RF ablation of fibroids under intrauterine sonographic guidance with the VizAblate system can be accomplished with a high degree of reliability and without adverse events.

Keywords Radiofrequency ablation · Fibroids · Intrauterine sonography · Myomata

Introduction

Uterine fibroids are the most prevalent benign uterine tumors and have an age-specific cumulative incidence in the USA that is nearly 70% among white women and greater than 80% among black women [1]. Uterine fibroids are estimated to occur in approximately 20–25% of adult women overall with symptoms that may involve menorrhagia and subfertility as well as bulk symptoms. Despite numerous alternatives to hysterectomy, over 200,000 hysterectomies are performed for fibroids annually in the USA [1, 2]. There is also a lack of consensus regarding optimal therapy for uterine fibroids, so that more than 150 years after the first abdominal hysterectomy for fibroids, there is no definitive clinical evidence for what constitutes the "best" treatment for fibroids [3].

J. G. Garza-Leal · I. H. León · L. C. Saenz
Universidad Autónoma de Nuevo León,
Monterrey, Nuevo Leon, Mexico

D. Toub (✉) · D. Uecker · M. Munrow · D. King · J. Bajor
Gynesonics, Inc,
604 Fifth Avenue, Suite D,
Redwood City, CA 94063, USA
e-mail: dtoub@gynesonics.com

J. Coad
West Virginia University,
Morgantown, WV, USA

Radiofrequency ablation (RFA) has been used as a fibroid treatment modality since the early 1990s, with multiple clinical studies confirming its safety and efficacy [4–9]. It has been shown that radiofrequency ablation results in heat/thermal fixation and coagulative necrosis within the treated fibroids [9, 10]. Recent studies have been performed using RFA in conjunction with simultaneous, real-time sonography to enable volumetric ablations that result in volume reduction and symptomatic relief [8, 9, 11].

Cho and colleagues performed transcervical fibroid RFA in 153 women who were followed up to 18 months post-treatment [8]. Symptomatic relief was assessed through the Uterine Fibroid Symptom-Quality of Life questionnaire; the authors reported a 91% reduction in symptoms and a 46% improvement in quality of life. They demonstrated a 73% mean reduction in fibroid volume with only 4.3% (6/153) of the women requiring reintervention. Ghezzi and colleagues performed percutaneous RFA on up to three fibroids per patient in 25 women and followed them for 12 to 36 months. These patients all demonstrated symptomatic improvement and showed a mean 59% improvement in their quality of life with a 4% (1/25) reintervention rate at 1 year and as much as an 84% reduction in mean fibroid volumes at 36 months [9].

The VizAblate System™ (Gynesonics; Redwood City, CA) is a novel transcervical device that combines radiofrequency ablation for treatment with intrauterine sonography for lesion targeting. The VizAblate System (Fig. 1) consists of an intrauterine ultrasound (IUUS) probe and a single-use, disposable articulating handpiece that are combined into a single treatment device (Fig. 2). Other components of the VizAblate System include a custom RF generator and an ultrasound system with a custom graphical user interface (GUI). These uniquely integrated components provide the gynecologist with a high-quality image-guided treatment system. The VizAblate IUUS probe is used to localize fibroids from within the uterine cavity and guide placement of the VizAblate needle electrodes into targeted fibroids. Once positioning has been confirmed, therapeutic RF energy is delivered to the fibroid according to a fixed treatment cycle that is dependent on the desired ablation size.

The VizAblate GUI incorporates a treatment overlay ("treatment guides"), consisting of several graphical elements intended to assist the physician with the proper introducer and electrode placement and achieve safe ablation of the targeted fibroid. These graphical elements include the ablation zone (a red oval), the thermal safety border (a green oval), and additional elements for alignment of the overlay with the actual introducer and electrode positions as visualized in the ultrasound image (Fig. 3). The Ablation Zone represents the dimensions of an average ablation generated for the selected electrode deployment size. The thermal safety border represents the distance from the needle electrode beyond which tissue is safe from potential thermal damage; this is important from a safety perspective as there will be thermal heating of tissue beyond the area of the ablation that is represented by the ablation zone. The ablation zone and thermal safety border overlays have been validated through bench investigations of bovine muscle, direct uterine serosal temperature measurements using thermocouples and infrared thermography, and subsequent pathological analysis. The VizAblate GUI guides the physician through the prescribed procedure workflow, requiring specific steps in order to initiate RF treatment. This enables the gynecologist to select the appropriate needle electrode deployment width that

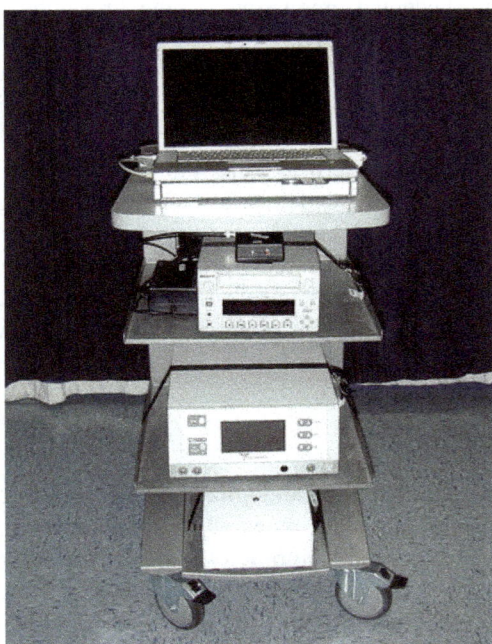

Fig. 1 The VizAblate System. The ultrasound display is provided by the laptop, while the RF generator resides on the second shelf from the bottom

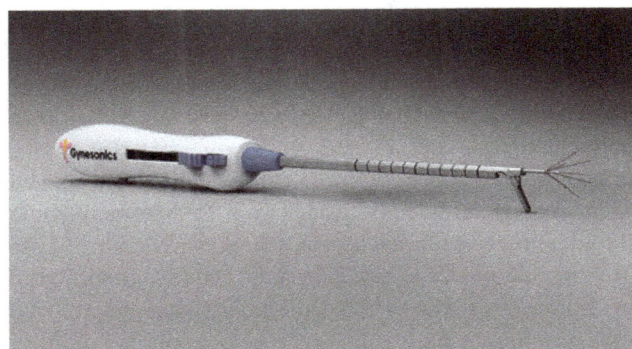

Fig. 2 The VizAblate treatment device

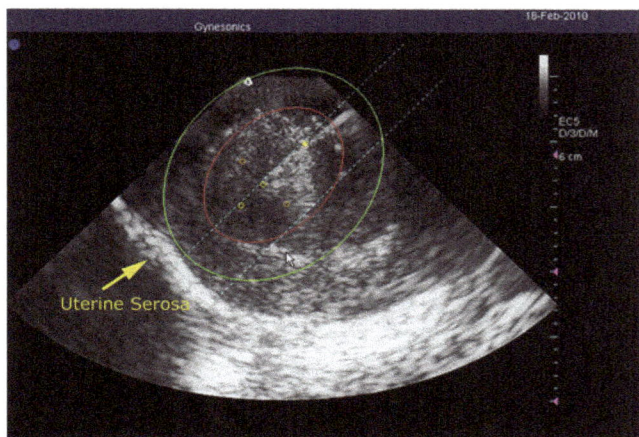

Fig. 3 IUUS image of a submucosal fibroid with the VizAblate treatment guides (ablation zone in *red*, thermal safety border in *green*) indicated. The mean region treatment delineates where the ablation will occur and the thermal safety border demarcates the extent of thermal spread beyond the ablation. The serosa is visible as an echogenic border around the uterus (*yellow* arrow)

maximizes ablation volume while avoiding thermal damage to the uterine serosal surface.

The shape of the ablations created by the VizAblate System are ellipsoidal, with an approximate maximum length of 5.0 cm and width of 4.0 cm. Single ablations with the current VizAblate System can ablate fibroids up to 5 cm in diameter. The ablation dimensions depend on how deeply the needle electrodes are deployed as well as the treatment time at temperature (105°C). The ablation width is adjustable in half-centimeter increments between 1.0 and 4.0 cm. The system automatically modulates RF power to maintain the target temperature for a prescribed duration, depending on the size of the desired ablation. The user simply matches the size of the Ablation Zone to that of the targeted fibroid, and ensures that the Thermal Safety Border is within the serosal margin at all times; the software algorithm then selects the duration of treatment by design based on the size of the Ablation Zone. Four minutes at temperature is used to ablate fibroids from 1 to 2 cm in diameter, 6 min is necessary to ablate fibroids greater than 2 cm up to 3.5 cm in diameter, and 9 min is required to ablate fibroids 3.5 cm or larger. These capabilities allow the physician to safely tailor the ablation position and volume to the particular fibroid and its location relative to the serosa. In many cases, a fibroid can be completely ablated when situated sufficiently distant from the serosa. When a fibroid is too close to the serosa, the physician can still use the treatment guides to safely ablate a significant portion of the fibroid's volume while still maintaining safety with respect to the serosa.

The VizAblate System has been developed in an open abdomen, perihysterectomy setting involving 89 treated

subjects. The use of concurrent laparotomy in that work enabled serosal temperature monitoring and also permitted the packing of bowel out of harm's way. In actual use, the VizAblate System would be introduced into the endometrial cavity via a transcervical approach in order to ablate submucosal, intramural, and transmural fibroids without incisions and without a requirement for general anesthesia.

This report describes the initial safety, tolerability, and procedure times of the VizAblate System when used under conditions for its anticipated use, in a closed abdomen setting, in women with uterine fibroids.

Materials and methods

Patient selection

This study was a prospective, non-randomized, single-arm, single-site trial (Canadian Task Force classification II-2) involving subjects with uterine fibroids who had elected to undergo hysterectomy for menorrhagia and other uterine symptomatology. The initial protocol and subsequent revisions were approved by the Ethics Committee of the Universidad Autónoma de Nuevo León Facultad de Medicina in Monterrey, Mexico. The procedures followed were in accordance with the ethical standards of the national responsible committee on human experimentation (Comisión Federal para la Protección contra Riesgos Sanitarios/Federal Commission for the Protection against Sanitary Risk; COFEPRIS) and with the Helsinki Declaration of 1975, as revised in 2000. All enrolled subjects provided written informed consent for treatment with the VizAblate System prior to hysterectomy.

Each subject underwent screening that included transvaginal sonography, endometrial biopsy, and a pregnancy test. Women were eligible for inclusion if they were 25 years of age or older, had previously agreed to undergo elective hysterectomy, and had between one and five fibroids ranging from 1 to 5 cm in diameter on a screening sonographic examination.

Procedure

There were two non-randomized subject cohorts: the acute group (subjects received hysterectomy immediately after closed abdomen use of the VizAblate System) and the subacute group (subjects underwent delayed hysterectomy on postablation days 16 and 17). On the procedure date, subjects in the acute group underwent epidural catheter placement for regional anesthesia as they were to undergo total abdominal hysterectomy immediately following transcervical radiofrequency ablation.

The women in the subacute group who were to undergo a delayed hysterectomy received conscious sedation (intravenous midazolam and fentanyl) with paracervical blockade (lidocaine) at the time of transcervical radiofrequency ablation. For both groups, a dispersive electrode pad was placed bilaterally on the anterior thighs with a thermocouple positioned at each leading edge for skin temperature monitoring. Intraoperative evaluation included transvaginal sonography to confirm the presence, location, and fibroid sizes present within the uterus.

After achieving cervical dilatation to 8 mm, the VizAblate articulating handpiece containing the IUUS probe was inserted transcervically into the subject's uterus. Several milliliters (generally 10–15 ml) of hypotonic fluid in the form of 1.5% glycine were infused through the device for acoustic coupling. Leiomyomata were then visualized and mapped in a systematic fashion within the uterus.

Throughout this study, the investigator was asked to treat fibroids in a manner consistent with his expected "real world" clinical use. That is, to ablate those fibroids having a reasonable probability of being symptomatic, while ensuring subject safety and attempting to ablate at least 50% of each fibroid's volume. In doing so, the investigator determined the best ablation size and location for each individual fibroid, and whether one or more ablations should be performed.

The treated fibroids each received from one to two volumetric ablations, ranging from 1 to 4 cm in width (in half-centimeter increments) using radiofrequency energy (maximum output 150 W) for 4–9 min at steady temperature of 105°C. As indicated, ablation dimensions are a function of both the needle electrode deployment width and treatment time.

All subjects were treated with the VizAblate System by a single surgeon. After treatment with VizAblate, the women underwent total abdominal hysterectomy either immediately (acute group) or just over 2 weeks later (subacute group). Following immediate or delayed hysterectomy, uteri were sectioned and stained for viability with TTC (Fig. 4) to quantify the fibroid ablation dimensions and the percentage of the fibroid volume that was ablated.

Procedure times were recorded for all subjects in the subacute group based on real-time videos of each procedure; these times were taken from the start of transvaginal sonography to the end of RF ablation with the VizAblate System. Procedure times for women in the acute group were not considered because of confounding ancillary measurements, image optimization procedures as part of the device development process at that time, and additional delays owing to the need for subsequent laparotomy in these subjects. Subjects in the subacute group were interviewed regarding pain during the VizAblate procedure and recovery using a 10-point numeric variable analog

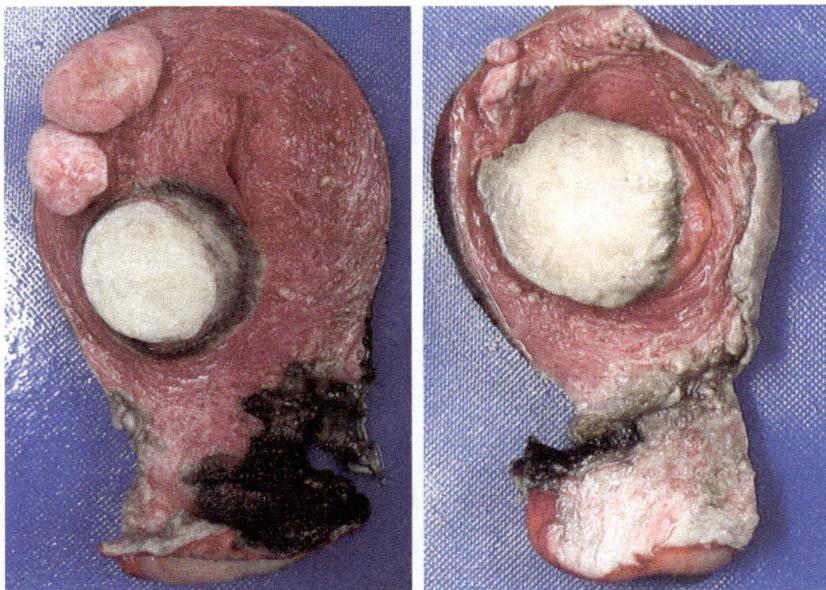

Fig. 4 TTC-stained hysterectomy specimen from a subject in the subacute group with two ablated intramural fibroids in the same uterus. The *pink* tissue represents viable, non-ablated tissue, whereas the *white region* indicates the ablation. The fibroid on the left is a 2.8×2.5×2.1-cm intramural leiomyoma in which 100% of the fibroid volume has been ablated. The fibroid on the *right* is a 4.1×3.7×3.8- cm intramural fibroid; 90% of the fibroid's volume was ablated. There is *black ink* on the anterior surface applied by the pathologist, seen here below the peritoneal reflection, indicating the anterior surface of the uterus to maintain the orientation during subsequent pathological analysis

scale (VAS) before discharge from the hospital after their VizAblate procedure and again when they returned for their hysterectomy; the latter interview covered the interval between the VizAblate procedure and the hysterectomy over 2 weeks later.

Findings

Acute group

A total of 13 subjects were enrolled and 12 were treated. One enrolled subject was not treated with the VizAblate system due to the presence of apparent adenomyosis upon sonography in the operating room, with uncertainty as to whether the visualized lesion represented a fibroid or an adenomyotic cyst. She underwent her scheduled hysterectomy where pathologic evaluation demonstrated adenomyosis and a small fibroid.

Of the 12 treated subjects, one was found on pathology examination to have had adenomyosis rather than a fibroid; the screening transvaginal ultrasound results were not suggestive of adenomyosis, even in retrospect. This subject was excluded from the ablation percentage results, as precise tissue boundaries for the region of adenomyosis were not obtainable. In all, a total of 13 individual lesions were treated, representing 12 fibroids and one region of adenomyosis. There were 14 ablations in total; one of the 12 fibroids received two ablations and one subject had two fibroids that each received single ablations.

The maximum treated fibroid dimensions, based on measurements from the hysterectomy specimens, ranged from 0.8 cm (0.3 cm^3) to 5.1 cm (69.5 cm^3) in diameter. All targeted fibroids contained volumetric ablations ranging from 1.9 cm (1.8 cm^3) to 4.0 cm (30.9 cm^3; dual overlapping ablations) in diameter, depending on the clinically selected ablation size. The needle electrode deployment sizes selected during the procedures ranged from 1 to 3.5 cm in width.

The mean percentage of ablated fibroid volume in the 11 treated fibroids≤5.0 cm in diameter was 62.3%±27.6% (range 15–100%; median 60%). In five of these 11 fibroids (45.5%), at least 75% of the fibroid volume was ablated. The mean percentage ablation in all 12 treated fibroids, irrespective of fibroid size, was 62.1%±26.3% (range 15–100%; median 60%).

With regard to serosal safety, no thermal injury to the uterine serosa was associated with any of the 13 fibroid ablations, either upon gross inspection at the time of hysterectomy or after pathologic examination. The maximum dispersive electrode pad temperature was 37.6°C. There were no complications and all subjects were discharged in good condition after hysterectomy.

Subacute group

Thirteen subjects were enrolled in the subacute group and seven were treated. A total of eight fibroids each received a single ablation with the clinically selected treatments ranging from 1.5 to 4.0 cm in width using radiofrequency energy (maximum output 150 W) for up to 9 min at a constant temperature of 105°C.

One enrolled subject withdrew early in order to pursue pharmacologic treatment, while another did not show up on the day of the procedure. Four additional subjects were not treated due to pathology detected on imaging findings in the operating room that were not amenable to treatment; one subject had imaging that was suggestive for adenomyosis; two subjects had purely subserosal myomata that could not be safely treated in a closed abdomen setting; one had a fibroid whose diameter measured considerably above the upper limit of 5.0 cm for inclusion within the study.

The maximum diameter of treated fibroids ranged from 1.6 to 7.4 cm (hysterectomy specimen measurements). Six of the eight fibroids were less than 5.0 cm in maximum diameter. All eight targeted fibroids contained volumetric ablations ranging from 2.5 cm^3 (1.7 cm diameter) to 36.2 cm^3 (4.1 cm diameter), depending on the clinically desired ablation size.

For all six treated fibroids≤5 cm in diameter, the mean percentage of the fibroid that was ablated was 76.3%±25.5% (range 40–100%; median 85%). In four of these six fibroids (66.7%), at least 75% of the fibroid volume was ablated. The mean percentage ablation in all eight treated fibroids, irrespective of fibroid size, was 62.9%±33.3% (range 20–100%; median 65%).

The mean procedure duration from the start of transvaginal sonography to the end of RF ablation was 25.8 min ±6.0 min (range 18–32 min) for the six procedures involving single fibroid ablations. The procedure time was 39 min for the one subject who had two separate fibroids ablated; each ablation involved 6 min of steady-state ablation at 105°C.

As with the acute group, none of the eight fibroid ablations had any evidence of serosal injury at laparotomy or at the time of pathologic evaluation. There were no immediate complications and all subjects were ambulatory and discharged in good condition within 2 h of the VizAblate procedure. The maximum dispersive electrode pad temperature was 36.5°C. Between the VizAblate procedure and hysterectomy 16–17 days later, there were no adverse events reported other than anticipated common side effects (cramping, spotting, and discharge). Six of seven (85.7%) subjects experienced a total of 13 instances of minor side effects such as spotting (four subjects), continuous bleeding for 6–10 days post-treatment (two subjects), clear discharge in three subjects and cramping in four subjects.

Procedure-associated pain levels (10-point VAS scale) averaged 0.9±1.1 (range 0–3) and were similar during immediate recovery and at discharge after the VizAblate procedure. Return to normal activity averaged 3.3±3.2 days (range 0.3–8 days), and the mean pain level from the time of the procedure to hysterectomy was 3.0±2.1 (range 0–5). Table 1 lists the results for the recovery questionnaire.

Pooled data

For the acute and subacute groups combined, a total of 26 subjects were enrolled. Twenty-two ablations were performed on 20 fibroids in 19 subjects.

Uterine weights ranged from 103 to 513 g. The treated fibroid diameters ranged from 0.8 to 7.4 cm and the ablation volume ranged from 1.8 to 36.2 ml, depending on desired ablation size

For the 17 treated fibroids≤5 cm in diameter that were treated in the acute and subacute substudies, the average pooled percentage of ablated fibroid volume was 67.2%± 27.0% (range 15–100%; median 75%). At least 75% of the fibroid volume was ablated in nine of these 17 fibroids (52.9%). The mean percentage of ablated fibroid volume in all 20 fibroids treated for both groups, regardless of size, was 62.4%±28.3% (range 15–100%; median 60%). Grouped as well as pooled ablation results may be found in Table 2.

Discussion

Since the 1990s, several new modalities to treat uterine fibroids have emerged, including uterine artery embolization and magnetic resonance-guided focused ultrasound (MRgFUS). Uterine artery embolization is effective treatment, with a 20–28.4% failure rate after 5 years [12, 13]. Nonetheless, it is not considered appropriate for women who desire future fecundity and has been associated with postembolization syndrome and premature ovarian failure [13–18]. MR-guided focused ultrasound, like radiofrequency ablation methods, ablates fibroids using energy to generate hyperthermic tissue temperatures. Based on the published MRgFUS and RFA literatures, hyperthermic ablation leads to tissue necrosis, reduction in fibroid volume, and symptomatic relief [7–10, 19, 20]. MRgFUS, however, is not widely available and requires up to 3 h per treatment.

Radiofrequency energy and sonography are familiar to most gynecologists. In the past, attempts to ablate fibroids with radiofrequency energy ("myolysis") were limited by the lack of concurrent imaging that necessitated multiple transserosal passes via laparoscopy or laparotomy in an attempt to effectively coagulate the myoma.

The VizAblate System uses a transcervical approach, in which fibroid ablation takes place under real-time visualization as an intrauterine sonography probe is built into the device. This built-in imaging removes the need for the physician to coordinate more than one device. The graphical interface delineates the boundaries of both ablation and thermal spread, enabling the gynecologist to avoid thermal injury to the serosa with its potential for adhesiogenesis and injury to bowel or bladder. Ablation volume is a function of time at temperature (105°C) and electrode deployment, so the gynecologist can choose the electrode deployment (which corresponds to a treatment time of 4, 6, or 9 min) that optimizes the fibroid ablation volume while maintaining safety.

As indicated, a single ablation with the VizAblate System can treat a fibroid up to 5 cm in diameter, although multiple ablations may be used to manage larger fibroids. For the 17 fibroids in this study that were no more than 5 cm in diameter, an average of 67.2%±27.0% of a targeted fibroid's volume was ablated (range 15–100%; median 75%). There was a large range in ablation percentage, but in most cases, a significant portion (up to 100%) of a targeted fibroid was successfully targeted and ablated. This percentage is under direct control of the gynecologist and depends on the placement of the treatment guides, and therefore the electrodes, within the target fibroid. Fibroids that lie closer to the endometrial cavity, namely submucous and many intramural fibroids, may be completely ablated through the use of the VizAblate System, depending on their size and location. Such fibroids are believed to be chiefly responsible for menorrhagia [21, 22]. For fibroids that lie close to the uterine serosa, the geometry may be such that the treating gynecologist will not necessarily

Table 1 Recovery questionnaire results for the subacute group

	Procedure pain[a]	Recovery pain[a]	Pain at discharge[a]	Return to normal activity (days)	Worst pain from procedure to hysterectomy[a]
Mean±SD	0.9±1.1	0.4±0.8	0.3±0.8	3.3±3.2	3.0±2.1
Maximum	3.0	2.0	2.0	8.0	5.0
Minimum	0.0	0.0	0.0	0.3	0.0

[a] 10-point scale

Table 2 Ablation results

Group	No. of treated subjects	No. of treated fibroids	No. of ablations	Fibroid diameter range	Mean percentage of fibroid ablation[a]
Acute	121	12	14[b]	0.8–5.1 cm	62.3%±27.6%; range 15–100% median 60%
Subacute	7	8	8[c]	1.6–7.4 cm	76.3%±25.5%; range 40–100% median 85%
Pooled	19	20	22	0.8–7.4 cm	67.2%±27.0%; range 15–100% median 75%

[a] For fibroids≤5.0 cm in maximum diameter

[b] Includes one fibroid that received two ablations, one subject with two fibroids that each received single ablations, and one ablation in pathology-confirmed adenomyosis

[c] One subject had two fibroids, each of which received a single ablation

ablate 100% of the fibroid's volume. This is dictated by the need to avoid thermal injury to the serosal surface, both to prevent adhesiogenesis as well as injury to adjacent viscera. The thermal safety border thus constrains the size and position of the fibroid ablation. However, it has been reported in the MRgFUS literature that it is not necessary to ablate 100% of a fibroid in order to provide fibroid volume reduction and durable symptomatic improvement [20, 23].

Previous to the work described in this report, the VizAblate System was safely used in 89 women who underwent fibroid ablation in an open abdomen setting. This permitted the bowel to be packed out of harm's way, and also enabled the recording of serosal temperatures during ablation through the use of thermocouples as well as an infrared camera. Unlike the previous work involving concurrent laparotomy, this current study examined the safety, tolerability, and procedure duration for the VizAblate System when used in a manner approaching real-world conditions in a closed abdomen setting. The initial cases (acute group) involved women who underwent hysterectomy immediately after fibroid ablation with the VizAblate System. This enabled assessment of the serosal surface, both intraoperatively and in the pathology laboratory, along with evaluation for any suspected thermal injury to adjacent bowel.

After demonstrating safety in the acute group, the VizAblate System was used in women who underwent a delayed hysterectomy (subacute group), 16–17 days post-ablation. These subjects also provided information relative to their recovery over the 2-week interval between the ablation and hysterectomy; such information would have been confounded by the performance of immediate hysterectomy in the acute group.

This study found no complications associated with closed abdomen use of the VizAblate System. In every subject, there was no evidence of thermal serosal injury at the time of hysterectomy or on pathologic examination of the extirpated uteri. No subject required readmission for any reason, nor did any subject need to return to the operating room. Not unexpectedly, some subjects experienced cramping, bleeding, and spotting over the 2 weeks following the procedure.

Pain scores in the subacute group following the procedure suggest that the VizAblate System may be successfully used with conscious sedation and paracervical blockade. Overall, the procedure was well tolerated, with minimal pain levels associated with fibroid ablation, and pain scores for the interval from the ablation procedure to hysterectomy averaging 3.0±2.1 (range 0–5) out of a maximum of 10.

All treatments for uterine fibroids have their relative advantages. The VizAblate System does not involve uterine distension; only 10–15 ml of hypotonic fluid are required for acoustic coupling, similar to the volumes required for saline infusion sonography. Furthermore, there is no need to increase intrauterine pressures above mean arterial pressure. The combination of imaging and treatment in one device does not require the gynecologist to coordinate a separate ultrasound probe with the treatment device. In addition, intrauterine sonography may provide a higher resolution view of the uterus than that of standard transvaginal ultrasound. The gynecologist can also readily select ablation sizes to match those of the symptomatic fibroids, providing flexibility in creating volumetric ablations. The graphical user interface delineates the boundaries of the expected ablation and indicates the margins of thermal spread for the selected ablation size; this permits the gynecologist to constrain the ablation to the fibroid and avoid thermal damage to the serosa and adjacent structures. Use of the transcervical route avoids the need for laparoscopy and suggests this treatment modality could be suitable for an office setting. Procedure times, generally 30 min or less, are somewhat less than what has been reported on average for hysteroscopic myomectomy using a resectoscope (42.2 min; CI 39.7–44.7 min) [24].

There are some limitations to this study. Subjects were not screened for preexisting pelvic pain nor were many potential etiologies of menorrhagia (such as anovulation) excluded prior to enrollment, so the observed presence of post-procedure cramping and spotting in the subacute group may overestimate the true minor side effect incidence associated with transcervical radiofrequency ablation of fibroids. This study also did not assess the efficacy of treatment with the VizAblate System with regard to menorrhagia symptoms. A forthcoming, 48-subject trial will examine the efficacy of transcervical, intrauterine ultrasound-guided fibroid ablation with the VizAblate System and accrue additional safety and tolerability data.

Conclusions

The VizAblate System was used to safely target and ablate fibroids in 19 treated women who underwent a total of 22 radiofrequency ablations in a closed abdomen setting. VizAblate was well tolerated when used with conscious sedation and paracervical blockade, supporting its potential future use in an office setting. Procedure times were on the order of 30 min or less. The coupling of intrauterine sonography with radiofrequency ablation in a single device enables imaging, precise fibroid targeting, and treatment in one minimally invasive procedure.

Declaration of interest Dr. Garza is a consultant for Gynesonics and has stock options. Dr. Coad is a consultant for Gynesonics. Drs. León and Saenz have no conflicts to disclose. The remaining authors are employees of Gynesonics and have stock options. The Universidad Autónoma de Nuevo León received remuneration for patient treatment and West Virginia University received compensation for pathologic analysis of hysterectomy specimens. The authors alone are responsible for the content and writing of the paper.

References

1. Day Baird D, Dunson DB, Hill MC et al (2003) High cumulative incidence of uterine leiomyoma in black and white women: ultrasound evidence. Am J Obstet Gynecol 188(1):100–107
2. Dembek CJ, Pelletier EM, Isaacson KB et al (2007) Payer costs in patients undergoing uterine artery embolization, hysterectomy, or myomectomy for treatment of uterine fibroids. J Vasc Interv Radiol 18(10):1207–1213
3. Manyonda I, Sinthamoney E, Belli AM (2004) Controversies and challenges in the modern management of uterine fibroids. BJOG 111(2):95–102
4. Goldfarb HA (1992) Avoiding hysterectomy: Nd:YAG laser and bipolar coagulating needle. Clin Laser Mon 10(12):191–193
5. Goldfarb HA (1995) Bipolar laparoscopic needles for myoma coagulation. J Am Assoc Gynecol Laparosc 2(2):175–179
6. Bergamini V, Ghezzi F, Cromi A et al (2005) Laparoscopic radiofrequency thermal ablation: a new approach to symptomatic uterine myomas. Am J Obstet Gynecol 192(3):768–773
7. Carrafiello G, Recaldini C, Fontana F et al (2009) Ultrasound-guided radiofrequency thermal ablation of uterine fibroids: medium-term follow-up. Cardiovasc Intervent Radiol 33(1):113–119. doi:10.1007/s00270-009-9707-3
8. Cho HH, Kim JH, Kim MR (2008) Transvaginal radiofrequency thermal ablation: a day-care approach to symptomatic uterine myomas. Aust N Z J Obstet Gynaecol 48(3):296–301
9. Ghezzi F, Cromi A, Bergamini V et al (2007) Midterm outcome of radiofrequency thermal ablation for symptomatic uterine myomas. Surg Endosc 21(11):2081–2085
10. Luo X, Shen Y, Song W et al (2007) Pathologic evaluation of uterine leiomyoma treated with radiofrequency ablation. Int J Gynecol Obstet 99(1):9–13
11. Iversen H, Lenz S (2008) Percutaneous ultrasound guided radio-frequency thermal ablation for uterine fibroids: a new gynecological approach. Ultrasound Obstet Gynecol 32(3):325
12. Kooij SM, Hehenkamp WJ, Volkers NA et al (2010) Uterine artery embolization vs hysterectomy in the treatment of symptomatic uterine fibroids: 5-year outcome from the randomized EMMY trial. Am J Obstet Gynecol 203(2):105.e1–105.e13
13. Spies JB, Bruno J, Czeyda-Pommersheim F et al (2005) Long-term outcome of uterine artery embolization of leiomyomata. Obstet Gynecol 106(5 Pt 1):933–939
14. Homer H, Saridogan E (2009) Uterine artery embolization for fibroids is associated with an increased risk of miscarriage. Fertil Steril 94(1):324–330
15. ACOG Committee Opinion (2004) Uterine artery embolization. Obstet Gynecol 103(2):403–404
16. Usadi RS, Marshburn PB (2007) The impact of uterine artery embolization on fertility and pregnancy outcome. Curr Opin Obstet Gynecol 19(3):279–283
17. Bradley LD (2009) Uterine fibroid embolization: a viable alternative to hysterectomy. Am J Obstet Gynecol 201(2):127–135
18. Katsumori T, Kasahara T, Tsuchida Y et al (2008) Amenorrhea and resumption of menstruation after uterine artery embolization for fibroids. Int J Gynaecol Obstet 103(3):217–221
19. Morita Y, Ito N, Hikida H et al (2007) Non-invasive magnetic resonance imaging-guided focused ultrasound treatment for uterine fibroids—early experience. Eur J Obstet Gynecol Reprod Biol 139(2):199–203
20. Stewart EA, Gostout B, Rabinovici J et al (2007) Sustained relief of leiomyoma symptoms by using focused ultrasound surgery. Obstet Gynecol 110(2 Pt 1):279–287
21. Clevenger-Hoeft M, Syrop CH, Stovall DW et al (1999) Sonohysterography in premenopausal women with and without abnormal bleeding. Obstet Gynecol 94(4):516–520
22. Sulaiman S, Khaund A, McMillan N et al (2004) Uterine fibroids —do size and location determine menstrual blood loss? Eur J Obstet Gynecol Reprod Biol 115(1):85–89
23. Funaki K, Fukunishi H, Sawada K (2009) Clinical outcomes of magnetic resonance-guided focused ultrasound surgery for uterine myomas: 24-month follow-up. Ultrasound Obstet Gynecol 34 (5):584–589
24. Emanuel MH, Wamsteker K (2005) The intra uterine morcellator: a new hysteroscopic operating technique to remove intrauterine polyps and myomas. J Minim Invasive Gynecol 12(1):62–66

26

The hysteroscopic view of infertility: the mid-secretory endometrium and treatment success towards pregnancy

A. Santi · R. Felser · N. A. Bersinger · D. M. Wunder ·
B. McKinnon · M. D. Mueller

Abstract The purpose of this study was the analysis of a correlation, in infertile patients, between the quality of the endometrium based on its vascularisation and the chances of conception. Hysteroscopy was carried out to determine the quality of the endometrial surface using the Sakumoto–Masamoto classification ("good" vs. "poor" endometrium) in the secretory phase of the menstrual cycle. The results were set in relation to the outcome of the subsequent infertility treatment, i.e. the establishment of a pregnancy within the study period (4 years). In 108 (67%) of the 162 followed-up patients, the endometrium was endoscopically classified as "good", while in 54 (33%) the result was "poor". The overall pregnancy rate was 37% (60 patients); 47 of all pregnancies (78%) occurred in women with a "good" endometrium while 13 (22%) had a "poor" classification. This positive association between the establishment of a pregnancy in the follow-up and a "good" classification of the endometrial vasculature in the group with a "good" endometrium was significant ($P=0.0165$, Fisher's exact test). This study confirms the usefulness of endometrial evaluation by hysteroscopy as a diagnostic instrument for providing a prognosis of the chance for the patients to become pregnant.

Keywords Endometrium · Embryo implantation · Infertility · Hysteroscopy

A. Santi · R. Felser · N. A. Bersinger (✉) · D. M. Wunder ·
M. D. Mueller
Department of Obstetrics and Gynaecology, Inselspital,
University of Berne,
DKF Murtenstrasse 35,
Berne CH-3010, Switzerland
e-mail: nick.bersinger@dkf.unibe.ch

B. McKinnon
Department of Clinical Research, University of Berne,
Berne, Switzerland

D. M. Wunder
Department of Obstetrics and Gynaecology, Centre Hospitalier
Universitaire Vaudois, University of Lausanne,
Lausanne, Switzerland

Background

One of the most difficult questions put forward by patients after the failure of a fertility therapy such as in vitro fertilisation (IVF) and intra-cytoplasmic sperm injection (ICSI) is related to the lack of success. The implantation rate per transferred embryo normally does not exceed 30%. Often the failure of "embryo implantation" is given as an explanation as the failure in one of the most critical stages at the beginning of conception, i.e. when apposition and implantation has to occur inside the uterine cavity. Current knowledge about the mechanism of these interactions is still difficult to interpret [1].

Various different suggestions have been made for investigating these mechanisms and attempting to understand which would be the characteristic elements of the endometrium that ensure ideal conditions for the embryo; but they have until today been limited to the so-called theory of the endometrial "opportunity window" [2] and did not offer effective clinical instruments for understanding which groups of patients would be at an increased risk of embryo implantation failure [3]. By using hysteroscopy as a diagnostic procedure for the assessment of pathologies inside the uterine cavity, it has, however, been shown that the differential characterisation of the endometrial surface could be a helpful tool for evaluating the in vivo vascularisation of the uterine mucosa. Already, Sakumoto et al. in 1992 in the first place [4], and after him Masamoto

Fig. 1 Endoscopic examination of the endometrial surface and scoring. **a** "Masamoto good": ring-type glandular openings and well-developed vascular networks are visible. **b** "Masamoto poor": glandular openings are punctate typed, and the visible vasculature is sparse

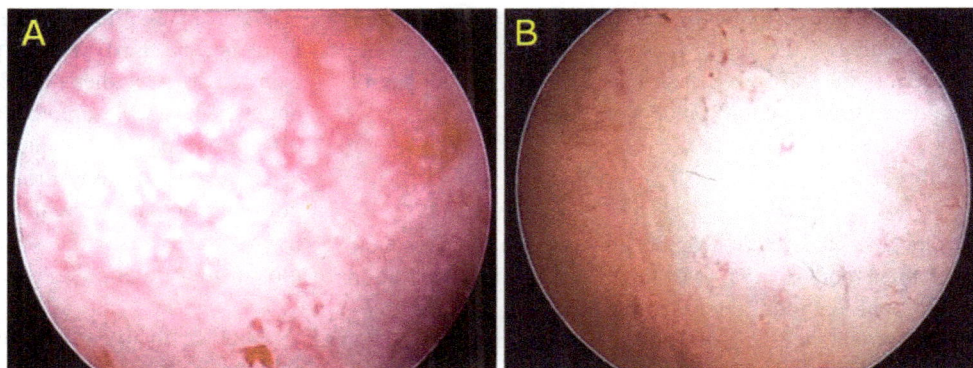

et al. in 2000 [5], have described the technique and used this differentiation in order to demonstrate that the endometrium could be classified into two distinct groups: a "good" endometrium, which has circular gland openings and an intense vascular ramification on one hand, and a "poor" endometrium, which is characterised by a surface with a lower gland and vascular density on the other.

The purpose of this study was to demonstrate the impact of the hysteroscopy, according to this vascularisation-based staging, and to investigate whether this endometrium quality could be used as a tool to assess the potential to achieve a pregnancy irrespective of the chosen type of infertility treatment.

Materials and methods

All infertile patients attending our fertility centre and with a regular menstrual cycle were asked to participate in this comparative, prospective study. They underwent a pre-operative transvaginal sonography (TVS), a full hormonal assessment (FSH, LH, 17β-estradiol, thyroid-stimulating hormone and prolactin) in the serum on cycle days 3 to 5 and then a hysteroscopy in the second part of the menstrual cycle for evaluating the vascularisation of the endometrium. Informed, written consent was obtained from the patients after explanation of the study by the clinician prior to the procedure, and they were asked to avoid a pregnancy in the examination cycle. The study protocol was approved by the local ethical committee.

The inclusion criteria were infertility (absence of conception after 12 months of regular, unprotected intercourse), age less than 43 years, regular cycles (25–31 days) and normal hormonal values (including FSH <12 mU/mL)

had to be fulfilled. All partners provided a spermiogram for the exclusion of male factor infertility. Further exclusion criteria were known causes of uterine malformations, endometrial adhesions and hormonal therapy such as oral contraceptives or other oestrogen–progesterone medications within the last 3 months before hysteroscopy. If necessary, the procedure was combined with a laparoscopy to test the tubal patency, and the hysteroscopy was done in most cases during the same operating session and under general anaesthesia. The ultrasonographers were located in the same university department, but not involved in the surgical procedure, and the surgeon was blinded to the TVS findings.

The endometrial surface was evaluated according to the Sakumoto–Masamoto grading ("good" vs. "poor"). Endoscopic findings were categorised as "good" with an appearance representing ring-type glandular openings and maximal glandular secretion or "poor" with a low development level of vessel networks on the endometrial surface. This is illustrated in Fig.1. Hysteroscopic procedures were carried out when indicated (e.g. polyps, myomas, adhesions, septa). The diagnostic hysteroscopy was performed with a 5-mm-outer diameter scope (30°, Karl Storz) connected to a standard endoscopic camera, and a saline solution at low pressure (not higher than 60 mmHg) was used for the distension of the uterine cavity. Hysteroscopic findings were observed and analysed by three gynaecologists using videotape records.

The follow-up interval lasted for 12 months from hysteroscopy. Data were recorded and analysed for a correlation between the vascularisation score of the endometrium and the occurrence of embryo implantation (spontaneous pregnancy, successful outcome after hormonal stimulation with or without intrauterine insemination or

Table 1 A 2×2 contingency table for endometrium evaluation and pregnancy outcome

Outcome	Endometrium "good"	Endometrium "poor"	Total
Pregnant	47	13	60
Not pregnant	61	41	102
Total	108	54	162

$P=0.0165$ by Fisher's exact test

successful IVF/ICSI-embryo transfer treatment). For statistical evaluation, the Fisher's exact test was applied using GraphPad Prism Software (San Diego, USA). For alpha, we considered 0.05 as cutoff value to avoid type I error.

Findings

A total of 178 infertile women underwent a hysteroscopic assessment, and 162 (91%) of them could be followed up in our hospital. A "good" endometrium according to Sakumoto–Masamoto staging was diagnosed in 108 of them (67%), while 54 (33%) patients were graded as "poor". No differences in the distribution pattern of the causes and duration of infertility, the age of the patients (mean 33.8 years in the "good" and 33.6 in the "poor" group) or the pre-treatment day 3 serum level of follicle-stimulating hormone (6.8 and 7.4 U/L) were observed between these two groups.

A normal uterine cavity was reported in 133 (83%) women, while endometrial polyps, submucosal fibroids, adhesions or uterine malformations were found in 29 cases (17%). On the other hand, the pre-operative TVS indicated intrauterine pathologies in 15 cases (9.3%). The overall pregnancy rate was 37% (60 women); 15 women became pregnant spontaneously, 22 patients succeeded after follicular stimulation with recombinant gonadotropins (rFSH) and 23 after treatment with in vitro fertilisation and embryo transfer including ICSI.

In the total pregnancy group ($N=60$), a "good" endometrium was found in 47 women (78%) while this was the case in 61 patients (60%) of the group who did not achieve a pregnancy. Forty-one patients with a "poor" endometrium did not succeed in getting pregnant. Only 13 patients with a "poor" endometrium did succeed in establishing pregnancy in the follow-up. The association between endometrium quality by Sakumoto–Masamoto classification and pregnancy outcome was statistically significant ($P=0.0165$, OR$=2.43$, CI$=1.17$–5.05); the contingency matrix for the pregnancy outcome is shown in Table 1.

Conclusion

Our results confirm those of the studies carried out by Sakumoto and Masamoto [4, 5], indicating that a hysteroscopic examination of the mid-secretory endometrium can be a reliable instrument for determining the chances of a patient to become pregnant. The classification in "good" and "poor" is leading to the conclusion that a poorly vascularised endometrium with limited glandular (secretory) structures may result in a tissue which is not suitable for a correct embryo implantation and endometrial development, and this irrespective of other factors of sterility.

Nevertheless, our results showed a lower fraction of patients (one third) with a "poor" endometrium in comparison to earlier studies (45.9% in the study of Sakumoto [4] and 61.3% in Masamoto et al. [5]): we believe that this difference can be explained with a different patient selection in the study groups. As a matter of fact, we did not focus on patients with a history of repeated abortions as it was the case in the study of Masamoto [5], but on a global infertile population.

Another clearly interesting but only partially surprising finding is the high percentage (17.2%) of intrauterine pathologies that have been diagnosed in the hysteroscopic examination when compared to the total number of patients with suspected intracavitary problems found in the pre-operative sonography (9.3% of all women, and this in spite of all ultrasound examinations having been carried out by the same team of experienced gynaecologists). These results, nevertheless, are in large agreement with previously published studies [6, 7].

We therefore conclude that a hysteroscopic examination, particularly in cases of idiopathic infertility or after several unsuccessful treatment cycles with in vitro fertilisation [8], is strongly indicated [9] and has the added benefit of providing a prognostic measure for determining the chances of the patient to become pregnant, in the future, in addition to its diagnostic significance [10].

Declaration of interest The authors report no conflicts of interest. The authors alone are responsible for the content and writing of the paper.

References

1. Cakmak H, Taylor HS (2010) Implantation failure: molecular mechanisms and clinical treatment. Hum Reprod Update 17:252–253
2. Tabibzadeh S (1999) Molecular control of the implantation window. Hum Reprod Update 5:373–385
3. Diedrich K, Fauser BC, Devroey P, Griesinger G (2010) The role of the endometrium and embryo in human implantation. Hum Reprod Update 13:365–377
4. Sakumoto T, Sakumoto T, Inafuku K, Miyara M, Takamiyagi N, Miyake A, Shinkawa T, Nakayama M (1992) Hysteroscopic assessment of midsecretory-phase endometrium, with special reference to the luteal-phase defect. Horm Res 37:48–52
5. Masamoto H, Nakama K, Kanazawa K (2000) Hysteroscopic appearance of the mid-secretory endometrium: relationship to early phase pregnancy outcome after implantation. Hum Reprod 15:2112–2118
6. Grimbizis GF, Tsolakidis D, Mikos T, Anagnostou E, Asimakopoulos E, Stamatopoulos P, Tarlatzis BC (2010) A prospective comparison of transvaginal ultrasound, saline infusion sonohysterography, and diagnostic hysteroscopy in the evaluation of endometrial pathology. Fertil Steril 94:2720–2725

7. Kelecsi S, Kelekci S, Kaya E, Alan M, Alan Y, Bilge U, Mollamahmutoglu L (2005) Comparison of transvaginal sonography, saline infusion sonography, and office hysteroscopy in reproductive-aged women with or without abnormal uterine bleeding. Fertil Steril 84:682–686

8. Bozdag G, Aksan G, Esinler I, Yarali H (2008) What is the role of office hysteroscopy in women with failed IVF cycles? Reprod Biomed Online 17:410–415

9. Lorusso F, Ceci O, Bettocchi S, Lamanna G, Costantino A, Serrati G, Depalo R (2008) Office hysteroscopy in an in vitro fertilization program. Gynecol Endocrinol 24:465–469

10. Makrakis E, Makrakis E, Hassiakos D, Stathis D, Vaxevanoglou T, Orfanoudaki E, Pantos K (2009) Hysteroscopy in women with implantation failures after in vitro fertilization: findings and effect on subsequent pregnancy rates. J Minim Invasive Gynecol 16:181–187

27

Nomegestrol acetate versus combined oral contraceptive as rapid endometrial preparation for operative hysteroscopy

Liliana Mereu · Giuliana Giunta · Giada Carri ·
Claudia Prasciolu · Edmundo Daniel Albis Florez ·
Luca Mencaglia

Keywords Hysteroscopy · Nomegestrol
acetate · Endometrial preparation · Ethinyl estradiol and
gestodene oral contraceptive

Introduction

Hysteroscopy is now the established "gold standard" for the assessment and treatment of intrauterine pathology such as fibroids, polyps, synechiae, septa and endometrial resection and/or destruction, and is regarded as a safe, acceptable and well-tolerated procedure [1–5]. In fertile women, hysteroscopic

L. Mereu (✉) · G. Giunta · G. Carri · C. Prasciolu ·
E. D. Albis Florez · L. Mencaglia
Division of Gynaecology, Centro Oncologico Fiorentino,
Sesto Fiorentino, Italy
e-mail: liliana.mereu@lacittadellasalute.it

G. Giunta
Department of Maternal Infant and Radiological Sciences,
University Hospital G. Rodolico,
Catania, Italy

G. Carri
Department of Obstetrics and Gynaecology,
Catholic University of Sacred Heart,
Rome, Italy

C. Prasciolu
Division of Gynaecology, Obstetrics and Pathophysiology
of Human Reproduction, University of Cagliari,
Cagliari, Italy

E. D. Albis Florez
Department of Obstetrics and Gynaecology, University El Bosque,
Bogotà, Colombia

procedures are best performed when the endometrium is thin because the operating time is lessened and fluid absorption decreases, making surgery easier [6–9]. For these reasons, the days immediately after menstruation are the best period for hysteroscopy. Scheduling surgery during the early follicular phase is not always possible, so several drugs have been proposed to reduce endometrial thickness, intra-operative bleeding, surgical difficulties and duration of surgery [6, 10, 11]. Even if preoperative treatment with gonadotropin-releasing hormone analogues (GnRH-a) or danazol for 2 or 3 months has been recommended to remove large intramural sub-mucous myomas or perform endometrial resection [9], they are not as often used for procedure preparation especially in case of minor hysteroscopy. GnRH-a result in a state of temporary menopause and are expensive, while danazol induces unfavourable side effects including weight gain, growth of hair, acne and general malaise [12]. Several studies have reported that gestrinone also is capable of reducing uterine volume, menorrhagia and endometrial thickness [13–15].

A limiting factor existing among the previous treatments is the long time required to reduce the endometrium. Recently, to speed up endometrial preparation, other original treatments have been proposed as oral progestins and vaginal raloxifen [16], nomegestrol acetate [17] and oral contraceptives [18], and they obtained good results in terms of preparation of the endometrium, cost and acceptability. Shortening the preparation time before surgery may improve patient compliance and work organization [19].

The aim of this prospective, randomised study was to compare the effectiveness of nomegestrol acetate versus combined oral contraceptive treatments as short preoperative endometrial preparation before hysteroscopic surgery.

Materials and methods

Between February and July 2011, 42 pre-menopausal women were prospectively enrolled in the study. The inclusion criteria were: hysteroscopic diagnosis of endocavitary pathologies and regular menstrual cycle rhythms for the previous 6 months. Exclusion criteria were: age <18 and >45, hormonal therapies in the previous 12 weeks, previous uterine surgery, concomitant adnexal pathologies, endometriosis and cardio-vascular, hepatic or renal impairment.

The study protocol was conformed to the ethical guidelines of the 1975 Helsinki Declaration, and the Institutional Review Board of the department approved it. Written informed consent was obtained from each female patient upon enrolment.

Before treatment (day 14 of the menstrual cycle), each woman received a trans-vaginal ultrasound (TVUS) evaluation to measure endometrial thickness, ovarian size and number of ovarian follicles. On day 1 of the menstrual cycle, patients were randomised to receive 3 weeks of therapy with 5 mg of nomegestrol acetate daily (group A, $n=21$) or 20 µg of ethinyl estradiol/75 mg gestodene daily (group B, $n=21$). Allocation to one of the two parallel treatment groups (21 in each) was performed using the SPSS v 17.0 randomisation program (SPSS Inc., Chicago, IL). Both surgeons were not aware of the therapy at the time of surgery.

Surgery was performed the day after the last assumption of hormonal medicament. Patients were hospitalized the same day of surgery. Preoperative exams as TVUS, ECG and routine blood test were performed in the early morning, and side effects experienced by the patients during treatment were recorded. The effectiveness of the therapy was intraoperatively evaluated by assessing the visibility of the uterine cavity, the endometrial features, the difficulty of the procedure and the success of surgery. Hormonal effects of the studied drugs are evaluated by assessing endometrial thickness and number and size of ovarian follicles.

Operative hysteroscopy was performed under general anaesthesia by two expert endoscopic surgeons (L.M. and L.M.), using a bipolar resectoscope. More specifically, after the tenaculum was placed and the cervix dilated to Hegar 8, the procedure used a 22-Fr continuous-flow resectoscope fitted with a cutting loop electrode at a power setting of 120-W cutting current. A sterile saline solution was used for uterine distension.

To evaluate the visibility, we assigned a score from 0 to 1 for each of the five following parameters: left ostium, right ostium, fundus, anterior wall and posterior wall. A score from 0 to 2 was classified as "bad visibility", a score of 3 was classified as "moderate visibility" and a score from 4 to 5 was rated as "good visibility".

The endometrial features assessed by direct vision during hysteroscopic procedure were classified according to Baggish and Barbott as: "atrophic" when the endometrium was thin,

Table 1 Patients' main characteristics

	Group A ($n=21$), NOMAC	Group B ($n=21$), EE/GSD	P value
Age (median, SD; years)	35±6	37±7	0.35
BMI (median, SD; kg/m^2)	22±2	21±3	0.22
Parity (median, range; number)	1 (0–2)	1 (0–2)	0.8

NOMAC 5 mg nomegestrol acetate, *EE/GSD* 20 µg ethinyl estradiol/75 mg gestodene, *BMI* body mass index

regular and pale; "normal" when the endometrial appearance was compatible with the proliferative phase; "normal with small hyperplastic areas" when only small focused areas of thickness were present and "hyperplastic" when a diffuse thick polypoid endometrium was found [6].

The difficulty of the procedure and the success of surgery were evaluated by the surgeon marking two separated 100-mm visual analogue scale from 0 (minimum) to 100 (maximum). One month after surgery, women underwent a diagnostic hysteroscopy to confirm the completeness of the treatment.

Statistical analysis was performed with SPSS 11 (SPSS, Chicago, IL). Data were expressed as mean±SD (range) or as number (percent) of cases. To compare data between the two groups, a Student's t test was used for parametric data and the Mann–Whitney test for non-parametric data. Dichotomous variables were analysed with the χ^2 test and the Fischer exact test, when appropriate. A P value of <0.05 was considered statistically significant.

Results

Between February to July 2011, we identified 42 pre-menopausal women who were consecutively enrolled in

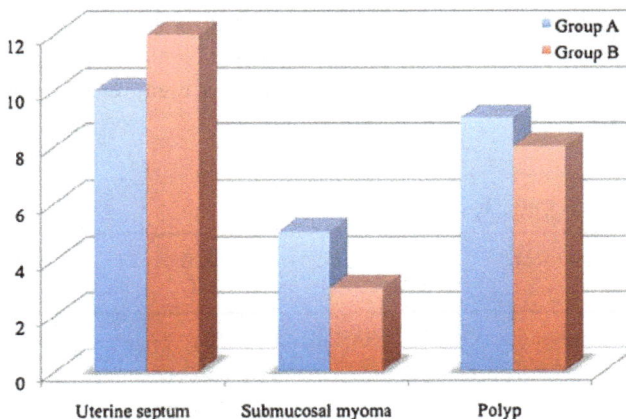

Fig. 1 Prevalence of endocavitary pathologies. NOMAC: 5 mg nomegestrol acetate; EE/EGST: 20 µg ethinyl estradiol/75 mg gestodene

Table 2 Endometrial and follicle pattern before and after treatment

	Group A, NOMAC	Group B, EE/GSD	P value (inter-group)
Endometrial thikness before treatment (median, SD; mm)	7.2±1.2	6.9±0.9	0.08
Endometrial thikness after treatment	4.6±2.0	3.9±0.2	0.001
P value (intra group)	.001	.0001	
Mean diameter of dominant follicle before treatment (median, SD; mm)	14.8±0.4	15.0±0.4	0.07
Mean diameter of dominant follicle after treatment (median, SD; mm)	9.5±1.0	6.4±0.9	0.0001
P value (intra group)	0.0001	0.0001	

NOMAC 5 mg nomegestrol acetate, *EE/GSD* 20 μg ethinyl estradiol/75 mg gestodene

the study. The two study groups were similar for age, parity and body mass index (BMI) (Table 1), as well as for prevalence of uterine endocavitary pathologies (Fig. 1). No differences were retrieved at enrolment between groups in terms of endometrial thickness (group A, 7.2±1.2 mm; group B, 6.9±0.9 mm; $P=0.08$) and mean follicular diameter ($P=0.07$) (Table 2).

The reduction in endometrial thickness in group B (EE/GSD) was statistically significantly greater than in group A (NOMAC) ($P<0.001$) as well as the ovarian dominant follicle mean diameter ($P<0.0001$) (Table 2).

An assessment of the endometrium during surgery showed that all patients responded to the treatment with a significant difference between groups. Surgeon satisfaction in terms of endometrial preparation was higher for women of group B compared with group A (83.4 % "good visibility" group B vs 57.5 % group A) (Table 3). At hysteroscopy, the endometrial mucosa appeared to be very thin, hypotrophic, regular and pale in all of the women of the two groups. However, we observed some cases of "hyperplastic endometrial features" in group A; the endometrial surface was high and irregular, with areas of stromal oedema and glandular development (Fig. 2).

Difficulty to perform hysteroscopic surgery was greater in group A, mean 5 (range 3–9), than with group B, mean 2 (range 0–6), $P<0.001$. No significant differences emerged in relation to time taken for cervical dilatation, operating time, postoperative complications and completeness of surgery.

Table 3 Visibility score

Visibility score	Group A (n=21), NOMAC	Group B (n=21), EE/GSD	P value
Bad visibility	3 (14 %)	0 (0 %)	0.06
Moderate visibility	6 (28 %)	3 (14 %)	0.08
Good visibility	12 (58 %)	18 (86 %)	0.002

NOMAC 5 μg nomegestrol acetate, *EE/GSD* 20μg ethinyl estradiol/75 mg gestodene

Discussion

The success of hysteroscopic surgery is related to good and constant visibility during the procedure, bearing in mind that the surgical field is extremely limited and very often narrowed by endometrial thickness and by the endouterine pathology itself [20]. With a prepared endometrium, the uterine cavity became easier to explore, and endocavitary pathologies are easy to detect and treat. A preoperative pharmacological treatment for endometrial mucosa thinning is recommended to achieve the best conditions of visibility [21, 22]. The efficacy of GnRH agonists and danazol administration for thinning the endometrium before hysteroscopic surgery has been reported by several investigators [9, 12]. However, they are expensive drugs with many side effects, and they require a long time to thin the endometrium.

Oral contraceptives and progestogens have been also proposed as a rapid treatment before hysteroscopic surgery, but only few randomised data are available to assess their effectiveness as endometrial thinning agents [15–18].

Shortening the preparation time before surgery may increase patients' compliance and improve work organization. The results of this study demonstrate that a short treatment

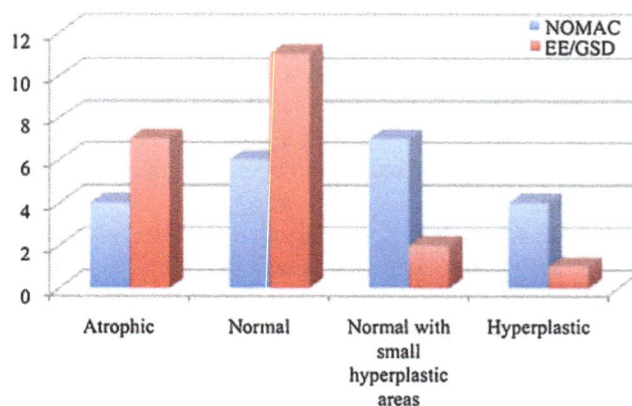

Fig. 2 Endometrial features during hysterosocopy. *NOMAC* 5 mg nomegestrol acetate, *EE/EGST* 20 μg ethinyl estradiol/75 mg gestodene

with both 5 mg of nomegestrol acetate and 20 µg of ethinyl estradiol/75 mg gestodene before operative hysteroscopy provides a very fast and effective endometrial suppression.

According to TVUS evaluation, the endometrial features under direct hysteroscopic exploration of the cavity demonstrated that endometrial preparation was better in group B than in group A. Indeed, all group B women had very thin, pale and regular endometrium. In contrast, in group A in some cases, the endometrial surface was high and irregular, with areas of stromal oedema and glandular development probably related to the progestin-induced decidualization. Accordingly, surgeon satisfaction was significantly greater for group B. Side effects, owing to the short period over which the two drugs were administered, were infrequent in both treatments, without significant differences between the two groups. Limitations of this trial were the limited number of cases and the presupposition that no variation occurs in endometrial features in the natural menstrual cycle; nevertheless, it is unlikely that the natural variations could significantly affect the study results.

Conclusions

In conclusion, our data suggest that both treatments, used for a brief period, are good ways to prepare the endometrium before hysteroscopic surgery. Satisfactory endometrial preparation can be obtained with only 3 weeks of treatment, and this improves acceptability and scheduling for hysteroscopic treatment. However, the endometrial preparation with 5 mg nomegestrol acetate appears to be less comfortable for the surgeon in terms of visibility of the uterine cavity than 20 µg ethinyl estradiol/75 mg gestodene endometrial preparation. No differences in completeness of surgery, operative time and intraoperative complications were noticed.

Conflict of interest The authors report no conflicts of interest. The authors alone are responsible for the content and writing of the paper.

References

1. Gimpelson RJ, Whalen TR (1995) Hysteroscopy as gold standard for evaluation of abnormal uterine bleeding. Am J Obstet Gynecol 173:1637–1638
2. Sutton C (2006) Hysteroscopic surgery. Best Pract Res Clin Obstet Gynaecol 20:105–137
3. Bosteels J, Weyers S, Puttemans P, Panayotidis C, Van Herendael B, Gomel V, Mol BW, Mathieu C, D'Hooghe T (2010) The effectiveness of hysteroscopy in improving pregnancy rates in subfertile women without other gynaecological symptoms: a systematic review. Hum Reprod Update 16:1–11
4. Di Spiezio SA, Mazzon I, Bramante S, Bettocchi S, Bifulco G, Guida M, Nappi C (2008) Hysteroscopic myomectomy: a comprehensive review of surgical techniques. Hum Reprod Update 14:101–119
5. Goldstein SR (2009) The role of transvaginal ultrasound or endometrial biopsy in the evaluation of the menopausal endometrium. Am J Obstet Gynecol 201:5–11
6. Rai VS, Gillmer MD, Gray W (2000) Is endometrial pre-treatment of value in improving the outcome of transcervical resection of the endometrium? Hum Reprod 15:1989–1992
7. Römer T, Schmidt T, Foth D (2000) Pre- and postoperative hormonal treatment in patients with hysteroscopic surgery. Contrib Gynecol Obstet 20:1–12
8. Brooks PG, Serden SP, Davos I (1991) Hormonal inhibition of the endometrium for resectoscopic endometrial ablation. Am J Obstet Gynecol 164:1601–1606
9. Parazzini F, Vercellini P, De Giorgi O, Pesole A, Ricci E, Crosignani PG (1998) Efficacy of preoperative medical treatment in facilitating hysteroscopic endometrial resection, myomectomy and metroplasty: literature review. Hum Reprod 13:2592–2597
10. Vercellini P, Perino A, Consonni R, Trespidi L, Parazzini F, Crosignani PG (1996) Treatment with a gonadotrophin releasing hormone agonist before endometrial resection: a multicentre, randomised controlled trial. Br J Obstet Gynaecol 103:562–568
11. Donnez J, Vilos G, Gannon MJ, Stampe-Sorensen S, Klinte I, Miller RM (1997) Goserelin acetate (Zoladex) plus endometrial ablation for dysfunctional uterine bleeding: a large randomized, double-blind study. Fertil Steril 68:29–36
12. Sowter MC, Lethaby A, Singla AA (2002) Pre-operative endometrial thinning agents before endometrial destruction for heavy menstrual bleeding. Cochrane Database Syst 3:CD001124
13. Fedele L, Bianchi S, Gruft L, Bigatti G, Busacca M (1996) Danazol versus a gonadotropin-releasing hormone agonist as preoperative preparation for hysteroscopic metroplasty. Fertil Steril 65:186–188
14. Marchini M, Fedele L, Bianchi S, Di Nola G, Nava S, Vercellini P (1992) Endometrial patterns during therapy with danazol or gestrinone for endometriosis: structural and ultrastructural study. Hum Pathol 23:51–56
15. Triolo O, De Vivo A, Benedetto V, Falcone S, Antico F (2006) Gestrinone versus danazol as preoperative treatment for hysteroscopic surgery: a prospective, randomized evaluation. Fertil Steril 85:1027–1031
16. Cicinelli E, Pinto V, Tinelli R, Saliani N, De Leo V, Cianci A (2007) Rapid endometrial preparation for hysteroscopic surgery with oral desogestrel plus vaginal raloxifene: a prospective, randomized pilot study. Fertil Steril 88:698–701
17. Florio P, Imperatore A, Litta P, Franchini M, Calzolari S, Angioni S, Gabbanini M, Bruni L, Petraglia F (2010) The use of nomegestrol acetate in rapid preparation of endometrium before operative hysteroscopy in pre-menopausal women. Steroids 12:912–917
18. Grow DR, Iromloo K (2006) Oral contraceptives maintain a very thin endometrium before operative hysteroscopy. Fertil Steril 85:204–207
19. Heinonen PK, Helin R (2009) Endometrial resection following levonorgestrel intrauterine system treatment for menorrhagia. Gynecol Surgery 9:245–249
20. Panayotidis C, Weyers S, Bosteels J, Van Herendael B (2009) Intrauterine adhesions (IUA): has there been progress in understanding and treatment over the last 20 years? Gynecol Surgery 6:197–211
21. Lewis BV (1994) Guidelines for endometrial ablation. British Society of Gynaecological Endoscopy. Br J Obstet Gynaecol 101:470–473
22. Nicolaou D, Salman G, Richardson R (2009) Operative hysteroscopy in the outpatient setting: its role within a gynaecology service. Gynecol Surgery 6:21–24

28

The efficacy of hysteroscopy in diagnosis and treatment of endometrial pathology

Andreia Alexandra Rocha Antunes

Abstract Hysteroscopy has become the first choice approach for patients with suspicion for intrauterine lesions. The one-stop approach in which diagnosis and hysteroscopic treatment is performed in one session has been described as being highly appreciated by the patient, has a low risk profile, and is a cost-efficient approach. This study addresses the value of hysteroscopy on diagnostic accuracy and its effectiveness to the one-stop therapeutic approach. This is a prospective study of patients admitted in the ambulatory surgery unit of the Sto. André–Leiria Hospital (Portugal) from February 2005 to February 2008 for a one-stop diagnostic and therapeutic approach. Patient selection was done on transvaginal ultrasound findings or on clinical pathology. Depending on the transvaginal ultrasound report and the clinical data, the instrumentation and analgesia for the one-stop approach was defined. The average age was 54 years (range24–87 years). The majority of patients (96.2%) presented with a transvaginal ultrasonographic lesion. The hysteroscopic evaluation characterized the hysteroscopic findings in two groups: the "uterine cavity lesions" (endometrial and cervical polyps, myomas, malignant smooth muscle tumor, placenta or first trimester debris, bone, adhesions or septum, lost IUD, or no lesion) and "the endometrial characterization" (which include functional atrophic or thin endometrium, dysfunctional, endometritis, cystic atrophy, hyperplasia, polypoid, and carcinoma). We concluded that the ambulatory performance of direct visualization of uterine cavity by hysteroscopy guarantees a high diagnostic accuracy, allowing the simultaneous accomplishment of biopsies and surgical treatment of the visualized lesions.

Keywords Hysteroscopy · Histology · Endometrial pathology · Uterine lesions

Background

Since the beginning we felt that the certification of each exam should be a priority, so we decided to biopsy every endometrium and every lesion, to compare the diagnostic accuracy of hysteroscopy with the pathologic exam. To prove the efficacy of this technique, we decided to include in this prospective study only the procedures where hysteroscopy diagnosis and treatment were performed in one single session. Diagnostic accuracy and effectiveness of hysteroscopy were evaluated.

Subjects and methods

A prospective study was carried out at the day surgery unit of the gynecology department from Santo André Hospital, which is a public care unit in Leiria (Portugal), from February 2005 to February 2008. All patients referred with either abnormal ultrasound findings, abnormal uterine bleeding, infertility, abnormal cells in cervix cytology, or cervical polyps were admitted to the one-stop procedure in the outpatient department after informed consent of the patient. Hysteroscopic examination and hysteroscopic surgery or biopsies were performed to every patient, and pathological investigations were carried out. Postmenopausal patients were given 400 mg transvaginal mysoprostol the night before hysteroscopy.

Hysteroscopy was performed using either rigid panoramic type 30° telescopes of 2 and 3 mm with continuous irrigation sheath with five French working channels or the

A. A. R. Antunes (✉)
Hospital de Santo André, S.A,
Rua das Olhalvas–Pousos,
2410-197 Leiria, Portugal
e-mail: Andreia.antunes@sapo.pt

4-mm forward 0° and 30° lenses (Karl Storz, Tuttlingen, Germany). Uterine distention was provided by using the continuous flow and pressure-controlled pump system after J. Hamou (Karl Storz). For the hysteroscopic surgical procedures done with the 5 mm instruments and the bipolar needle, we used saline solution as distension medium. For the monopolar resectoscopy, we used sorbitol solution as the distension medium. The electric generator used was an autocon II 400 (Karl Storz). The monopolar setting for cutting was 80–100 W, and the bipolar setting for cutting at 40–60 W power. The procedure to follow and the choice of instrumentation used depend on the preclinical information provided. When the sonographic parameters showed a uterine length less than 9 cm, an endometrial thickness less than 9 mm, or one single lesion (polyp or myoma) less than 9 mm, the procedure was started without any analgesic procedure and with the small-bored instruments.

In case major pathology was expected and the use of the resectoscope was scheduled, the patients underwent some kind of anesthesia (propofol sedation or spinal anesthesia). In this case the kind of anesthetic procedure was decided in the operating room by the anesthetist according the clinical characteristics of the patient and the estimated time of procedure by the hysteroscopist. In this case the patient was admitted in a recovery room with a nurse in constant surveillance during 6 h postoperative procedure.

The diagnostic hysteroscopy was performed following the vagino-cervical route under direct vision. After entering the uterine cavity, the tubal ostia were identified as the anatomical landmarks and a systematic examination was performed. Hysteroscopic findings were allocated either to "the uterine cavity lesions" or "the endometrial aspect." In the uterine cavity, lesion groups could be found: endometrial polyp, cervical polyp, myoma, cyst, malignant smooth muscle tumor, placenta rest, abortion debris, endometrial ossification, adhesions, congenital malformation, and lost IUD. In the endometrial aspect characterization group, we differentiated between functional, atrophic or thin endometrium, dysfunctional, endometritis, cystic atrophy, hyperplasia, polypoid, and carcinoma.

The hysteroscopic observation was documented, and an endometrial biopsy and/or the removal of the pathology were performed. The histopathological results were used as gold standard and compared with the hysteroscopic documented observation. The sensitivity, specificity, and predictive value of hysteroscopy were calculated.

Results

Four hundred nineteen women fulfilled the inclusion criteria. The average age was 54 years (range 24–87 years), of which 43.9% were menopausal.

The referral cause was for the majority of patients (96.2%) an abnormal results in the sonographic examination such as endometrial thickness, endometrial irregularity, endometrium heterogeneity, endometrium liquid, polyps, myomas, IUD, foreign body, and placental or fetal debris. Only 3.8% of patients had a normal sonographic exam, being in these patients the referral causes: one case of infertility, others of endometrial cells on cervix cytology, two cases of cervical polyps, five cases of post menopausal metrorrhagia, and six cases of menorrhagia.

We divided the hysteroscopic findings in two groups:

1. The uterine cavity lesions—those included 19 cases of uterine adhesions, 1 of which was associated with a myoma, another with a cervical and endometrial polyp, and 5 with endometrial polyps. Twelve cases of septate uterus were found, associated to endometrial cyst in 1 case, 3 cases to endometrial polyps, 1 to complex hyperplasia, and 2 to endometrial adenocarcinoma. A total of 247 endometrial polyps were diagnosed, 1 with adenocarcinoma, 8 were associated with cervical polyps, and 11 to myomas. There were 15 cervical polyps, 8 of which associated to endometrial polyps, and another to myoma and uterine adhesion. Submucous myomas were found in 42 patients. The other diagnostic lesions included three cases of endometrial cysts, six cases of abortion debris retention, one of placental retention, one case of malignant smooth muscle tissue, one case of residual endometrial ossification, and six of intrauterine retention of IUD, one of these associated to an endometrial polyp. The remainder 97 cases did not have any uterine lesion.

2. The endometrial aspect characterization—we detected 2 cases of endometrial carcinoma, 41 cases of endometrial hyperplasia, 45 cases of dysfunctional endometrium, 23 of polypoid endometrium, 4 cases of endometritis, and 6 cases of cystic atrophic endometrium. Functional endometrium was found in 109 cases, thin endometrium in 2 cases, and in 166, there was an atrophic endometrium. In 21 cases no endometrial biopsies were made. All of this included thin or atrophic endometrium in asymptomatic postmenopausal woman with concordant diagnosis of polyps on sonographic and hysteroscopic evaluation. In these patients only the polypectomy was performed.

When compared to histopathologic analysis as gold standard, hysteroscopy failed the diagnosis of the following uterine lesions: one case of myoma that was really a polyp, two cases considered without endometrial lesions that had polyps on histopathologic exam, and 2 polyps that were myomas after all (see Table 1). The hysteroscopy also failed in the endometrial characterization of the following cases: one complex hyperplasia (focal) wrongly classified as atrophic endometrium, two cases of dysfunctional endometrium, and

Table 1 The uterine cavity lesions: hysteroscopic and histopathologic characterization

Uterine lesion	Hysteroscopic exam	Histopathologic exam
Endometrial polyp	247[a] (1 carcinoma)	248 (1 carcinoma)
Cervical polyp	15	15
Myoma	42[b]	40
Cyst	4	3
Malignant smooth muscle tumor	1	1
Placenta	1	1
Abortion first trimester debris	6	6
Bone (residual endometrial ossification)	1	1
Endometrial adhesions	19	–
Septate uterus	12	–
IUD	6	–
No. of lesion	97[c]	126[d]

[a] FP-2 cases were myomas

[b] FP-1 case was a polyp

[c] FN-2 cases were polyps

[d] Includes the 12 cases of isolated adhesions, 8 of isolated septate uterus, 5 of isolated lost IUD without other injuries associated, and still 1 case of cyst that had been destroyed and 4 of type 2 myomas which were not submitted to biopsy

two other of polyploid endometrium (Table 2). The hysteroscopic evaluation was characterized as functional endometrium, dysfunctional endometrium in 12 cases, polyploid endometrium in 4, simple hyperplasia in 1 case, and complex hyperplasia in another. Two cases classified as focal complex hyperplasia in septate uterus were in the end endometrium adenocarcinomas. Considering the 22 false-positive diagnosis, these include 2 cases of focal hyperplasia that were atrophic endometrium, 5 cases of polyploid endometrium, 6 cases of dysfunctional endometrium, and 9 of hyperplasia that were all functional endometrium (see Tables 3 and 4).

Table 2 The endometrial aspect characterization by hysteroscopy and histopathologic exam

Endometrium characterization	Hysteroscopic exam	Histopathologic exam
Functional, atrophic, or thin endometrium	298	276+21 no biopsy
Dysfunctional	45	53
Endometritis	4	4
Cystic atrophy	6	6
Hyperplasia	41	31
Polyploid	23	24
Carcinoma	2	4

Table 3 Failure of endometrial diagnosis of endometrial characterization (false negative)

Hysteroscopic exam	Histopathologic exam	False negative
Hyperplasia	Carcinoma	2
Functional	Polyploid	4
Functional	Hyperplasia (1 simple, 1 complex)	2
Functional	Dysfunctional	12
Atrophic	Dysfunctional	2
Atrophic	Polyploid	2
Atrophic	Complex hyperplasia	1

Considering the diagnostic accuracy of hysteroscopy in the evaluation of intra-cavity lesions, the sensitivity, specificity, positive and negative predictive values were respectively 99.3%, 97.7%, 98.9%, and 98.5%. The values of the same parameters regarding the characterization of endometrium were as follows: 79.8%, 91.97%, 81.8%, and 90.97%. The diagnostic accuracy was 98.8% for endometrial lesions diagnosis and 88.8% for endometrial characterization.

The incidence of endometrial adenocarcinoma was 1.2%, and the sensitivity and specificity of hysteroscopy were respectively 60% and 99.5%, with a diagnostic accuracy of 99.5%. The incidence of endometrial hyperplasia was 9.8%. The hysteroscopy had a sensibility of 90% and a specificity of 97% for the diagnosis of this pathology, and the diagnostic accuracy was 64%.

The complication rate was 3.3%, including 2 cases of postoperative hemorrhage that were inpatient for 24-h surveillance and were discharged after that and 12 cases of some kind of perforation or false route. Only half of these patients stood for 24-h inpatient surveillance and were dismissed with no other complication, except one case of uterine perforation during a myomectomy of a 4-cm myoma in a postmenopausal woman, which became the most serious complication because the resectoscope hook entered in the abdominal cavity and so laparotomy was performed to exclude abdominal injury and hysterectomy was performed at the same time.

The five endometrial carcinomas (one in a polyp lesion) were submitted to a gynecology oncologic committee

Table 4 Failure of endometrial diagnosis of endometrial characterization (false positive)

Hysteroscopic exam	Histopathologic exam	False positive
Hyperplasia	Functional	9
Polyploid	Functional	5
Dysfunctional	Functional	6
Hyperplasia	Atrophic	2

which selected the final treatment, and all cases submitted to hysterectomy: two cases were endometrioid adenocarcinoma in situ (stage T1is) and three cases were well-differentiated, invasive endometrioid adenocarcinomas with less than half myometrium invasion, i.e., T1N0M0.

Discussion

Transvaginal sonography is a valuable method to identify women at risk for endometrial disease, not only by measuring endometrium thickness but also by accessing focal abnormalities within the endometrial cavity. But, its value is limited in the endometrial characterization because the image of endometrium is given in a gray scale which makes interpretation difficult and less accurate, and also because although in post menopausal women the presence of thick endometrium (i.e., more than 5 mm) may predict some kind of pathology [1–3], the exact lesion cannot most of times be discriminated. Transvaginal ultrasound fails to differentiate intrauterine abnormalities (i.e., myomas, polyps, hyperplasia, etc.), so having a low diagnostic sensitivity ranging from 76% to 96% [4, 5]. Visualization of the endometrial echo or endomyometrial complex may also be limited by the uterine position, myometrial lesions that distort endometrial line, and by the resolution of the imaging technology. The accuracy of this modality is also related to the timing of the menstrual period or menopausal status. It is also notable that polyps and myomas less than 1 cm in diameter cannot be detected by transvaginal sonography [6].

Hysteroscopic inspection of uterine cavity is a simple, outpatient and well-accepted method for investigation of intrauterine pathology [7]. The direct visualization in vivo, real-time, real-color, hydrated, well-illuminated, and augmented vision of the uterine cavity make this diagnostic tool very accurate to detect minute focal endometrial pathology and small lesions otherwise not possible, complemented to the ability of performing guided direct biopsies and treatment on the same diagnostic procedure [8, 9].

Hysteroscopic examination may predict endometrial lesions with a good accuracy as well as endometrial aspect characterization, adopting a nomenclature similar to that used by the pathologist. This approach makes correlation between hysteroscopic findings and histopathologic results easier, as well as the dialogue between others investigators; the use of a universal language is the best way to achieve concordant and consistent results.

Comparing our results with other studies, we conclude that diagnostic power of hysteroscopy is very different among the various studies in medical literature (see Table 5). Various factors are implicated in these different results, including the hysteroscopist experience, quality of equipment, distension source, quality of the endometrial sampling, focus population including (pre- or postmenopausal), and patient selection (clinical symptoms, sonography suspected) [10].

The accuracy of hysteroscopy to diagnose uterine lesions is better than that of endometrial characterization (98.8% versus 88.8%). The false diagnoses were lower and include: one case of hysteroscopic diagnosis of myoma that was a polyp, a fibrous polyp with a very round shape may macroscopically simulate a polyp, and two cases of polyps that were myomas on histopathologic exam; myomas type 1 or 2 with a secretor endometrium covering its surface;

Table 5 Comparing studies in accessing sensitivity and specificity of hysteroscopy for diagnose endometrial pathology

Author (reference)	Year	No. of women	Hormonal state	Focus	Sensitivity	Specificity
Gezer et al. [20]	2004	385	Pre/postmenopausal	AUB/polyps	83.9	63.9
Gezer et al. [20]	2004	385	Pre/postmenopausal	AUB/myomas	80	92
Feng and Li [4]	2002	112	Pre/postmenopausal	PMM/abnormal US	92.3	97.4
Tinelli et al. [21]	2008	752	Postmenopausal	PMM	98	91
Angioni et al. [22]	2008	319	Postmenopausal	PMM/polyps	100	97
Angioni et al. [22]	2008	319	Postmenopausal	PMM/myomas	100	98
Loverro et al. [6]	1999	106	Postmenopausal	PMM (no HRT)	97.5	100
Sousa et al. [23]	2001	200	Postmenopausal	PMM	88.9	98.3
Cordeiro et al. [24]	2009	245	Postmenopausal	Abnormal TUS/benign polyps	98.7	72.7
Cordeiro et al. [24]	2009	245	Postmenopausal	Abnormal TUS/adenocarcinoma	94.1	98.9
Antunes	2010	419	Pre/postmenopausal	Abnormal TUS or clinics/ uterine lesions	99.3	97.7
Antunes	2010	419	Pre/postmenopausal	Abnormal TUS or clinics/ endometrium characterization	79.8	91.7

AUB abnormal uterine bleeding, *PMM* postmenopausal metrorrhagia, *TUS* transvaginal ultrasound

and the two false negative include two focal thicker lesions interpreted as dysfunctional endometrium that were polyps on histopathologic exam.

The false diagnosis on endometrium characterization is a concern, particularly the false negative; 12 cases of dysfunctional endometrium were misdiagnosed as functional endometrium. Dysfunctional endometrium traduces a discordant maturation between endometrium and the hormonal cycle, or a focal discordance with focal areas in various phases of endometrial cycle at the same time. The estrogen and progesterone receptors' distribution on the endometrium layer is irregular, varying from one region to one other, with the day of the cycle and is dependent on the presence of "accidents" on the endometrial cavity like myomas, polyps, and septate [11]. Those lesions may be very subtle and we may not interpret them; in these cases, the use of a colorant might help us. Only seriated biopsies can help us to diagnose these subtle lesions. The above commentary is extensive to the other cases of "innocent" endometrium (functional or atrophic) and that the biopsy revealed polypoid or hyperplasic endometrium [12–14].

We found a higher incidence of carcinomas on septate uterus 16.7% versus 1.2% on the total studied population. These uteri have a greater endometrial surface and a congenital intra-cavity accident, so might be more susceptible to endometrial proliferative disease including carcinoma. This must be confirmed with more investigation.

The two false negative (for carcinoma) occurred with septate uterus in two postmenopausal patients. In one case, the hysteroscopic exam revealed complex hyperplasia and the histopathologic exam revealed well-differentiated, invasive adenocarcinoma (T1N0M0); the other case was a hysteroscopic diagnosis of simple focal hyperplasia, and the biopsy revealed complex atypical hyperplasia with focus of adenocarcinoma. After hysterectomy the histopathologic examination showed in an area of 3 mm (corresponding to the biopsied area) in situ endometrioid adenocarcinoma. Hysteroscopic guided biopsy permitted the correct histopathologic diagnose.

It is understood that preoperative blind biopsies specimens are insufficient for diagnosis in women with intrauterine lesions which include neoplasias [15]. Furthermore, investigators have reported that hysteroscopy had failed to detect endometrial adenocarcinoma and stromal cancer [16], also a well-recognized complex hyperplasia and has a very similar hysteroscopic image to carcinoma [17, 18]. Combined hysteroscopy and biopsy leads to almost 100% accuracy in diagnosis of carcinoma and its precursors [18]. Hysteroscopists, whatever their experience, should not ever forget this complementary procedure, the hysteroscopic guided biopsy whatever for benign or malignant pathology [19].

We recommend that all patients should have a transvaginal sonographic exam performed previously to the hysteroscopy, the sonographic findings plus the clinical data permit to select the correct hysteroscopic material (2, 3, or 4-mm scopes) and well planning the exam (with or without cervical preparation, with or without anesthesia). Hysteroscopy exam should include a detailed inspection for 15–20 min of the total uterine cavity and several biopsies of every suspicious lesion and should include all endometrial layers. We recommend the use of scissors to catch a sufficiently profound and large specimen, instead of using the biopsy forceps alone. The specimen should be placed directly on the formol container to avoid material fragmentation. Lastly and very important is the continuous dialogue with the pathologist and constant auto critics comparing every hysteroscopic findings with the histopathologic exam, and is from this reflection that we may offer the patient and our colleges the best we can.

Conclusion

The hysteroscopy allows direct visualization of uterine cavity, and this particularity confers it a high diagnostic acuity, that associated to the possibility of simultaneous treatment or biopsy procedures gives it an irreplaceable value in the diagnosis and treatment of intrauterine diseases.

Conflict of interest   No payment or support was received in kind for any aspect of the submitted work (including but not limited to grants, data monitoring board, study design, manuscript preparation, statistical analysis, etc.). There have been no financial relationships (regardless of amount of compensation) with any entities that have an interest related to the submitted work. There have been no financial associations or interests (personal, professional, political, institutional, and religious or others) that a reasonable reader would want to know about in relation to the submitted work. The above declaration is signed by the author.

References

1. Smith-Bindman R, Kerlikowske K, Feldstein VA et al (1998) Endovaginal ultrasound to exclude endometrial cancer and other endometrial abnormalities. J Am Med Assoc 280:1510–1517

2. Bree RL, Carlos R (1995) US for postmenopausal bleeding consensus development and patient-centered outcomes. Radiology 222:595–598

3. Karlsson B, Granberg S, Wikland M et al (1995) Transvaginal ultrasonography of the endometrium in woman with postmenopausal bleeding—a Nordic multicenter study. Am J Obstet Gynecol 172:1488–1494

4. Feng L, Li D (2002) Evaluation of intrauterine disorders by hysteroscopy and transvaginal sonography. Gynecol Endosc 11:401–404

5. Gibbs Henson J, Hawkins K (2004) A retrospective analysis of the role of transvaginal sonography in the evaluation of patients with abnormal postmenopausal bleeding. BMUS J 12(4):218–221

6. Loverro G, Bettochi S, Cormio G, Nicolardi V et al (1999) Transvaginal sonography and hysteroscopy in postmenopausal uterine bleeding. Maturitas 33(2):139–144

7. Paschopoulos EB, ParasKevaidiis E, Stefanidis K et al (1997) Vaginoscopy approach to outpatient hysteroscopy. J Am Assoc Gynecol Laparosc 4:13–15

8. Pasqualotto EB, Margossian H, Price LL et al (2000) Accuracy of preoperative diagnostic tools and outcome of hysteroscopic management of menstrual dysfunction. J Am Assoc Gynecol Laparosc 7:201–209

9. Pal L, Lapensee L, Toth TL et al (1996) Comparison of office hysteroscopy, transvaginal ultrasonography in the diagnosis of endometrial abnormalities. Obstet Gynecol 87:345–349

10. Bruno E, Gama CR (2003) Hipertrofia endometrial. In: Crispi CP, Oliveira FMM, Errico G, Damian Junior JC (eds) Tratado de Videoendoscopia Ginecologica. Atheneu, São Paulo, pp 1021–1032

11. Miyahira H (1995) Analise crítica do diagnostic histeroscopico endometrial (1995) In Tese de Doutorado em Medicina (Ginecologia), UFRJ:10–30

12. Silveira LP (1998) Análise do valor preditivo do diagnóstico histeroscópico de endométrio hipertrófico. In Tese de mestrado em Medicina (Ginecologia), UFR:15–22

13. Fay TN, Khanen N, Hosking D (1999) Out-patient hysteroscopy in asymptomatic postmenopausal women. Climacteric 2:263–267

14. Clark TJ, Voit D, Gupta JK et al (2002) Accuracy of hysteroscopy in the diagnosis of endometrial cancer and hyperplasia: a systematic quantitative review. J Am Med Assoc 288(13):1610–1621

15. Kent AS, Haines P, Manners TB et al (1996) Blind endometrial biopsies: insufficient for diagnosis in woman with intra-uterine pathology. Gynecol Endosc 7:273–278

16. Colafranceschi M, Bettochi S, Mencaglia L et al (1996) Missed hysteroscopic detection of uterine carcinoma before endometrial resection: report of three cases. Gynecol Oncol 62(2):298–300

17. Mencaglia L (1995) Hysteroscopy and adenocarcinoma. Obstet Gynecol Clin North Am 22(3):573–579

18. Mencaglia L, Valle RF, Perino A, Guilard G (1990) Endometrial carcinoma and its precursors: early detection and treatment. Int J Gynecol Obstet 31:107–116

19. Gasparri F, Scarselli G, Mencaglia L (1984) Studio pilota periáttuazione dello screening per il carcinoma dell'endométrio. Oncol Gynecol 3:50

20. Gezer A, Saar A, Demirkiran F, Benian A et al (2004) The efficacy of hysteroscopy for endometrial pathology: the experience of a university clinic on diagnostic accuracy and the comparison with the other methods. Gynecol Surg 1(4):227–230

21. Tinelli R, Tinelli FG, Cicinelli E, Malvasi A, Tinelli A (2008) The role of hysteroscopy with eye-directed biopsy in postmenopausal woman with uterine bleeding and endometrial atrophy. Menopause 15(4 Pt 1):737–742

22. Angioni S, Loddo A, Milano F, Piras B et al (2008) Detection of benign intracavitary lesions in postmenopausal woman with abnormal uterine bleeding: a prospective comparative study on outpatient hysteroscopy and blind biopsy. J Minim Invasive Gynecol 15(1):87–91

23. Sousa R, Silvestre M, Sousa LA, Falcão F et al (2001) Transvaginal ultrasonography and hysteroscopy in post menopausal bleeding: a prospective study. Acta Obstet Gynecol Scand 80:856–862

24. Cordeiro A, Condeço R, Leitão C et al (2009) Office hysteroscopy after ultrasonographic diagnosis of thickened endometrium in postmenopausal patients. Gynecol Surg 6:317–322

29

Broad ligament fibroids—a radiological and surgical challenge

Lindsay M. Kindinger · Thomas E. Setchell · Tariq S. Miskry

Abstract Currently, there is limited data on the ease of imaging of broad ligament fibroids and their safe laparoscopic management. We aimed to review all laparoscopic myomectomies over an 8-year period, focusing on intraoperative findings and corresponding pre-operative imaging. All laparoscopic myomectomies performed between 2004 and 2012 were reviewed. Cases with broad ligament fibroids were identified. Presenting symptoms, imaging, intraoperative findings, complications and 6-month follow-up were noted. Ten broad ligament fibroids were identified from 185 cases of laparoscopic myomectomies. Mean broad ligament fibroid diameter was 8.1 cm, and the largest was 15 cm. Mean combined fibroid weight was 267 g (range 30–560 g). Blood loss was associated with the total number of fibroids excised rather than the diameter of the broad ligament fibroid (range 30–400 ml). Accurate pre-operative diagnosis at imaging was made in only one of the ten broad ligament fibroids. Of the remainder, one was thought to be an ovarian mass, one fibroid was missed entirely and seven were reported non-specifically as 'lateral'. This case series indicates the challenge posed by broad ligament fibroids at pre-operative imaging. Underreporting may reflect a lack of awareness of the surgical significance of broad ligament fibroids. There should be a high level of suspicion for location within the broad ligament if a fibroid reported is as lateral. With adequate operator experience, large fibroid size should not contraindicate laparoscopic management of broad ligament fibroids.

Keywords Fibroid · Myoma · Broad ligament · Laparoscopy · Myomectomy · Ultrasound

Background

Uterine fibroids are commonly intramural, submucosal or subserosal. Less frequently subserous or pedunculated fibroids may extend into the peritoneal folds of the broad ligaments to form an intraligamentous fibroid. These broad ligament fibroids are of clinical and surgical importance. Their anatomical location may cause local pressure effects including ureteric obstruction [1]. Excision, however, is associated with risk of surgical complications particularly ureteric and uterine vessel injuries [2] and concealed haematoma formation [3].

Broad ligament fibroids also present a diagnostic challenge on imaging. Appearing adnexal in location, they may be confused with ovarian tumours [4, 5] or may have an alternative histological diagnosis following myomectomy; a suspected broad ligament fibroid was reported as a pelvic schwannoma at histology [6].

With well-established advantages over laparotomy, growing surgical expertise has enabled laparoscopic excision of increasingly large fibroids [7]. There is a paucity of literature on the laparoscopic management of fibroids within the broad ligament however [8]. The probability of complications arising at myomectomy for intraligamentous fibroids is increased compared to fibroids in other locations. Sizzi et al. indicated an 18.8 % complication rate, reporting an odds ratio of 2.43 for developing any complication [2].

Within our unit, several cases of fibroid location within the broad ligament, revealed for the first time intraoperatively, were noted to be inconsistent with their pre-operative imaging

---

Synopsis The anatomical location of the broad ligament fibroid presents a challenge for the unprepared laparoscopic surgeon. This series indicates the radiological challenge in identifying these fibroids pre-operatively.

L. M. Kindinger (✉) · T. E. Setchell · T. S. Miskry
Department of Gynaecology, St Mary's Hospital,
Imperial College Healthcare NHS Trust,
Praed StreetPaddington London W2 1NY, UK
e-mail: lindsay.kindinger@nhs.net

reports. Given the potential complications of intraligamentous myomectomy [2], surgical anticipation is crucial, particularly for the inexperienced laparoscopic surgeon. We therefore aimed to assess the accuracy of pre-operative imaging for broad ligament fibroids within our unit, as well as our associated complication rate at laparoscopic myomectomy.

Methods

All laparoscopic myomectomies performed between September 2004 and 2012 within a single unit were reviewed. Case notes with broad ligament fibroids were identified. Intraoperative findings were noted, particularly operative time, blood loss, combined fibroid weight and intra- and post-operative complications. Fibroid location at laparoscopy was compared to pre-operative imaging reports, where imaging modality and grade of operator were noted.

Symptoms at presentation and at a 6-month follow-up were documented. All procedures followed were in accordance with the ethical standards of the responsible committee on human experimentation (institutional and national) and with the Helsinki Declaration of 1975, as revised in 2000.

Operative technique

All laparoscopic myomectomies were performed under general anaesthesia. A standard three-port laparoscopy was performed. Intraoperative measures were taken to reduce complications. The ureter was observed closely throughout the procedure. Vasopressin was routinely injected into the broad ligament fibroid to reduce intraoperative bleeding [9]. Depending on the location of the fibroid in relation to the uterine vessels and the ureter, an incision was made on the anterior or posterior leaf of the broad ligament. Blunt dissection was used in combination with careful monopolar and bipolar electrosurgery for coagulation. Care was taken to minimise the risk of thermal injury to surrounding structures, particularly the uterine vessels and ureter.

Following fibroid enucleation, the area was washed to observe haemostasis. Laparoscopic suturing within the broad ligament was limited. Peritoneal closure of the broad ligament was not routinely performed. GnRH analogues were not used. In two cases, due to concern over haematoma development, an absorbable haemostatic cellulose polymer Surgicel® (Ethicon Inc., Johnson & Johnson, USA) was placed into the enucleated cavity. No subsequent complications were reported.

Findings

Of the 185 laparoscopic myomectomies, ten women with broad ligament fibroids were identified. Mean age was 36 years (ranging from 27 to 52 years; a hysterectomy was culturally unacceptable to the 52-year-old—she felt she could not await menopause due to severe pressure symptoms from a 130-mm fibroid). Median BMI was 24.2 (range 20–29). Most common symptoms included pelvic pain (40 %), pressure symptoms (40 %) and subfertility (20 %). Eight were nulliparous, one had a single vaginal delivery and one had two vaginal deliveries.

All ten women underwent pre-operative ultrasound imaging for fibroid mapping. Only one broad ligament fibroid was reported as situated within the broad ligament. Seven broad ligament fibroids were reported as 'lateral' or 'lateral pedunculated' (Table 1). Of the 185 cases, an additional 35 fibroids reported as lateral were located outside the broad ligament. There were no false positive reports.

Seniority of the reporting radiologist and route of ultrasound did not improve the detection of the broad ligament fibroids. The majority had a transabdominal ultrasound (81 %, $n=153$), whereas 12 % had both transvaginal and transabdominal. The ultrasound route was not specified in the remainder.

Three women with broad ligament fibroids went on to have a pelvis MRI due to uncertainty of the pelvic mass. One broad ligament fibroid was reported as an ovarian mass on MRI and was booked for a salpingo-ophrectomy. One 60-mm broad

	Fibroid diameter (mm)	Fibroid reported on imaging	Imaging modality	Grade of reporter
Table 1 Pre-operative ultrasound imaging for fibroid mapping	50	Broad ligament	US and MRI	Radiology consultant
	60	Ovarian mass	US and MRI	Radiology consultant
	60	Missed on US	US	Radiology consultant
	60	Lateral subserosal	US	Radiology consultant
	60	Lateral	US and MRI	Radiology consultant
	65	Lateral pedunculated	US	Ultrasonographer
	70	Lateral pedunculated	US	Ultrasonographer
	100	Lateral	US	Radiology consultant
	130	Lateral pedunculated	US	Radiology consultant
	150	Lateral	US	Radiology consultant

Table 2 Operative findings at laparoscopic myomectomy for broad ligament fibroids

Broad ligament myomectomy operative findings	Average (mean)	Minimum	Maximum
Blood loss (ml)	136	30	400
Number of fibroids present	1.8	1	16
Fibroid diameter (mm)	81	50	150
Fibroid weight (g)	267	30	560
Operating time (min)	105	50	180
Inpatient stay (days)	1.6	1	2

ligament fibroid was considered to be missed on ultrasound as it was not reported. There were no false positive reports of a broad ligament fibroid.

The operative findings at laparoscopic myomectomy for broad ligament fibroids are detailed in Table 2. One third of operations were for multiple myomectomies. No women had more than one broad ligament fibroid.

Figure 1 demonstrates an association between *blood loss* (dashed red line) and the *number* of fibroids *excised* (grey column). There does not appear to be any correlation between blood loss and the diameter of the broad ligament fibroid (dotted blue line). No blood transfusions were required, and there were no conversions to laparotomy. There were no complications, minor or major.

At 6-month follow-up, symptoms were noted in eight of the ten women. Seven of the eight had complete symptomatic improvement. The presenting complaint in the woman without symptomatic improvement was subfertility; she was yet to conceive at 6-month follow-up. In this case, a total of three subserosal myomas were excised including a 10-cm broad ligament fibroid.

Discussion

Anatomical location within the broad ligament has previously been associated with an increased complication risk at myomectomy [2]. Ultrasound, as the first-line imaging tool for uterine structural abnormalities such as fibroids [10], plays an important role in pre-operative planning for such procedures.

This case series indicates the challenge posed on ultrasound in accurately identifying fibroids within the broad ligament. We illustrate general underreporting of broad ligament fibroids; of the 185 cases, there were no false positive reports. This may reflect a lack of awareness among radiologists of the surgical significance of broad ligament location. Standardising ultrasound criteria for broad ligament fibroids may improve detection. Various standards can be applied to adnexal masses that are suspected to be broad ligament fibroids, such as size, vascularity and anatomical relationship to the uterine arteries or other pelvic sidewall structures. Ultimately though, the rarity of broad ligament fibroids, and the potential for misdiagnosis as ovarian or retroperitoneal tumours [4–6], makes the development of standardised ultrasound criteria extremely difficult.

In the future, it may be useful to regard 'lateral fibroids' with suspicion for location within the broad ligament; seven of the ten broad ligament fibroids were reported as lateral (the remaining 35 of the total 42 lateral fibroids were outside the broad ligament). If reported as lateral, one may further direct radiologists to specifically look for broad ligament fibroids on ultrasound or MRI. In these cases, standardising ultrasound technique with a combined use of transvaginal and abdominal ultrasounds, with the use of colour imaging, would be recommended.

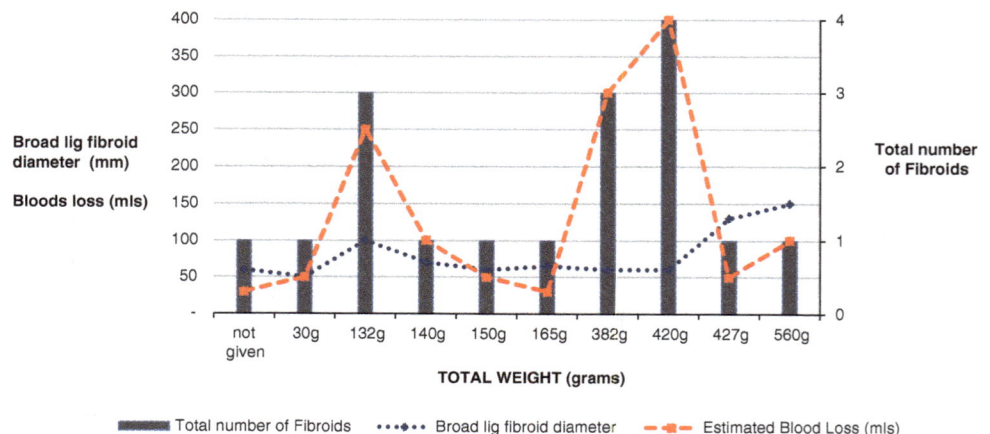

Fig. 1 Total specimen weight (*x-axis*) compared to blood loss and broad ligament fibroid size (*primary y-axis*) and total number of fibroids (*secondary y-axis*)

An assessment of improvement in the reporting of broad ligament fibroids following these implementations may be of interest. Alternatively, given the superior sensitivity of MRI in assessing uterine fibroids [11], a prospective study evaluating all lateral fibroids by MRI may improve the positive predictive value for broad ligament fibroids.

The limitations of our study are its small cohort size and retrospective analysis of a relatively uncommon condition. Our complication rates can therefore not be extrapolated to larger populations. This case series does, however, illustrate that the complication risk may not be as high as previously suggested [2], with the prerequisite of an experienced laparoscopic surgeon and adequate intraoperative precautions.

In addition, multiple ultrasound machines were used and replaced over the 8 years. We therefore are unable to comment on the effect of specific technologies on the accuracy and sensitivity of identifying fibroids within the broad ligament. Conclusions could not be drawn on the influence of the seniority of the reporting radiologist, the ultrasound route or the accuracy of MRI modality on the detection of broad ligament fibroids.

Conclusion

This case series highlights two main learning points:

1. Broad ligament fibroids are frequently underreported at pre-operative ultrasound. There should be a level of suspicion of broad ligament location if a fibroid is reported as lateral. Discussion with a radiologist may be considered.
2. Broad ligament fibroids can be managed laparoscopically given adequate operator expertise. Large size should contradict laparoscopic myomectomy of a broad ligament fibroid [8].

Conflict of interest   The authors declare that they have no conflict of interest.

References

1. Brown RS, Marley JL, Cassoni AM (1998) Pseudo-Meigs' syndrome due to broad ligament leiomyoma: a mimic of metastatic ovarian carcinoma. Clin Oncol (R Coll Radiol) 10(3):198–201
2. Sizzi O, Rossetti A, Malzoni M, Minelli L, La Grotta F, Soranna L et al (2007) Italian multicenter study on complications of laparoscopic myomectomy. J Minim Invasive Gynecol 14(4):453–462
3. Sinha R, Hegde A, Warty N, Patil N (2003) Laparoscopic excision of very large myomas. J Am Assoc Gynecol Laparosc 10(4):461–468
4. Yıldız P, Cengiz H, Yıldız G, Sam AD, Yavuzcan A, Çelikbaş B, Sahin L (2012) Two unusual clinical presentations of broad-ligament leiomyomas: a report of two cases. Medicina (Kaunas) 48(3):163–165
5. Rajanna DK, Pandey V, Janardhan S, Datti SN (2013) Broad ligament fibroid mimicking as ovarian tumor on ultrasonography and computed tomography scan. J Clin Imaging Sci 3:8
6. Sinha R, Sundaram M, Hegde A, Mahajan C (2008) Pelvic schwannoma masquerading as broad ligament myoma. J Minim Invasive Gynecol 15(2):217–219
7. Mais V, Ajossa S, Guerriero S, Mascia M, Solla E, Melis GB (1996) Laparoscopic versus abdominal myomectomy: a prospective, randomized trial to evaluate benefits in early outcome. Am J Obstet Gynecol 174(2):654–658
8. Theodoridis TD, Zepiridis L, Grimbizis G, Bontis J (2005) Laparoscopic management of broad ligament leiomyoma. J Minim Invasive Gynecol 12(6):469
9. Kongnyuy EJ, Wiysonge CS (2009) Interventions to reduce haemorrhage during myomectomy for fibroids. Cochrane Database Syst Rev 8(3):CD00535
10. National Institute of Clinical Excellence. NICE clinical guideline 44—heavy menstrual bleeding. http://www.nice.org.uk/nicemedia/pdf/CG44FullGuideline.pdf. Published 2007, UK. Accessed May 2013
11. Levens ED, Wesley R, Premkumar A, Blocker W, Nieman LK (2009) Magnetic resonance imaging and transvaginal ultrasound for determining fibroid burden: implications for clinical research. Am J Obstet Gynecol 200(5):537.e1–7

30

Ultrasound examination before, during, and after office endometrial sampling

Thierry Van den Bosch · Dominique Van Schoubroeck ·
Dirk Timmerman

Abstract Office endometrial sampling is widely used as the first diagnostic test in women with abnormal uterine bleeding. Because office sampling is a blind procedure, the lesion causing the symptoms may be missed. The use of ultrasound before, during, and after office endometrial sampling improves relevant tissue yield. The measurement of the endometrial thickness informs if sampling is indicated. The evaluation of ultrasound features (without or with fluid instillation) may suggest a focal intracavitary lesion necessitating operative hysteroscopy. The knowledge of the uterine cavity length, shape, and flexion may avoid nonrepresentative sampling. The concordance between the tissue yield and the ultrasound findings reflects the reliability of the sampling. If not concordant, further diagnostic steps such as fluid instillation sonography or hysteroscopy are indicated. We conclude that integrating ultrasound in the diagnostic algorithm for uterine intracavitary pathology optimizes office endometrial sampling.

Keywords Ultrasonography · Uterus · Endometrium · Leiomyoma · Metrorrhagia

T. Van den Bosch · D. Van Schoubroeck · D. Timmerman
Department of Development and Regeneration, KU Leuven,
3000 Leuven, Belgium

T. Van den Bosch
Department of Obstetrics and Gynecology, RZTienen, 3300 Tienen,
Belgium

T. Van den Bosch (✉)
KU Leuven Department of Development and Regeneration,
University Hospitals Leuven, Herestraat 49, 3000 Leuven, Belgium
e-mail: thierry.van.den.bosch@skynet.be

Background

Most practitioners favor office endometrial sampling as the first diagnostic test in women with abnormal uterine bleeding. The main reason is that tissue diagnosis is considered pivotal. Depending on the histology of the endometrial sample, further management is planned. The alleged medico legal value of a pathology report is an additional reason in favor of endometrial biopsy. However, because office sampling is a blind procedure, there is no control that the tissue yielded is representative for the patient's problem. If a relevant lesion is missed, management is likely to be inappropriate.

Compared with other office sampling devices such as the Novak or the Vabra curette, the Pipelle® de Cornier [1] has been reported to cause less procedure-related pain while offering a similar diagnostic accuracy [2, 3]. The popularity of the Pipelle® for office endometrial sampling dates from the early 1990s. Stovall et al. [4] reported in 1991 a 97.5 % sensitivity of Pipelle® sampling for endometrial cancer. This study is not very robust since only 40 patients with known endometrial cancer were included. In 1993, Rodrigues et al. [5] measured the endometrial denudation by office sampling in hysterectomy specimens. By Pipelle®, only 4.2 % of the total endometrial surface was sampled and they conclude the method to be unreliable. In 2002, a systematic review by Clark et al. [6], on the accuracy of outpatient endometrial biopsy in the diagnosis of endometrial cancer, reported an excellent positive likelihood ratio of 66.5 (95 % CI, 30.0–147.1) and a good negative likelihood ratio of 0.14 (95 % CI, 0.1–0.3). A possible explanation for the apparent contradiction between Rodrigues' and Clark's conclusions may be the tissue characteristics of endometrial cancer. Malignant endometrial tissue not only tends to protrude into the uterine cavity, it is also more friable because of less intercellular cohesion (Fig. 1). Tumor tissue is thus more prone to be aspirated during Pipelle® sampling.

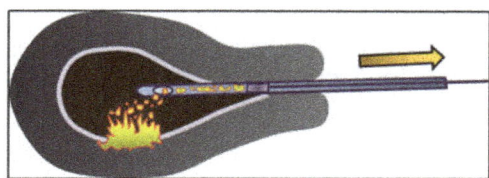

Fig. 1 Pipelle® aspiration biopsie of a focal malignant lesion

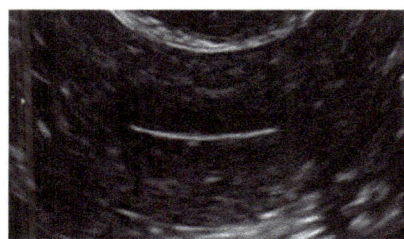

Fig. 3 Ultrasound image of a uniform thin endometrium

Endometrial cancer can be missed by office sampling [7]: small tumors or lesions hidden behind a benign focal lesion may escape the sampler. In the presence of intracavitary fluid or blood, the aspirated material may contain little or no endometrial cells (Fig. 2).

Many benign focal intracavitary lesions, such as endometrial polyps or intracavitary fibroids will not be picked-up by office sampling [8]. Although they are not life threatening, polyps and fibroids cause abnormal bleeding both before and after menopause. It is therefore relevant not to overlook benign focal lesions.

The value of ultrasound before, during, and after office endometrial sampling to improve relevant tissue yield will be discussed in this paper.

Ultrasonography before endometrial sampling

The indication for further testing in case of abnormal bleeding depends on different parameters: in postmenopausal women endometrial investigation may be indicated after a single episode of bleeding, whereas in younger women expectant management may be justified. After menopause, endometrial cancer is to be excluded first, whereas before menopause endometrial malignancy is much less likely. In women of reproductive age presenting with recurrent or persistent abnormal uterine bleeding, endometrial sampling may evidence endometrial hyperplasia, subacute endometritis or luteal dysfunction. However, this issue is beyond the scope of this paper. In this paper, it is assumed that further testing is clinically indicated. In case of (recurrent) abnormal uterine bleeding, the endometrial thickness is measured at transvaginal ultrasonography. If the endometrium is thin and uniform (Fig. 3), endometrial pathology is unlikely [9]. In those cases, endometrial sampling may not be necessary. The proposed threshold

for total endometrial thickness above which further testing is indicated ranges from 3 to 5 mm [10–12].

The evaluation of the endometrium by ultrasound is not limited to an endometrial thickness measurement, but should include a detailed evaluation of the endometrial features at unenhanced ultrasonography, color Doppler imaging, and, if indicated, fluid instillation sonography (FIS), according the International Endometrial Tumor Analysis terms and definitions [13]. If a focal intracavitary lesion is seen, blind sampling is not the diagnostic test of choice because most endometrial polyps and intracavitary fibroids are missed at office sampling [8]. A hysteroscopical resection of these lesions is a more appropriate approach (Fig. 4).

If a diffuse thickening of the endometrium is seen or if endometrial cancer is suspected, office endometrial sampling is indicated. The endometrial thickness at ultrasonography should be correlated with the tissue yield at sampling: the thicker the endometrium, the higher the tissue yield is expected to be [14]. The tissue yield is related to the histology: the highest tissue yield in endometrial cancer, and the lowest tissue yield in endometrial atrophy [14]. To obtain a representative endometrial biopsy, the uterine cavity should be sampled, from the fundus to the endocervical canal. Although the clinician usually feels when the tip of the device touches the fundus, there are some pitfalls. A cesarean section scar defect, extreme uterine retroversion, or an intracavitary fibroid may misleadingly give the impression that the tip of the sampling device touches the fundus (Fig. 5).

The uterine cavity length, the uterine flexion, and the possible presence of an intracavitary fibroid or a cesarean section scar defect assessed by transvaginal ultrasound enable the clinician to ascertain that the sampling device will be introduced deep enough and that the endometrial sample will be representative. One should be aware that sampling disturbs the ultrasound features of the endometrium [15]. The

Fig. 2 Endometrial cancer missed by Pipelle® sampling in case of **a** a small lesion hidden behind a benign focal lesion and **b** in case of intracavitary fluid

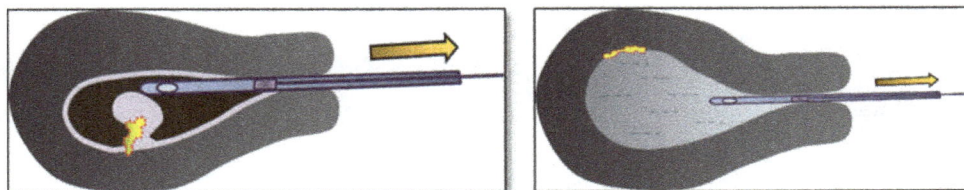

Fig. 4 Diagnostic algorithm

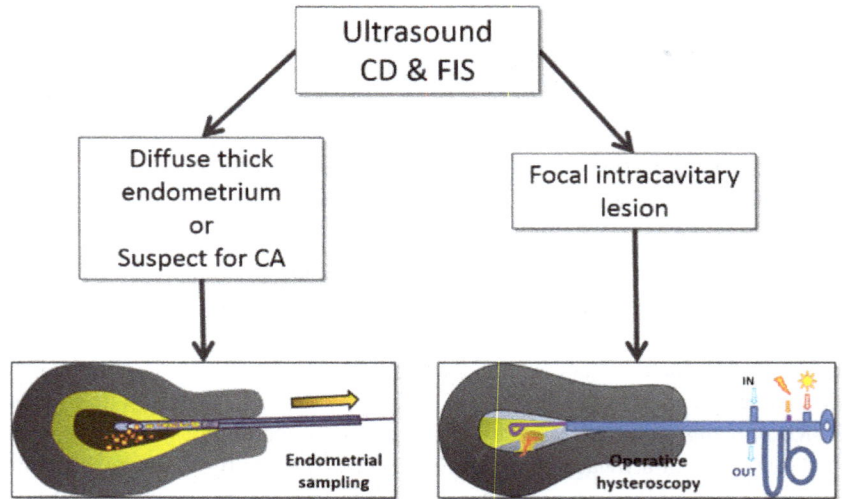

Fig. 5 Incomplete endometrial sampling in case of **a** cesarean scar defect, **b** severe uterine retroflection, **c** proximal benign focal intracavitary lesion

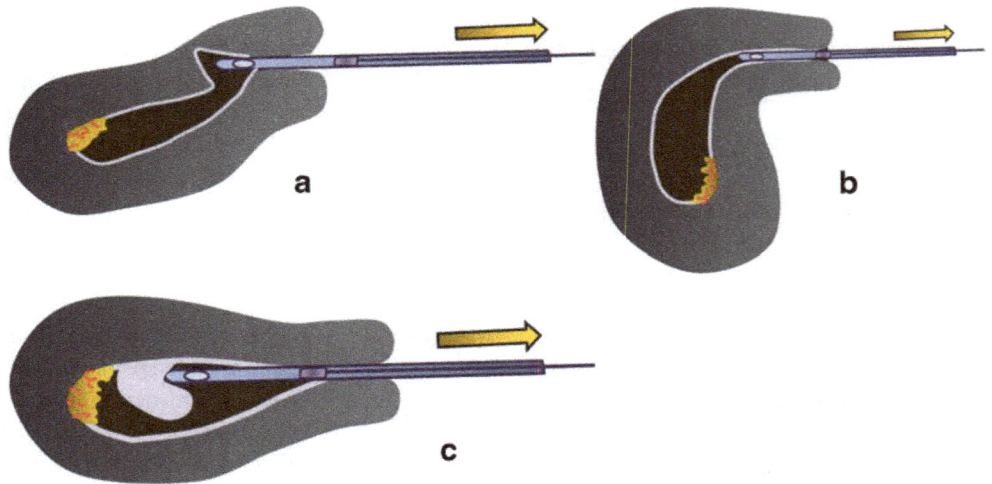

endometrial thickness, as well as other ultrasound characteristics such as the endometrial outline or the echogenicity of the endometrium is altered by the sampling procedure. This is another incentive to perform an ultrasound examination before proceeding with office endometrial biopsy.

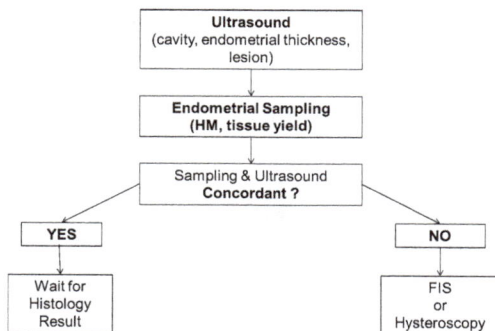

Fig. 6 Diagnostic algorithm based on ultrasound features and findings at endometrial sampling

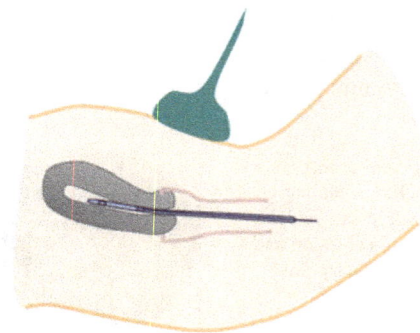

Fig. 7 Endometrial sampling under transabdominal ultrasound guidance

Fig. 8 Pipelle sampling in case of intracavitary fluid

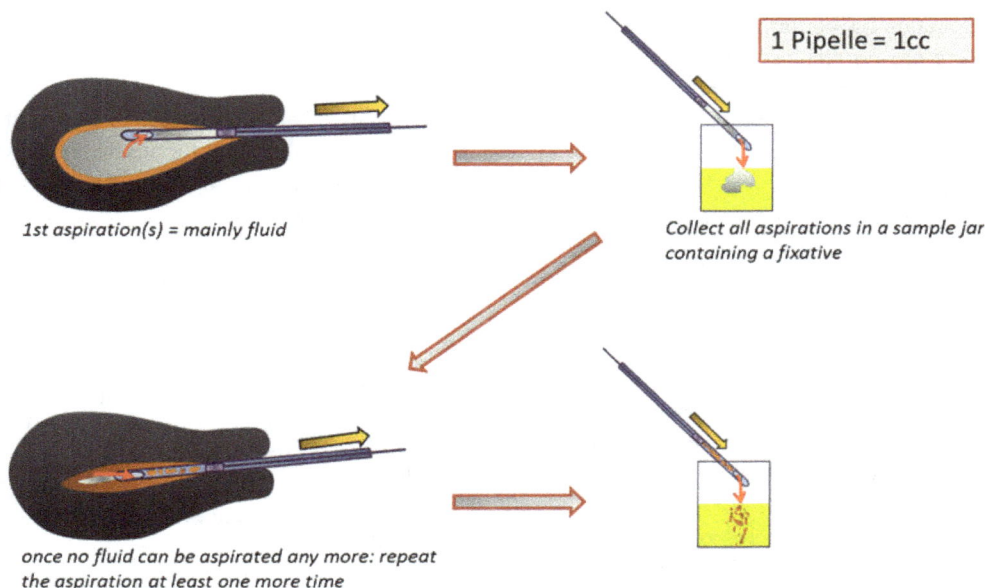

1st aspiration(s) = mainly fluid

Collect all aspirations in a sample jar containing a fixative

1 Pipelle = 1cc

once no fluid can be aspirated any more: repeat the aspiration at least one more time

Ultrasonography during endometrial sampling

After having checked that the hysterometry on the sampling device matches the presampling ultrasound cavity length estimation, the actual tissue aspiration can be started. A Pipelle® sampler is a transparent device, allowing the estimation of the tissue yield during aspiration [14]. Endometrial tissue is visible as small whitish lumps, and can usually easily be differentiated from blood, pus, or mucus within the sampling device. The estimation of the amount of tissue retrieved during sampling correlates well with the tissue yield estimation of the pathologist [14]. Implementing a strict procedure for endometrium biopsy, including presampling ultrasound examination and assessment of the tissue yield during sampling (scored from 1 to 4), in 257 consecutive women with abnormal bleeding, the median endometrial thickness at ultrasound and the median tissue yield score was 18.3 mm and score 4 in the endometrial cancer cases, compared with 11.5 mm and score 2 in endometrial polyp cases, and 3.9 mm and score 1 in endometrial atrophy [14]. If the tissue yield is concordant with the ultrasound findings (e.g., a thick endometrium and a high tissue yield), the histology result will most probably be reliable. If, on the other hand, the tissue yield is low in a patient with a thickened endometrium at ultrasonography, the lesion could have been missed and one cannot rely upon the histology result. Further testing, such as FIS with saline (SIS) or gel (GIS) [16], or hysteroscopy is needed (Fig. 6).

The insertion of the sampler may be difficult at times. This can be secondary to previous cervical surgery or due to retroversion of the uterus or to a cesarean section scar defect. In order to avoid a "fausse route" and to minimize patient's discomfort, endometrial sampling can be performed under ultrasound guidance. The direction of the sampler's insertion path is guided through transabdominal ultrasound (Fig. 7). This may be easier to do if the woman has some bladder filling.

Ultrasonography after endometrial sampling

Ultrasound examination after sampling should confirm the presampling ultrasound diagnosis: e.g., if the ultrasound image before sampling suggested the presence of blood or clots in the uterine cavity, an ultrasound examination after Pipelle®

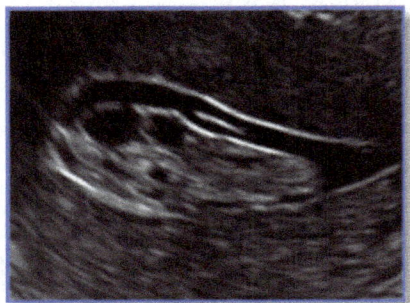

Fig. 9 Endometrial polyp diagnosed at fluid instillation sonography (FIS)

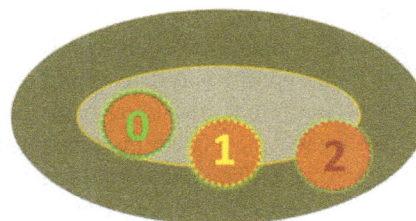

Fig. 10 Grading of intracavitary fibroids [13]

aspiration can confirm that the clots have disappeared and that there are no residual focal lesions. In case of intracavitary fluid, it is important that the sampling is repeated till no fluid can be aspirated any more. Thereafter, at least one additional aspiration is performed for endometrial tissue sampling (Fig. 8).

The woman will hardly experience pain as long as the tip of the sampler is surrounded by fluid and does not touch the cavity wall. When there is no fluid in the cavity anymore, the endometrial mucosa will be sucked against the tip of the sampler, causing patient's discomfort or pain, especially if the endometrium is thin. In case of a thick endometrium at ultrasound and low tissue yield during sampling, a missed focal intracavitary lesion is to be suspected. One can immediately proceed with FIS to detect or exclude a focal lesion (Fig. 9).

Both FIS and hysteroscopy have a similar diagnostic accuracy for the detection of endometrial polyps and intracavitary fibroids [17].

In case of a focal intracavitary lesion, the ultrasound report should also provide additional information to tailor the operation. If one or more polyps are diagnosed, their size and number may determine whether a resection is to be performed as an outpatient's procedure or in theater under general anesthesia or sedation. If one or more fibroids are diagnosed, each lesions' size, grade (Fig. 10), and number should be documented accurately to allow estimation of the technical complexity of the resection procedure [18–25].

A fibroid larger than 2 cm or protruding less than 50 % into the uterine cavity (grade 2) as well as the presence of more than one lesion are known to be technically challenging for the operative hysteroscopist. Ultrasound can give valuable information improving further management planning, such as the need for sedation or anesthesia, the expected operation time, and for informing the patient about the expected procedure's success rate (one or two step procedure).

Conclusion

Transvaginal ultrasound assessment of the uterine cavity informs the clinician if office endometrial sampling is indicated. If the endometrium is very thin and uniform, further testing may not be necessary. If a focal intracavitary lesion is detected, an operative hysteroscopy is warranted—not office sampling. The ultrasound examination also provides valuable information to plan the operative hysteroscopy. If endometrial sampling is to be performed, the ultrasound findings will improve sample quality. Incomplete insertion of the device can be avoided and the tissue yield during sampling can be anticipated by the endometrial thickness measured at ultrasound examination. The added value of ultrasound before,

during, and after endometrial sampling should be validated in future studies.

We conclude that integrating ultrasound in the diagnostic algorithm for uterine intracavitary pathology optimizes endometrial sampling and allows quality control of the sampling procedure.

Conflict of interest Thierry Van den Bosch, Dominique Van Schoubroeck, and Dirk Timmerman declare that they have no conflict of interest.

Declaration of interest The authors report no conflicts in interest. The authors alone are responsible for the content and writing of the paper.

References

1. Cornier E (1984) The Pipelle: a disposable device for endometrial biopsy. Am J Obstet Gynecol 148:109–110
2. Kaunitz AM, Masciello A, Ostrowski M, Rovira EZ (1988) Comparison of endometrial biopsy with the endometrial Pipelle and Vabra aspirator. J Reprod Med 33:427–431
3. Hill GA, Herbert CM 3rd, Parker RA, Wentz AC (1989) Comparison of late luteal phase endometrial biopsies using the Novak curette or PIPELLE endometrial suction curette. Obstet Gynecol 73:443–445
4. Stovall TG, Photopulos GJ, Poston WM, Ling FW, Sandles LG (1991) Pipelle endometrial sampling in patients with known endometrial carcinoma. Obstet Gynecol 77:954–956
5. Rodriguez GC, Yaqub N, King ME (1993) A comparison of the Pipelle device and the Vabra aspirator as measured by endometrial denudation in hysterectomy specimens: the Pipelle device samples significantly less of the endometrial surface than the Vabra aspirator. Am J Obstet Gynecol 168:55–59
6. Clark TJ, Mann CH, Shah HM, Khan KS, Song F, Gupta JK (2002) Accuracy of outpatient endometrial biopsy in the diagnosis of endometrial cancer: a systematic quantitative review. BJOG 109:313–321
7. Van den Bosch T, Cornelis A (1998) Endometrial malignancy missed by office sampling. Aust N Z J Obstet Gynaecol 38:1–2
8. Van den Bosch T, Vandendael A, Van Schoubroeck D, Wranz PAB, Lombard CJ (1995) Combining vaginal ultrasonography and office endometrial sampling in the diagnosis of endometrial disease in postmenopausal women. Obstet Gynecol 85:349–352
9. Van den Bosch T, Van Schoubroeck D, Vergote I, Moerman P, Amant F, Timmerman D (2007) A thin and regular endometrium on ultrasound is very unlikely in patients with endometrial malignancy. Ultrasound Obstet Gynecol 29:674–679
10. Smith-Bindman R, Kerlikowske K, Feldstein VA, Subak L, Scheidler J, Segal M, Brand R, Gracy D (1998) Endovaginal ultrasound to exclude endometrial cancer and other endometrial abnormalities. JAMA 280:1510–1517
11. Tabor A, Watt HC, Wald NJ (2002) Endometrial thickness as a test for endometrial cancer in women with postmenopausal vaginal bleeding. Obstet Gynecol 99:663–670
12. Timmermans A, Opmeer B, Khan K, Bachmann LM, Epstein E, Clark JT, Gupta JK, Bakour SH, Van den Bosch T, van Doorn HC, Cameron ST, Giusa MG, Dessole S, Dijkhuizen FPHLJ, ter Riet G, Mol WJ (2010) Endometrial thickness measurement for detecting endometrial cancer in women with postmenopausal bleeding: a systematic review and meta-analysis. Obstet Gynecol 116:160–167
13. Leone F, Timmerman D, Bourne T, Valentin L, Epstein E, Goldstein SR, Marret H, Parsons AK, Gull B, Istre O, Sepulveda W, Ferrazzi E,

Van den Bosch T (2010) Terms, definitions and measurements to describe the sonographic features of the endometrium and intrauterine lesions: a consensus opinion from the International Endometrial Tumor Analysis (IETA) group. Ultrasound Obstet Gynecol 35:103–112

14. Van den Bosch T, Van Schoubroeck D, Van Calster B, Cornelis A, Timmerman D (2012) Pre-sampling ultrasound evaluation and assessment of the tissue yield during sampling improves the diagnostic reliability of office endometrial biopsy. J Obstet Gynaecol 32:173–176

15. Van den Bosch T, Van Schoubroeck D, Timmerman D (2005) Ultrasound examination of the endometrium before and after Pipelle® endometrial sampling. Ultrasound Obstet Gynecol 26:283–286

16. Werbrouck E, Veldman J, Luts J, Van Huffel S, Van Schoubroeck D, Timmerman D, Van den Bosch T (2011) Detection of endometrial pathology using saline infusion sonography versus gel instillation sonography: a prospective cohort study. Fertil Steril 95:285–288

17. de Kroon C, De Bock GH, Dieben SWM, Jansen FW (2003) Saline contrast hydrosonography in abnormal uterine bleeding: a systematic review and metaanalysis. BJOG 110:938–947

18. Wamsteker K, Emanuel MH, de Kruif JH (1993) Transcervical hysteroscopic resection of submucous fibroids for abnormal uterine bleeding: results regarding the degree of intramural extension. Obstet Gynecol 82:736–740

19. Emanuel MH, Wamsteker K, Hart AA, Metz G, Lammes FB (1999) Long-term results of hysteroscopic myomectomy for abnormal uterine bleeding. Obstet Gynecol 93:743–748

20. Cravello L, Agostini A, Beerli M, Roger V, Bretelle F, Blanc B (2004) Results of hysteroscopic myomectomy. Gynecol Obstet Fertil 32:825–828, Article in French

21. Marret H, Cottier JP, Alonso AM, Giraudeau B, Body G, Herbreteau D (2005) Predictive factors for fibroids recurrence after uterine artery embolisation. BJOG 112:461–465

22. Di Spiezio SA, Mazzon I, Bramante S, Bettocchi S, Bifulco G, Guida M, Nappi C (2008) Hysteroscopic myomectomy: a comprehensive review of surgical techniques. Hum Reprod Update 14:101–119

23. Rovio PH, Helin R, Heinonen PK (2009) Long-term outcome of hysteroscopic endometrial resection with or without myomectomy in patients with menorrhagia. Arch Gynecol Obstet 279:159–163

24. Camanni M, Bonino L, Delpiano EM, Ferrero B, Migliaretti G, Deltetto F (2010) Hysteroscopic management of large symptomatic submucous uterine myomas. J Minim Invasive Gynecol 17:59–65

25. Lasmar RB, Xinmei Z, Indman PD, Celeste RK, Di Spiezio SA (2011) Feasibility of a new system of classification of submucous myomas: a multicenter study. Fertil Steril 95:2073–2077

31

Intraoperative transvaginal sonography: a novel approach for localization of deeper myomas during laparoscopic myomectomy

P .G Paul[1] · Dimple K. Ahluwalia[1] · Dhivya Narasimhan[1] · Gaurav Chopade[1] · Saurabh Patil[1] · Varsha Rengaraj[1] · Tanuka Das[1]

Abstract The aim of this study is to assess the use of intraoperative transvaginal ultrasonography (TVS) to locate deep myomas that were not identified on laparoscopic view. The design of this study is a prospective observational study. This study was conducted in private Advanced Endoscopy and Infertility Treatment Centre, Kerala, India. The study comprised of 84 patients who underwent laparoscopic myomectomy from January 2011 to December 2013 in whom intraoperative TVS was used as an intervention. The number of additional deeper myomas removed was calculated, and recurrence at 1 year was calculated. The total number of myomas enucleated was 390, and the additional myomas enucleated after intraoperative TVS were 94. The recurrence of myomas at 1-year follow-up was 7.1 %. Intraoperative TVS was helpful to the surgeon for identifying deeper myomas making the surgery more effective.

Keywords Myomas · Intraoperative TVS · Laparoscopic myomectomy

Introduction

Laparoscopic myomectomy was described for the first time in the late 1970s for subserous myomas [1]. In the early 1990s, the technique was developed to include removal of intramural myomas [2]. As endoscopic surgeons gained experience, they started performing laparoscopic myomectomy for multiple and larger myomas, irrespective of size, number, or location of myoma [3].

One of the difficulties of laparoscopic myomectomy is locating the deeper and smaller myomas especially those closer to the endometrium (type 3) according to the International Federation of Gynecology and Obstetrics (FIGO) classification [4]. Laparoscopic myomectomy carries increased risk of residual myomas because unlike laparotomy, the uterus cannot be palpated to locate very small myomas. Postoperative recurrence may be either due to enlarged residual myomas or newly formed myomas. There are studies that show increased risk of recurrence (16.7–51.4 %) after 5 years of laparoscopic myomectomy [5, 6]. This increases the chance of reoperation and decreases the chances of symptom relief after the surgery. Several studies have shown that large myomas are associated with significant reduction in pregnancy rate after IVF [7, 8]. Khalaf et al. showed that smaller myomas ($\leq$5 cm) not encroaching endometrial cavity were found to significantly reduce ongoing pregnancy rate at each cycle of IVF by 40 %; similarly, Stovall et al. concluded that implantation and pregnancy rates were one half that of matched controls [9, 10].

Technical problems in identifying deeper myomas lead to misplaced incision causing more blood loss, myometrial integrity, and increased operating time. Good preoperative myoma mapping is helpful, but it is difficult to locate deeper and smaller intramural myomas intraoperatively [11]. Intraoperative location of myomas with laparoscopic contact ultrasound probes can be done [12]. But it is costly and not available as standard ultrasound probes. To overcome this, we attempted to use intraoperative transvaginal ultrasonography (TVS) with

✉ P .G Paul
drpaulpg@gmail.com

[1] Centre for Advanced Endoscopy and Infertility, Paul's Hospital, Vattekkattu Road, Kaloor, Kochi, Kerala 682 017, India

a simultaneous laparoscopic view to locate deep-seated and smaller myomas and to enucleate additional residual myomas.

The primary aim of the study was to assess the effectiveness of intraoperative transvaginal ultrasonography to locate deeper and smaller myomas, which were not identified on laparoscopic view.

Material and methods

This was a prospective observational study of women who underwent laparoscopic myomectomy for uterine leiomyomas from January 2011 to December 2013 when intraoperative TVS was done to identify the additional myomas.

For all patients, preoperative TVS and transabdominal scans were performed, and inclusion criteria were:

1) Patients with four or more myomas.
2) Patients with type 3 myoma, irrespective of the number of myomas (myoma that contacts the endometrium and is 100 % intramural) according to the FIGO classification [4].

Exclusion criteria were:

1) Patients with other coexisting diseases like endometriosis and severe pelvic adhesion.
2) Patients with submucous myomas type 0, 1, and 2 according to FIGO classification.
3) Postmenopausal women.

Laparoscopic myomectomy was not limited by factors such as location (anterior/posterior wall) and depth (subserosal/intramural). Data was collected on demographic characteristics, and the chief indication and symptoms were analyzed. The study was approved by the ethical committee of Paul's Hospital for the intervention.

Preoperatively GnRH agonists were not used before surgery because we found that degeneration of the myoma made the surgical dissection difficult. Postoperative patients were followed up with TVS by the first author for recurrence of myomas at 1 year, and any myoma of more than 2 cm was considered as recurrence (Fig. 1).

Fig. 1 Flow chart of patients from selection to 1 year after myomectomy

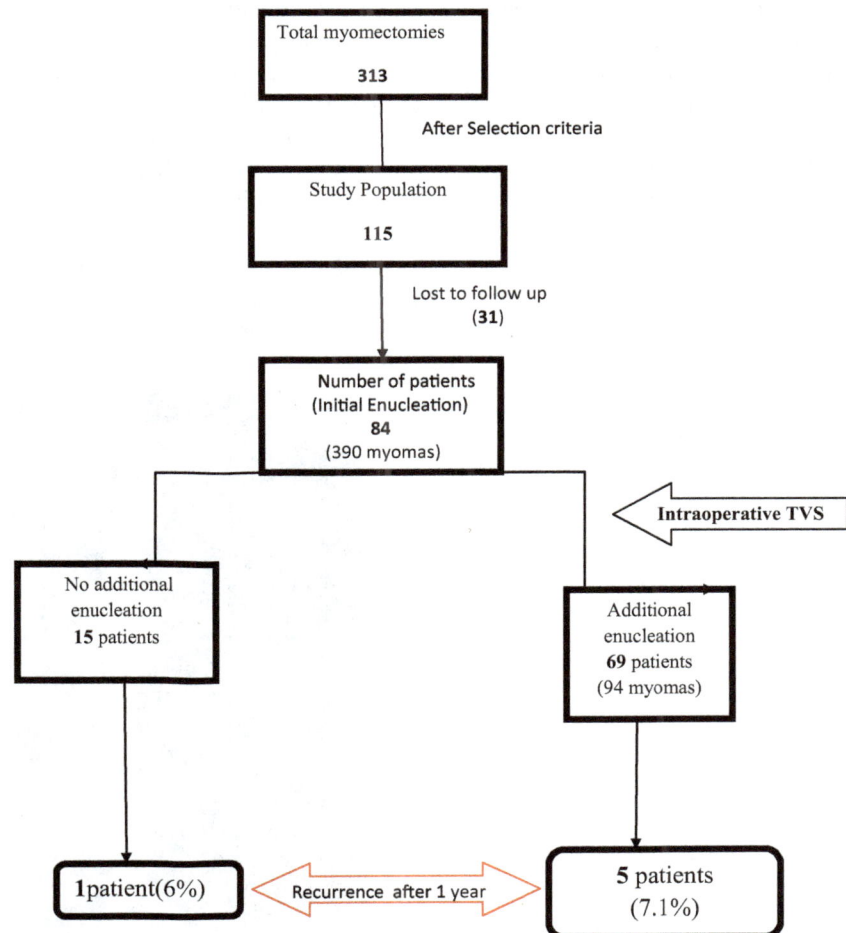

Fig. 2 Deep intramural myoma
mapped preoperatively

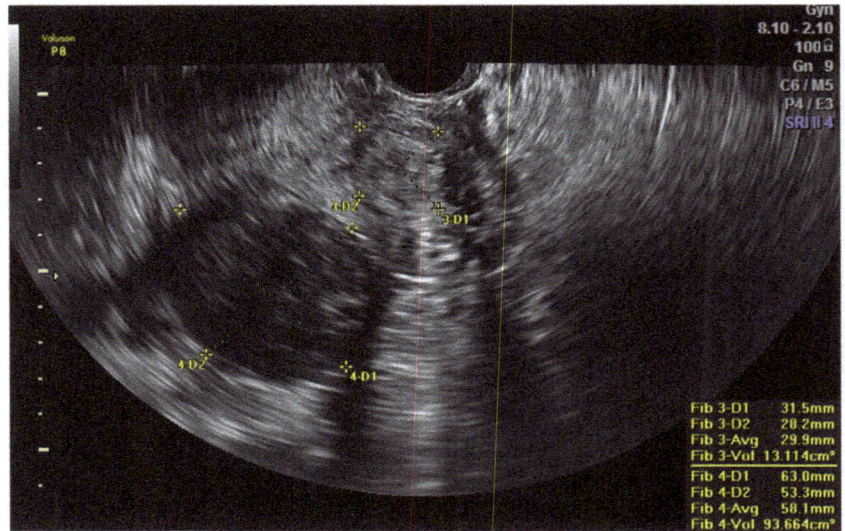

Surgical technique

All procedures were performed by the first author using similar technique under general anesthesia, as described in our previous publications [13, 14]. Hysteroscopy was performed to look for distortion of the endometrial cavity and to exclude any undiagnosed submucous myoma on ultrasonography. Entry into the abdominal cavity through an umbilical incision or a higher one in the case of larger uteri was accomplished using a 10-mm trocar. In patients with a previous history of an open surgery or in cases where intra-abdominal adhesions were suspected, entry under direct vision using a Ternamian Endotip (Karl Storz, Tuttlingen, Germany) was performed. Two ancillary 5-mm trocars lateral to the right and left epigastric vessels and a median supra-pubic trocar were inserted. Vasopressin 20 IU diluted in 60 ml of saline was infused into

the myometrium of the uterus to reduce the bleeding. A transverse or vertical incision was made over the myoma that was preoperatively mapped (Fig. 2) with Harmonic Ace (Ethicon Endosurgery, Cincinnati, Ohio).The myoma was kept under traction using myoma spiral and dissected with Harmonic Ace. The myomectomy site was sutured intracorporeally with polyglactin 910 (Vicryl, Ethicon, India) or 1-0 braided Lactomer (Polysorb, Tyco Healthcare) in single or double layers depending upon the depth of muscle defect. The myomas were removed with electromechanical morcellator (Karl Storz, Gynaecare, Tuttlingen, Germany). After enucleating all visible myomas, the intraoperative TVS was done, and additional myomas were identified.

Intraoperative TVS was done by either a second or third author and confirmed by an operating surgeon (first author). All preoperative TVS were done by the first author. We used

Fig. 3 Deep intramural myoma
identified by intraoperative
sonography

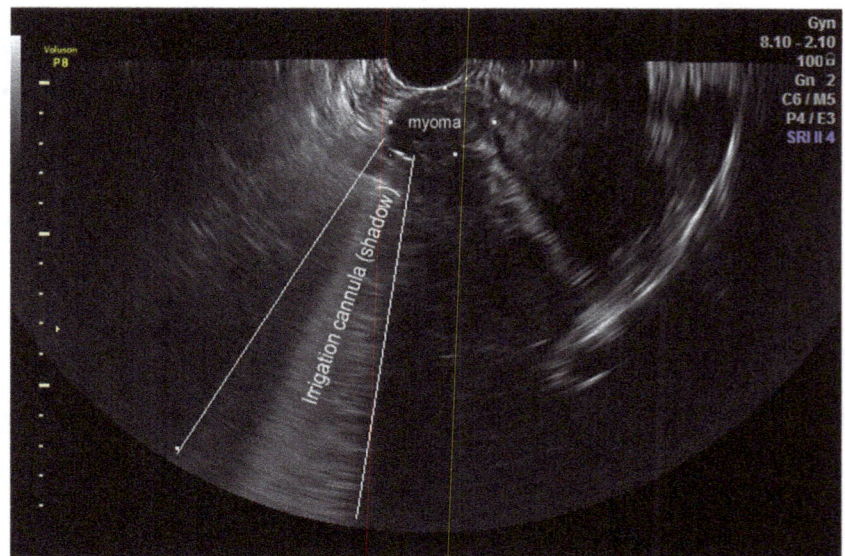

ultrasonic device Voluson E (GE Healthcare, Beethoven Street, 239 D m- 42,655, Solingen, Germany) with TVS probe RIC5-9W-RS/Gyn and detection frequency set at 8–14 MHz. The vaginal probe was covered with a sterile cover, and the whole uterus was scanned to identify any residual myoma. The laparoscopic surgeon (first author) filled the pouch of Douglas with normal saline to make an acoustic window for better ultrasonic visualization. The myoma identified on transvaginal ultrasound was located laparoscopically with a suction irrigation cannula by trial and error. The irrigating fluid from suction irrigation cannula seen as a comet shape on transvaginal ultrasound helps in the localization of the myoma (Fig. 3). The myoma thus identified was enucleated laparoscopically as described before (Fig. 4).

Results

The total number of myomectomies performed from January 2011 to December 2013 was 313. One hundred fifteen patients met inclusion criteria, but 31 patients were lost to follow-up; of these, 84 patients who met the inclusion criteria were included in the study. The mean age of our patients was 33.40 ± 5.13 and mean BMI was 32. The proportion of parity was 52 %. The primary preoperative indications were abdominal pain in 35 patients (41.7 %) followed by primary infertility in 22 patients (13.1 %) and menorrhagia in 14 patients (16.7 %) and as shown in Table 1.

The size of the myomas enucleated is shown in Table 2. The average number of myomas enucleated per patient was 4.64. Sixty-three patients had four or more myomas. Twenty-one patients had less than four myomas, but these were all type 3.

The total number of myomas removed was 390. The mean size of the myomas removed was 3.28 cm.

The average blood loss in milliliter was 163.86 ± 18.92 in patients with intraoperative TVS, whereas 148.18 ± 21.44

Table 1 Demographic characteristics/chief complaints

Demographic characteristics	
Age (years)	33.40 ± 5.13
BMI (mean)	32
Chief complaints	No. of patients
Abdominal pain	35 (41.7 %)
Primary infertility	22 (26.2 %)
Menorrhagia	14 (16.6 %)
Secondary infertility	4 (4.8 %)
Dysmenorrhea	5 (5.9 %)
Dysmenorrhea and menorrhagia	2 (2.4 %)
Irregular bleeding	2 (2.4 %)

without intraoperative TVS. The mean drop in hemoglobin concentration after surgery was 1 g%. The total time duration (induction to closure) was 134 ± 27.25 min in cases where intraoperative TVS was performed and 110 ± 21.02 min in cases without intraoperative TVS.

The additional myomas removed after performing intraoperative TVS were 94. These were visible during preoperative TVS also. Size (range) of the additional myomas removed was 2.5 (1.5–3.5 cm). Average number of additional myomas enucleated per patient was 1.1. Out of 94 additional myomas removed, 86 were FIGO type III and 8 were type IV. Recurrence of myoma at 1-year follow-up on ultrasound examination was 7.1 %.

Discussion

In patients with multiple myomas, an experienced laparoscopic surgeon can remove all visible myomas but identification of deeper and smaller myomas are difficult due to lack of tactile perception. The better way to overcome this limitation is the

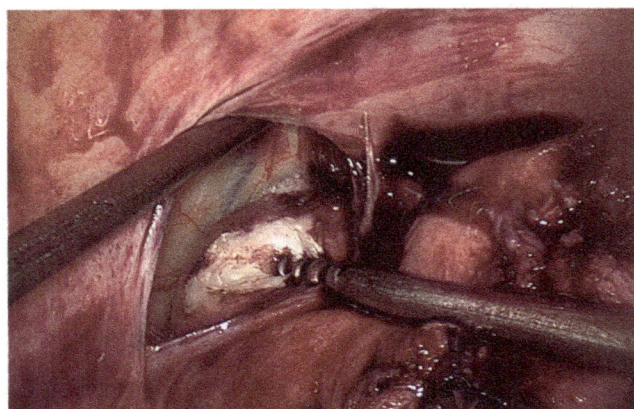

Fig. 4 Laparoscopic enucleation of deep intramural myoma

Table 2 Total number of myomas

Size (cm)	Number of myomas
<5	324 (83.08 %)
5–6	20 (5.13 %)
6–7	20 (5.13 %)
7–8	9 (2.31 %)
8	9 (2.31 %)
9	3 (0.77 %)
10	1 (0.26 %)
12	1 (0.26 %)
14	3 (0.77 %)
Mean size = 3.28 cm	Total—390 myomas

Table 3 Intraoperative findings

Intraoperative findings	With intraoperative TVS	Without intraoperative TVS
Total time duration (min)	134.63 ± 27.25	110 ± 21.02
Total blood loss (ml)	163.86 ± 18.92	148.18 ± 21.44
Number of additional myomas removed	1.1	

use of intraoperative ultrasonography. The aim of the study was to assess the effectiveness of intraoperative TVS to locate deeper and smaller myomas that were not identified on laparoscopic view. This is in contrast to a similar study where an intraoperative contact probe was used. However, this method is costly and not easily available [12]. To our knowledge, this is the first study where TVS is used intraoperatively to localize deep/hidden myomas.

In our study, mean size of myomas removed was 3.28 cm, which is not considered significant by Pritts et al. in his review article. Most of our patients were having a long duration of infertility and planning to go for IVF and that was the reason for removing smaller myomas. The size of the myomas removed is similar to other studies [9, 10, 15]. Additional myomas that were not visible laparoscopically were detected by intraoperative TVS in 69 of 84 patients. The mean size of the additional enucleated myomas was 2.5 (1.5 to 3.5 cm). In a similar study where intraoperative contact ultrasound probe was used, 25 additional myomas with a median diameter of 1.2 cm were enucleated in a group of 42 patients which is comparable to our study [12].

In our study, the operative time was more when intraoperative TVS was done due to the time taken for sonography and the surgical time for enucleating additional myomas. The blood loss was also more due to increased duration of the surgery. (Table 3) But blood loss was not clinically significant, and duration can be minimized with experience in intraoperative TVS.

Causes of postoperative recurrence are considered to be either enlargement of residual myomas or formation of new ones. Postoperative residual myomas greatly affect the recurrence rate. Some studies have reported that laparoscopic myomectomy is associated with a higher recurrence rate as compared with laparotomy recurrence rate [16, 17]. Doriot et al. and Hiroto Shimanuki et al. defined recurrence of a myoma >2 cm with transvaginal ultrasonography to be significant in their study after laparoscopic myomectomy [12]. In a study by Rossetti et al. which compares recurrence of myomas after 6 months in the abdominal and the laparoscopic group, there was a recurrence of 27 % in the laparoscopic group as compared to 23 % in the abdominal group [16]. In our study, recurrence at 1-year follow-up was 7.1 % that is lower than the above studies. In our study, recurrence was due to the formation of new ones as we had removed visible myomas.

The intraoperative ultrasound allowed precise localization of the myoma and determination of the best hysterotomy incision. A suboptimal incision would have caused greater trauma to the normal myometrium, as well as increased operating time for laparoscopic reconstruction of the uterus following the myomectomy. The other option would have been converting to an open procedure to enable palpation of the location of the known myomas and making an appropriate incision. Laparoscopic myomectomy is a well-accepted surgical approach for selected patients [16]. The intraoperative TVS allowed the surgeon to complete the myomectomy laparoscopically without tactile information.

Transvaginal sonography is a widely available imaging modality that every gynecologist is well versed with although there can be an interobserver variation. Its novel use intraoperatively to localize deep-seated myomas enables the surgeon to complete the myomectomy laparoscopically, despite the absence of tactile sensation. Limitation of the study was a lack of randomization and small sample size due to lost to follow-up (Fig. 1) and short follow-up time (1 year).

Conclusion

Intraoperative TVS is helpful to the surgeon for identifying deeper and smaller myomas, thus making the surgery more effective. Hence, intraoperative use of transvaginal sonography for patients with multiple and deep-seated myomas is advantageous.

Conflict of interest The authors declare that they have no competing interests. The authors alone handle the content and writing of the paper.

Informed consent All procedures followed were approved by the ethical standards of the responsible committee on human experimentation (institutional and national) and in accordance with the Helsinki Declaration of 1975, as revised in 2000(5). Informed consent was obtained from all patients for being included in the study.

Authors' contributions Dr. P.G Paul was the operating surgeon responsible for the planning and conduct of research work. Dr. Dimple K. Ahluwalia and Dr. Dhivya Narasimhan were the assistant surgeons assigned in performing ultrasound during surgeries and conducting studies. Dr. Gaurav Chopade performed statistical analysis and also helped in conducting studies. Dr. Saurabh Patil took charge of the reporting and review of literature. Dr. Varsha Rengaraj and Dr. Tanuka Das were responsible for the preparation of the manuscript.

References

1. Semm K, Mettler L, et al (1980) Technical progress in pelvic surgery via operative laparoscopy. Am J Obstet Gynecol 138:121–127

2. Daniell JF, Gurley LD, et al (1991) Laparoscopic treatment of clinically significant symptomatic uterine myomas. J Gynecol. Surg 7: 37–39

3. Sinha R, Hegde A, Mahajan C, Dubey N, Sundaram M (2008) Laparoscopic myomectomy: do size, number, and location of the myomas form limiting factors for laparoscopic myomectomy? J Minim Invasive Gynecol 15:292–300

4. Munro MG et al (2011) FIGO Working Group on Menstrual Disorders: FIGO classification system (PALM-COEIN) for causes of abnormal uterine bleeding in nongravid women of reproductive age. Int J of Gynecol & Obstet. 113:3–13. doi:10.1016/j.ijgo.2010.11.011

5. Doridot V, Dubisson J, Chapron C, et al (2001) Recurrence of leiomyomata after laparoscopic myomectomy. J Am Assoc Gynecol Laparosc 8:495–500

6. Nehzat FR, Roemisch M, Nezhat CH, et al (2001) Recurrence rate after laparoscopic myomectomy. J Am Assoc Gynecol Laparosc 8: 495–500

7. Benecke C, Kruger TF, Siebert TI, Van der Merwe JP, Steyn DW (2005) Effect of fibroids on fertility in patients undergoing assisted reproduction. A structured literature review. Gynecol Obstet Investig 59:225–230

8. Pritts EA, Parker WH, Olive DL (2009) Fibroids and infertility: an updated systematic review of the evidence. Fertil Steril 91:1215–1223

9. Khalaf Y, Ross C, El-Toukhy TH, Seed RP, Braude P, et al (2006) The effect of small intramural fibroids on the cumulative outcome of assisted conception. Hum Reprod 21:2640–2044

10. Stovall DW, Parrish SB, Van Voorhis BJ, et al (1998) Uterine leiomyomas reduce the efficacy of assisted reproduction cycles: results of a matched follow-up. Study; Hum Reprod vol.13(no.1): 192–197

11. Dubuisson JB, Fauconnier A (2007) Laparoscopic myomectomy. In: Atlas of operative laparoscopy and hysteroscopy. 3rd edn, Informa healthcare, U.K, p. 235

12. Shimanuki H et al (2006) Effectiveness of intraoperative ultrasound in reducing recurrent fibroids during laparoscopic myomectomy. J Reprod Med 51:683–688

13. Paul PG, Koshy A, Thomas T, et al (2006) Pregnancy outcomes following laparoscopic myomectomy and single layer myometrial closure. Hum Reprod 21:3278–3281

14. Paul PG, Koshy A, Thomas T, et al (2006) Laparoscopic myomectomy: feasibility and safety—a retrospective study of 762 cases. Gynecol Surg 3:97–102

15. Liselotte M, Thoralf Schollmeyer E, et al (2005) Update on laparoscopic myomectomy. Gynecol Surg 2:173–177

16. Rosette A, Sizzi O, et al (2001) Long-term results of laparoscopic myomectomy: recurrence rate in comparison with abdominal myomectomy. Hum Reprod 16:770–774

17. Miller CE et al (2000) Myomectomy. Comparison of open and laparoscopic techniques. Obstet Gynynecol Clin North Am 27: 407–420

32

Ultrasound-assisted intraoperative localization and laparoscopic management of a previously missed unruptured retroperitoneal ectopic pregnancy

Athanasios Protopapas · Nikolaos Akrivos · Stavros Athanasiou · Ioannis Chatzipapas · Aikaterini Domali · Dimitrios Loutradis

Abstract Primary retroperitoneal ectopic pregnancy represents an extremely unusual entity with a rather obscure pathogenesis. Implantation in the retroperitoneal space has been reported to occur both spontaneously and with use of assisted reproduction techniques. The pelvic and the upper retroperitoneum have both been involved, and implantation in the most unusual anatomic sites has been reported. The majority of retroperitoneal gestations are located close to large blood vessels, and laparotomy is performed because of the high risk of massive hemorrhage. Few cases have been treated with laparoscopy so far. We report the case of an early first-trimester retroperitoneal broad ligament live pregnancy occurring after spontaneous conception in a patient who had a history of an ipsilateral tubal ectopic pregnancy, previously treated with laparoscopic right salpingectomy. Current gestation had been missed during initial laparoscopy, and was located and removed during a repeat laparoscopic procedure under intraoperative ultrasonographic guidance.

Keywords Retroperitoneal pregnancy · Abdominal pregnancy · Ectopic pregnancy · Laparoscopy

Introduction

Ectopic pregnancy occurs in 1.5–2 % of all gestations, and is one of the major causes of maternal mortality during the first trimester of pregnancy, accounting for 6 % of all pregnancy-related deaths [1]. Most ectopic pregnancies (95 %) are located in the fallopian tubes, whereas the ovary and abdominal cavity are less frequently involved [1]. Abdominal pregnancy is the rarest form of ectopic pregnancy with an incidence of 1.3 % amongst all ectopics, and mortality rates are seven times higher than in non-abdominal cases [2, 3]. Abdominal pregnancies have been classified as either primary or secondary. Most abdominal pregnancies originate as tubal or ovarian pregnancies that rupture into the peritoneal cavity, where they re-implant [4]. A small fraction of the reported cases occur as a result of primary implantation either in the peritoneal cavity or the retroperitoneum [4].

The occurrence of an ectopic pregnancy in a retroperitoneal location is very rare. In 1938, the incidence of this condition had been reported to be 1 in 183,900 pregnancies [5]. To date, less than 25 well-documented cases of primary retroperitoneal pregnancy implantation have been reported in the medical literature. Development of an ectopic pregnancy in a retroperitoneal location has been reported to occur in the most unusual anatomic sites, such as the rectovaginal space [6], the obturator fossa [7], between the leaves of the broad ligament [8], at the level of the right paracolic sulcus [9], above the inferior vena cava [10], in the upper retroperitoneum [11], and even attached to the head of the pancreas [12]. Both spontaneous conception and assisted reproductive technologies (IUI and IVF-ET) have been implicated in the retroperitoneal development of ectopic pregnancies [6, 12–14]. Gestational age at first diagnosis and clinical presentations may vary considerably, from the asymptomatic woman in her early first trimester of pregnancy to the hemodynamically unstable patient with an advanced ruptured ectopic gestation presenting with life-threatening retroperitoneal hemorrhage. As a result, management strategies should be tailored to the individual patient. Laparotomy, laparoscopy, and medical treatment with

A. Protopapas (✉) · N. Akrivos · S. Athanasiou · I. Chatzipapas · A. Domali · D. Loutradis
1st University Department of Obstetrics and Gynecology of the University of Athens, "Alexandra" Hospital, 80 Queen Sophie Ave., 11528 Athens, Greece
e-mail: prototha@otenet.gr

methotrexate have all been used in the treatment of retroperitonal pregnancies of various locations.

We report the case of an early first trimester retroperitoneal pregnancy occurring after spontaneous conception in a patient who had a history of an ipsilateral tubal ectopic pregnancy, previously treated with laparoscopic right salpingectomy. The current ectopic was developing between the leaves of the right broad ligament. The living retroperitoneal gestation had been missed during initial laparoscopy, and was located and removed during a repeat laparoscopic procedure under intraoperative ultrasonographic guidance.

Case report

A 31-year-old woman presented to our department with a 6-week history of amenorrhea and a positive pregnancy test for routine antenatal care. Her medical history was unremarkable. Her obstetric history included a right tubal ectopic pregnancy managed by laparoscopic salpingectomy, followed by a term normal vaginal delivery of a healthy infant.

At presentation, the patient was asymptomatic and hemodynamically stable. Transvaginal sonography at 6^{+3} weeks, showed an empty uterine cavity. A gestational sac with embryonic heart activity was demonstrated to the right side of the uterus and in contact with the uterine fundus. On clinical examination, no vaginal bleeding was observed, and no lower abdominal or adnexal pain was elicited during bimanual examination. β-hCG levels were 7,450 mIU/ml, whereas her hemoglobin levels were within normal limits.

With the possible diagnosis of a right cornual pregnancy, the patient was scheduled for laparoscopic evaluation and management. At laparoscopy, the uterus was found slightly enlarged. The fundus was of normal shape and contour. The left adnexa and right ovary were normal. The right tube was found amputated at the level of the isthmus. No evidence of an ectopic intraperitoneal pregnancy was found anywhere in the pelvis, and the procedure was completed without any further intervention.

The following day, a repeat pelvic ultrasound confirmed once more the presence of an ongoing live pregnancy in contact with the right uterine cornu. Furthermore, levels of β-hCG were rising (9,832 mIU/ml). Assuming that we had failed to locate the pregnancy during our previous laparoscopy, we decided for a second attempt, and the patient was taken again to the operating theater.

At first, hysteroscopy was performed, but no pregnancy sac was seen in the uterine cavity or near the right ostium. Laparoscopy, this time under ultrasound guidance, followed. Initial laparoscopic findings were again identical to those described above (Fig. 1). With the aid of the transvaginal ultrasound probe, we identified once more the fetal sac to the right of the uterine fundus and managed to locate its exact position below and caudally to the right round ligament by carefully probing with a grasper the anterior leaf of the broad ligament, a maneuver that distorted the ultrasound image of the underlying pregnancy sac.

The round ligament and the anterior leaf of the broad ligament were opened above this area which was infiltrated with diluted vasopressin to reduce blood loss (Figs. 2 and 3). The reproperitoneal space was carefully dissected and a $3 \times 2.5 \times 2$ cm bulging mass was identified, arising from the right side of the uterine corpus (Figs. 4 and 5). Further dissection of the mass revealed the presence of a gestational sac (Figs. 6 and 7) through which an intact embryo could be clearly seen (Fig. 8). The sac was opened and the embryo along with the trophoblastic tissue were removed (Figs. 9 and 10). After evacuation of its trophoblastic contents, a fibrous capsule could be clearly identified. This structure had no communication with the uterine cavity (Fig. 11). Hemostasis was accomplished with bipolar diathermy and the broad and round ligaments were reconstructed with interrupted absorbable sutures (Fig. 12).

Our patient made an uneventful recovery and was discharged from our hospital on the second postoperative day. β-hCG levels were measured weekly and within 4 weeks they had returned to prepregnancy levels.

Discussion

Retroperitoneal ectopic pregnancy represents an extremely unusual entity with a rather obscure pathogenesis. Its incidence remains largely unknown mainly as a result of the frequent false reporting of abdominal intraperitoneal ectopic gestations with peritoneal invasion, as true retroperitoneal pregnancies. In the case of broad ligament ectopic pregnancy, according to Champion and Tessitore, the anatomical landmarks that surround the ectopic sac should include (a) the uterus medially, (b) the pelvic side walls laterally, (c) the pelvic floor inferiorly, and (d) the uterine tube or round ligament of the uterus superiorly [5]. These were exactly the boundaries in our case. To our opinion, the overlying peritoneum should also be found intact in order to confirm the diagnosis of a true retroperitoneal gestation.

Nevertheless, it is rather difficult to come up with a convincing explanation of how the embryo implanted in the retroperitoneal space in our case, as in others with similar locations. The patient conceived spontaneously and her only uterine surgery was a laparoscopic salpingectomy that preceded a normal-term vaginal delivery. The presence of a very small fistulous tract, resulting from past thermal injury during salpingectomy, cannot be entirely excluded as a causal factor. Nevertheless, the sac was found sufficiently distal to the tubal stump to support such a hypothesis. Another possible explanation, proposed by several investigators, is that the fertilized

Fig. 1–12 The film of
the procedure

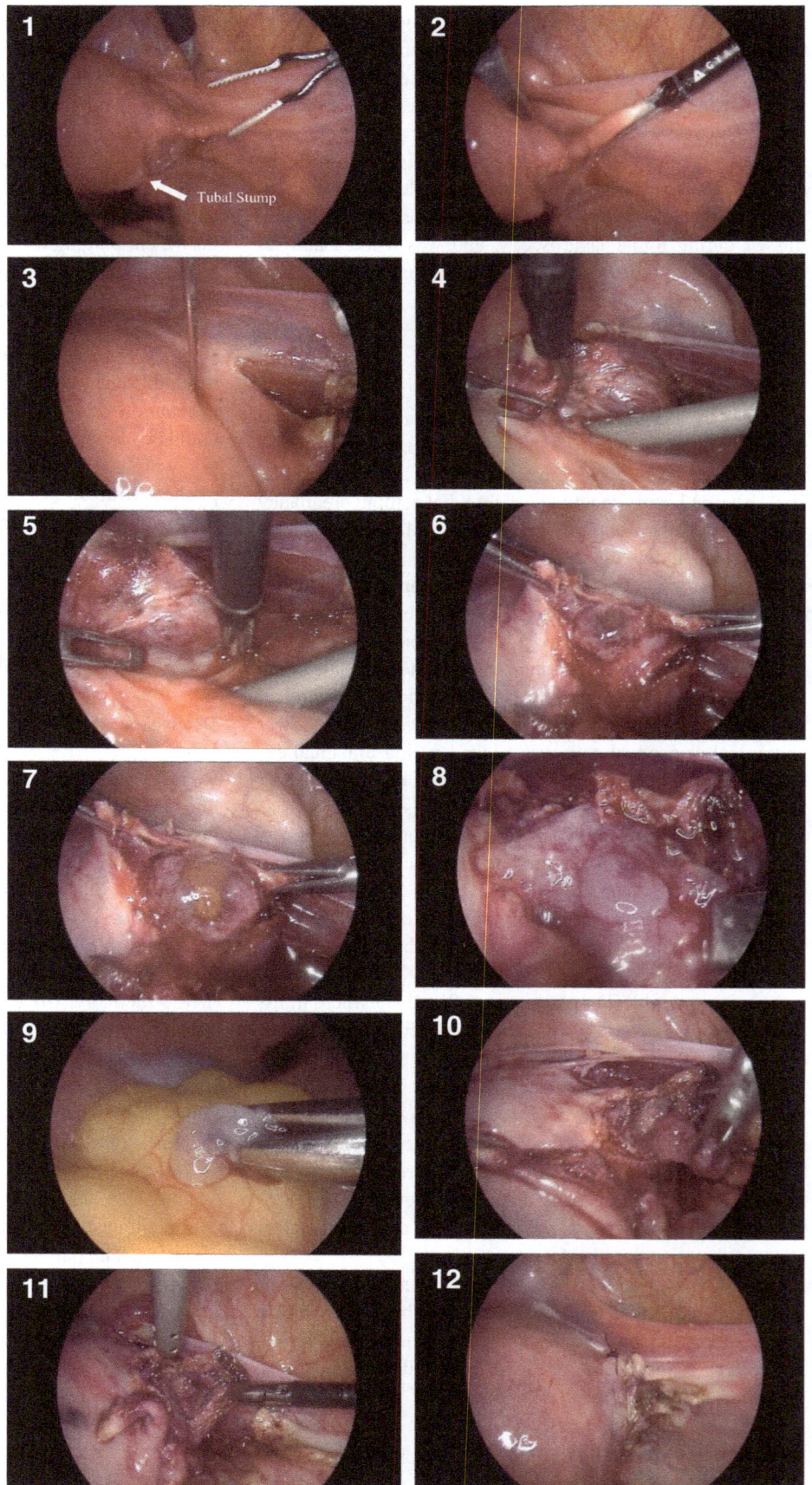

ovum may have reached the retroperitoneal space via the lymphatic system [7, 14, 15]. This hypothesis is supported by finding lymphatic tissue with the ectopic mass [15]. The transperitoneal route of implantation of the ectopic to the retroperitoneum through trophoblastic invasion provides a third yet not very convincing mechanism in our case, taking into account three factors: presence of an intact tubal stump, presence of healthy peritoneum above the sac, and conception occurring without use of assisted reproduction techniques.

Assisted reproductive techniques (both IVF-ET and IUI) appear to increase the risk of an ectopic pregnancy and thus implantation at unusual sites, which may be difficult to diagnose and have a high risk of life-threatening complications. Four mechanisms have been suggested for the abdominal location of an ectopic pregnancy in IVF-ET patients: spontaneous retrograde migration of the embryo after intrauterine transfer, iatrogenic placement of embryos in the retroperitoneal space at the time of transfer due to uterine perforation, retroperitoneal implantation through a fistulous tract, and transfer of the embryo from the uterine cavity to the retroperitoneal space through lymphatic channels [6, 7, 11].

Most of the reported cases of retroperitoneal pregnancies are located close to large blood vessels and the decision to dissect out the gestational tissue should not be taken without appropriate patient preparation and blood bank coverage. In the majority of such cases, laparotomy is performed because of the high risk of massive hemorrhage [11, 12, 16, 17]. The same applies naturally to cases with signs of acute and life-threatening intra-abdominal bleeding. Laparoscopic management has not been applied frequently, because of the risk of uncontrollable bleeding due to extensive trophoblastic invasion of the retroperitoneal vasculature. The incidence of deep trophoblastic infiltration of large retroperitoneal vessels has not been clearly reported in the existing literature. Nevertheless, there have been few reports of successful laparoscopic management of early retroperitoneal ectopic gestations, such as ours [3, 6, 10, 18], including a case with implantation of the sac on the inferior vena cava [19]. The laparoscopic approach is feasible and should be the treatment of choice, in hemodynamically stable patients without signs of rupture. Before attempting laparoscopic management of such cases, exclusion of large retroperitoneal vascular infiltration with the assistance of MRI may be necessary, especially in more advanced gestations. To our opinion, rupture of a retroperitoneal gestation is a contraindication for laparoscopic management as it results in a difficult to control, narrow operative field due to excessive bleeding from neovascularization. Injection of dilute vasopressin may assist in the dissection of the gestational sac, from surrounding structures, but one has to keep in mind that hemostasis should be meticulous, as the risk of a postoperative hematoma formation is high. Any gynecologist attempting such a procedure should be well-trained, have a thorough knowledge of the retroperitoneal anatomy, and be ready to convert to laparotomy in case of intraoperative complications or uncontrollable bleeding. Close cooperation with a general surgeon and/or an interventional radiologist may prove invaluable to safely conclude these procedures.

Adjuvant treatment with methotrexate, systemic or through selective arterial embolization has been suggested to control the risk of bleeding from the placental bed and to avoid the possibility of persistent trophoblastic tissue [3, 20]. Although surgery remains the mainstay of treatment for abdominal ectopic pregnancies, there are also case reports of early abdominal pregnancies being treated successfully with systemic methotrexate, leading to its resorption without the need for further surgery [21]. Factors that are associated with failure of medical management include initial β-hCG values greater than 5,000 mUI/mL, ultrasound detection of a moderate or large amount of free peritoneal fluid, the presence of fetal cardiac activity, and a pretreatment increase in the β-hCG level of more than 50 % over a 48-h period [1, 3, 5]. Our case presented with three out of four of the above-mentioned contraindications for medical management. Furthermore, the patient was hemodynamically stable, and this permitted the use of the transvaginal probe to assist in the exact localization of the ectopic gestation. Other preoperative imaging techniques, and in particular magnetic resonance imaging (MRI), may prove useful in guiding operative maneuvers but they are costly and not always readily available. It is very probable that the second laparoscopy would have been avoided if we had used intraoperative ultrasound during first surgery. We decided not to administer systemic methotrexate postoperatively, as removal of the trophoblastic tissue appeared complete. Indeed levels of β-hCG declined steeply postoperatively, indicating its complete excision.

In conclusion, although retroperitoneal pregnancy is an extremely rare condition, in a patient with clinical findings suggestive of ectopic pregnancy, if both the uterus and adnexa are normal during laparoscopic exploration, unusual locations such as the retroperitoneum should be carefully examined. Ipsilateral or bilateral salpingectomy does not exclude the occurrence of a parametrial pregnancy, and a clinician should be aware of such a possibility. Ultrasound should be used intraoperatively especially when we are dealing with a small and difficult-to-locate parametrial pregnancy

Informed consent All procedures followed were in accordance with the ethical standards of the responsible committee on human experimentation (institutional and national) and with the Helsinki Declaration of 1975, as revised in 2000. Informed consent was obtained from all patients for included in the study.

Conflict of interest All authors declare no conflict of interest.

References

1. Barnhart KT (2009) Ectopic pregnancy. N Engl J Med 361:379–387

2. Chetty M, Elson J (2009) Treating non-tubal ectopic pregnancy. Best Pract Res Clin Obstet Gynaecol 23:529–538

3. Tsudo T, Harada T, Yoshioka H, Terakawa N (1997) Laparoscopic management of early primary abdominal pregnancy. Obstet Gynecol 90:687–688

4. Lee JW, Sohn KM, Jung HS (2005) Retroperitoneal ectopic pregnancy. Am J Reprod 184:1600–1601

5. Champion PK, Tessitore NJ (1938) Intraligamentary pregnancy: a survey of all published cases of over 7 calendar months, with the discussion of an additional case. Am J Obstet Gynecol 36:281–293

6. Martinez-Varea A, Hidalgo-Mora JJ, Paya V, Morcillo I, Martin E, Pellicer A (2011) Retroperitoneal ectopic pregnancy after intrauterine insemination. Fertil Steril 95:2433e1–e3

7. Lin JX, Liu Q, Ju Y, Guan Q, Wu YZ, Zheng N (2008) Primary obturator foramen pregnancy: a case report and review of literature. Chin Med J 121:1328–1330

8. Abdul MA, Tabari AM, Kabiru D, Hamidu N (2008) Broad ligament pregnancy: a report of two cases. Ann Afr Med 7(2):86–87

9. Chang YL, Ko PC, Yen CF (2008) Retroperitoneal abdominal pregnancy at left parcolic sulcus. J Minim Invasive Gynecol 15:660–661

10. Bae SU, Kim CN, Hwang IT, Choi YJ, Lee MK, Cho BS, Kang Y, Park JS (2009) Laparoscopic treatment of early retroperitoneal abdominal pregnancy implanted on inferior vena cava. Surg Laparosc Endosc Percut Tech 19(4):e156–e158

11. Ferland RJ, Chadwick DA, O'Brien JA, Granai CO (1991) An ectopic pregnancy in the upper retroperitoneum following in vitro fertilization and embryo transfer. Obstet Gynecol 78:544–546

12. Dmowski WP, Rana N, Ding J, Wu WT (2002) Retroperitoneal subpancreatic ectopic pregnancy following in vitro fertilization in a patient with previous bilateral salpingectomy: how did it get there? J Assist Reprod Genet 19(2):90–93

13. Apantaku O, Rana P, Inglis T (2006) Broad ligament ectopic pregnancy following in-vitro fertilisation in a patient with previous bilateral salpingectomy. J Obstet Gynaecol 26(5):474

14. Iwama H, Tsutsumi S, Igarashi H, Takahashi K, Nakahara K, Kurachi H (2008) A case of retriperitoneal ectopic pregnancy following IVF-ET in a patient with previous bilateral salpingectomy. Am J Perinatol 25:33–36

15. Rersson J, Reynisson P, Masback A, Epstein E, Saldeen P (2010) Histopathology indicates lymphatic spread of a pelvic retroperitoneal ectopic pregnancy removed by robot-assisted laparoscopy with temporary occlusion of the blood supply. Acta Obstet Gynecol Scand 89(6):835–839

16. Hall JS, Harris M, Levy RC, Walrond ER (1973) Retroperitoneal ectopic pregnancy. J Obstet Gynaecol Br Commonw 80:92–94

17. Siow A, Chern B, Soong Y (2004) Successful laparoscopic treatment of an abdominal pregnancy in the broad ligament. Singap Med J 45(2):88–89

18. Olsen ME (1997) Laparoscopic treatment of intraligamentous pregnancy. Obstet Gynecol 89:862

19. Bae SU, Kim CN, Kim KH, Hwang IT, Choi YJ, Lee MK, Cho BS, Kang YJ, Park JS (2009) Laparoscopic treatment of early retroperitoneal abdominal pregnancy implanted on inferior vena cava. Surg Laparosc Endosc Percutan Tech 19(4):e156–e158

20. Parant O, Sarramon MF, Laffitte A, el Ghaoui A, Reme JM (1999) Parametrial pregnancy. Report of a case of "paracervical" pregnancy treated by medico-surgical management. J Gynecol Obstet Biol Reprod (Paris) 28(1):69–72

21. Okorie CO (2010) Retroperitoneal ectopic pregnancy: is there any place for non-surgical treatment with methotrexate? J Obstet Gynaecol Res 36(5):1133–1136

Permissions

List of Contributors

Michel P. H. Vleugels
Rivierenland Hospital, Tiel, Netherlands

Sergine Heckel
Centre Hospitalier St. Joseph St. Luc, Lyon, France

Sebastian Veersema
St. Antonius Hospital, Nieuwegein, Netherlands

Jean Bernard Engrand
Centre Hospitalier Général, Dunkerque, France

Vincent Villefranque
CHG René Dubos, Pontoise, France

Hervé Fernandez
CHU Kremlin Bicêtre, Paris, France

Pierre Panel
CHG André Mignot, Versailles, France

Daniele Bolla and René Hornung
Department of Obstetrics and Gynecology, Kantonsspital St. Gallen, Rorschacher Strasse 95, CH-9007, St. Gallen, Switzerland

Arthur von Hochstetter
Pathology Institute Enge Zurich, St. Gallen, Switzerland

Daniela Huber, Damien Robyr and Nicolas Schneider
Obstetrics and Gynecology, CHCV Sion Hospital, Rue Champsec 80, Sion 1950, Switzerland

Charalampos S. Siristatidis
Assisted Reproduction Unit, 3rd Department of Obstetrics and Gynecology, University of Athens, Athens, Attica, Greece

Dimitrios S. Miligkos
Department of Obstetrics and Gynecology, Princess Anne Hospital, Southampton University Hospitals, Southampton, UK

Igor V. Klyucharov
Department of Obstetrics and Gynecology No. 1, Kazan State Medical University, Republican Clinical Hospital, CCCH No. 18, CAC No. 2, Kazan, Russia

Nikos Vrachnis and Zoe Iliodromiti
2nd Department of Obstetrics and Gynecology, University of Athens Medical School, Aretaieio Hospital, Athens 11528, Greece

Charalampos Chrelias and Dimitrios Kassanos
2nd Department of Obstetrics and Gynecology, University of Athens Medical School, Aretaieio Hospital, Athens 11528, Greece

Johannes Bitzer
Department of Obstetrics and Gynecology, University Hospital Basel, Spitalstrasse 21, CH-4031, Basel, Switzerland

Stefano Bettocchi
First Unit of Obstetrics and Gynecology, Department of Biomedical Sciences and Human Oncology, University "Aldo Moro", Bari, Italy

G. Bigatti, C. Ferrario, M. Rosales and A. Baglioni
U.O. di Ostetricia e Ginecologia, Ospedale Classificato San Giuseppe Via San Vittore, 12-20123 Milan, Italy

S. Bianchi
Università degli Studi di Milano, Direttore dell'Unità Opertiva di Ostetricia e Ginecologia Ospedale Classificato San Giuseppe Via San Vittore, 12-20123 Milan, Italy

Dominique Van Schoubroeck, Thierry Van den Bosch, Lieveke Ameye, Thomas D'Hooghe and Dirk Timmerman
KU Leuven Department of Development and Regeneration, University Hospital Leuven, Herestraat 49, 3000 Leuven, Belgium

Tjalina Wibeke Oona Hamerlynck, Viviane Dietz and Benedictus Christiaan Schoot
Department of Obstetrics and Gynecology, Catharina Hospital Eindhoven, The Netherlands

G. Bigatti
U.O. di Ostetricia e Ginecologia, Ospedale Classificato San Giuseppe Via San Vittore, 12, 20123 Milan, Italy

Philippe R. Koninckx
University of KU Leuven, Leuven, Belgium
University of Oxford, Oxford, UK
Università Cattolica del Sacro Cuore, Rome, Italy
Vuilenbos 2, 3360 Bierbeek, Belgium
Gruppo Italo Belga, Heilig Hart, Leuven, Belgium

Leila Adamyan
Moscow State University, Moscow, Russia

Assia Stepanian
Villa del Rosario, Rome, Italy

Anastasia Ussia
Academia of Women's Health, Atlanta, GA, USA

Jacques Donnez
Université Catholique de Louvain, Woluwe, Brussels, Belgium

Arnaud Wattiez
University of Strassbourg, Strassbourg, France

Rudi Campo
European Academy for Gynecological Surgery, Scientific project on Female Genital Tract Congenital Anomalies, Diestsevest 43/0001, 3000 Leuven, Belgium

Grigoris F. Grimbizis
First Department of Obstetrics and Gynecology, Aristotle University of Thessaloniki, Tsimiski 51 Street, 54623 Thessaloniki, Greece

Lotte J. E. W. van Dijk
Department of Obstetrics & Gynecology, TweeSteden Hospital, Tilburg, The Netherlands

Maria C. Breijer, Ben W. J. Mol and Anne Timmermans
Department of Obstetrics & Gynecology, TweeSteden Hospital, Tilburg, The Netherlands

Sebastiaan Veersema
Department of Obstetrics & Gynecology, St. Antonius Hospital, Nieuwegein, The Netherlands

Ahmed Abdel-Gadir and Bina P. Chander
London Female and Male Fertility Centre, Highgate Hospital, 17-19 View Road, London N6 4DJ, UK

Oluseye O. Oyawoye
Department of Obstetrics and Gynaecology, Newham University Hospital, Glen Road, Plaistow, London E13 8SL, UK

Atef M. Darwish, Kamal M. Zahran, Mohammad A. Bedaiwi and Mahmoud S. Zakherah
Department of Obstetrics & Gynecology, Woman's Health University Hospital, 71111 Assiut ,Egypt

Daniela Huber and Nicolas Schneider
Obstetrics and Gynecology, CHCVs Sion Hospital, Rue Champsec 80, Sion 1950, Switzerland

Cristophe Duc
Pathology, ICHV Sion Hospital, Rue Champsec 80, Sion 1950, Switzerland

Dominique Fournier
Radiology, IRS Sion Radiologic Institute, Rue du Scex 2, Sion 1950, Switzerland

Fady M. Shawky Moiety and Amal Azzam
Department of Obstetrics and Gynecology, Shatby Maternity University Hospital, Shatby, Alexandria 21526, Egypt

Pietro Gambadauro
Centre for Reproduction, Department of Obstetrics and Gynaecology, Uppsala University Hospital, 751 85 Uppsala, Sweden

Rafael Torrejón
Department of Obstetrics and Gynaecology, "Puerta del Mar" University Hospital, University of Cádiz, Cádiz, Spain

Juliënne A. Janse and Sebastiaan Veersema
Department of Gynecology and Obstetrics, Sint Antonius Hospital Nieuwegein, Koekoekslaan 1, 3435 CM Nieuwegein, Netherlands

Frank J. Broekmans and Henk W. R. Schreuder
Division of Woman and Baby, University Medical Center Utrecht, 3508 GA Utrecht, Netherlands

A. B. Hooker and A. Thurkow
Department of Obstetrics and Gynaecology, Sint Lucas Andreas Hospital, Amsterdam, The Netherlands

Heleen van Dongen, Trudy Elskamp, Cor D. de Kroon and Frank Willem Jansen
Department of Gynaecology, Leiden University Medical Center, Albinusdreef 2, 2300 RC Leiden, The Netherlands

Anne Timmermans
Department of Gynaecology, University Medical Center Utrecht, Utrecht, The Netherlands

Cathrien E. Jacobi
Department of Medical Decision Making, Leiden University Medical Center, Leiden, The Netherlands

A. Pantelis, K. Dinas, T. Tantanasis, P. D. Loufopoulos and F. Carcea
Department of Obstetrics and Gynecology, Aristotle University of Thessaloniki, Evosmos, Greece

S. Angioni
Department of Obstetrics and Gynecology, University Hospital Don Calabria, Cagliari, Italy

Angelos Daniilidis
Department of Obstetrics and Gynecology, Aristotle University of Thessaloniki, 9 Smirnis, 56224, Evosmos, Thessaloniki, Greece

Atef M. Darwish, Ezzat H. Sayed, Safwat A. Mohammad and Ibraheem I. Mohammad
Department of Obstetrics and Gynecology, Woman's Health University Hospital, Egypt

Hoida I. Hassan
Department of Pathology, Faculty of Medicine, Assiut University Assiut, Egypt

Sharon P. Rodrigues, Kirsten J. de Burlet, Ellen Hiemstra, Andries R. H. Twijnstra, Trudy C. M. Trimbos-Kemper and Frank W. Jansen
Department of Gynecology, K6-76, Leiden University Medical Center, the Netherlands

Erik W. van Zwet
Department of Medical Statistics, Leiden University Medical Center, Leiden, The Netherlands

Hans Brölmann
Vrije Universiteit Medisch Centrum, Amsterdam, Netherlands

Marlies Bongers
Máxima Medisch Centrum, Veldhoven, Netherlands

José Gerardo Garza-Leal
Universidad Autónoma de Nuevo León, Monterrey, Nuevo Leon Mexico

Janesh Gupta
Birmingham Women's Hospital, Birmingham, UK

Sebastiaan Veersema
Sint Antonius Ziekenhuis, Nieuwegein, Netherlands

Rik Quartero
Medisch Spectrum Twente, Enschede, Netherlands

David Toub
Gynesonics, Inc., Redwood City, CA 94063, USA
Albert Einstein Medical Center, 5501 Old York Road, Philadelphia, PA 19141, USA

Pietro Litta
Department of Gynecological Science and Human Reproduction, University of Padua, Padua, Italy

Luigi Nappi
Department of Medical and Surgical Sciences, Institute of Obstetrics and Gynaecology, University of Foggia, Foggia, Italy

Pasquale Florio
U.O.C. Obstetrics & Gynecology, "San Giuseppe" Hospital, Empoli, Italy

Luca Mencaglia
Section of Gynecology, Centro Oncologico Fiorentino, Sesto Fiorentino, Italy

Mario Franchini
Palagi Freestanding Unit, Florence, Italy

Stefano Angioni
Department of Surgical Sciences, Section of Obstetrics & Gynecology, University of Cagliari, Azienda Ospedaliero Universitaria, Blocco Q, SS554, Monserrato, Cagliari, Italy

Jose Gerardo Garza-Leal, Iván Hernández León and Lorena Castillo Saenz
Universidad Autónoma de Nuevo León, Monterrey, Nuevo Leon, Mexico

David Toub, Darrin Uecker, Michael Munrow, Diane King and Jordan Bajor
Gynesonics, Inc, 604 Fifth Avenue, Suite D, Redwood City, CA 94063, USA

James Coad
West Virginia University, Morgantown, WV, USA

A. Santi, R. Felser, N. A. Bersinger, M. D. Mueller and D. M. Wunder
Department of Obstetrics and Gynaecology, Inselspital, University of Berne, DKF Murtenstrasse 35, Berne CH-3010, Switzerland

B. McKinnon
Department of Clinical Research, University of Berne, Berne, Switzerland

D. M. Wunder
Department of Obstetrics and Gynaecology, Centre Hospitalier Universitaire Vaudois, University of Lausanne, Lausanne, Switzerland

Liliana Mereu, Giuliana Giunta, Giada Carri, Luca Mencaglia and Edmundo Daniel Albis Florez
Division of Gynaecology, Centro Oncologico Fiorentino, Sesto Fiorentino, Italy

Giuliana Giunta
Department of Maternal Infant and Radiological Sciences, University Hospital G. Rodolico, Catania, Italy

Giada Carri
Department of Obstetrics and Gynaecology, Catholic University of Sacred Heart, Rome, Italy

Claudia Prasciolu
Division of Gynaecology, Obstetrics and Pathophysiology of Human Reproduction, University of Cagliari, Cagliari, Italy

Edmundo Daniel Albis Florez
Department of Obstetrics and Gynaecology, University El Bosque, Bogotà, Colombia

Andreia Alexandra Rocha Antunes
Hospital de Santo André, S.A, Rua das Olhalvas–Pousos, 2410-197 Leiria, Portugal

Lindsay M. Kindinger, Thomas E. Setchell and Tariq S. Miskry
Department of Gynaecology, St Mary's Hospital, Imperial College Healthcare NHS Trust, Praed StreetPaddington London W2 1NY, UK

Dominique Van Schoubroeck and Dirk Timmerman
Department of Development and Regeneration, KU Leuven, 3000 Leuven, Belgium

Thierry Van den Bosch
Department of Obstetrics and Gynecology, RZTienen, 3300 Tienen, Belgium
KU Leuven Department of Development and Regeneration, University Hospitals Leuven, Herestraat 49, 3000 Leuven, Belgium
Department of Development and Regeneration, KU Leuven, 3000 Leuven, Belgium

Athanasios Protopapas, Nikolaos Akrivos, Stavros Athanasiou, Ioannis Chatzipapas, Aikaterini Domali and Dimitrios Loutradis
University Department of Obstetrics and Gynecology of the University of Athens, "Alexandra" Hospital, 80 Queen Sophie Ave., 11528 Athens, Greece

Index